MOVING AHEAD

A Training Manual for Children with Motor Disorders

Springer

Singapore
Berlin
Heidelberg
New York
Barcelona
Budapest
Hong Kong
London
Milan
Paris
Tokyo

MOVING AHEAD

A Training Manual for Children with Motor Disorders

Joan O'Connor

The Hong Kong Society for Rehabilitation

Elsie Yu

Illustrations by
Lin Guohui, MD

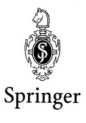

Springer

WHO Collaboration Centre for Rehabilitation
Hong Kong Society for Rehabilitation

The Spastics Association of Hong Kong

Joan O'Connor
(formerly)
The Hong Kong Society for Rehabilitation
WHO Collaborating Centre for Rehabilitation
7 Sha Wan Drive
Pokfulam
Hong Kong

Elsie Yu

Library of Congress Cataloging-in-Publication Data

O'Connor, J. (Joan) 1940-
Moving ahead : a training manual for children with motor disorders
/ J. O'Connor, E. Yu
Includes index.
ISBNB 9813083271
1. Movement disorders in children--Patients--Rehabilitation.
2. Psychomotor disorders in children--Patients--Rehabilitation.
3. Movement disorders in children--Patients--Education.
4. Psychomotor disorders in children--Patients--Education.
I. Yu, E. (Elsie), 1960-.   II. Title.
RJ496.M68036 1998
618.92'703--dc21   98-14892
                                      CIP

ISBN 981-3083-27-1

Typesetting: Typeset in Singapore by International Typesetters Pte Ltd
Printed in Singapore
SPIN 10636227   5 4 3 2 1 0

Joan O'Connor, SSC
Conductive Education Co-ordinator
WHO Collaborating Centre for Rehabilitation
Hong Kong Society for Rehabilitation
Hong Kong

Elsie Yu, PDOT, OTR
Occupational Therapist
Honorary Advisor, Jockey Club Conductive Learning Centre
The Spastics Association of Hong Kong
Hong Kong

Illustrator
Lin Guohui, MD
Rehabilitation Doctor
Rehabilitation Department
Chinese Seaman Guangzhou Sanatorium and
Guangzhou Geriatric Hospital of the People's Republic of China
Guangzhou City, Guangdong, People's Republic of China

The English songs were written and put to music by **June P.A. Rowlands** (Music Specialist), University of London 'Goldsmiths' College. Additional songs were written and put to music by **Jacqueline Gourlay Grant** (Head of Music and Performing Arts, Kennedy School-English Schools Foundation, Hong Kong).

The CD-Rom was made by **Jacqueline Gourlay Grant** and the **Childrens Choir of Kennedy School-English Schools Foundation, Hong Kong.**

Contents

Each child is special. Each child has a unique personality which develops week by week from birth onward. We watch over the child with care and with wonder as he or she achieves each new skill. The child turns to follow us with his eyes. He smiles. He reaches for a colorful object. He learns to grasp a toy and then to let go. The first time he sits by himself, the first time he pulls himself to standing, we are as excited as the child himself. We play and talk and help the child to learn. And as skills develop, the child takes the initiative, exploring his immediate world with his hands, feet and eyes. He talks to himself and to us about his small world and we respond. We soon know his likes and dislikes. We give him choices to make. We help him to understand good and bad. We give him opportunities to play with other children, learning about sharing, giving and receiving.

A disabled child is a very special child. The disabled child may see a plethora of experts. Soon a thick file follows him or her around filled with diagnostic tests and treatment suggestions for each part of the body and mind. Among all the appointments, parents and child care workers may find little time, energy or encouragement to give this special child the everyday opportunities that other children enjoy naturally. Children have the right to be loved. Children have the right to play. Children have the right to schooling.

This book is dedicated to giving the very special disabled child opportunities for learning the simple everyday acts of mobility, play, self care, communication, and socialising. When a child has disabilities, it is not always easy to know how to stimulate, encourage and guide him. This step-by-step training manual with its multiple drawings and songs will help parents and all who work daily with disabled children to uncover the abilities of children with special needs, and help these children discover and develop their own unique personalities.

I have known and worked closely with Joan O'Connor and Elsie Yu for many years. Their enthusiasm and commitment to helping our children is inspiring. With an equally devoted support team of illustrator and translator, they have produced a truly important book. I express my deep appreciation for their efforts.

Given the opportunity to work with children with motor disorders in China, the two authors of this manual quickly saw the need for assisting the front-line workers in their daily dealings with the children. So many of the care-givers would like to help the children to overcome some of their handicap. They do not feel that just feeding and cleaning the children is enough. But where to begin and what to aim for?

To help care-givers who ask themselves such questions, the authors have hit on the bold idea of creating this manual. Anyone who cares for these children can find answers here to the most elementary questions and find something they can do for and with the children. The tasks described here can give aim and purpose to the daily dealings with these children. This benefits the children, of course, but it also benefits the care-givers, who can feel they are now really supporting the children.

The two authors built their instructions on their own experience over many years with Chinese children, first in Hong Kong and later in China. They have read widely and gained experience in several countries, including Hungary, the United Kingdom and Japan. Patiently they have adapted the overseas model and ideas to fit into Chinese Society. So they know it works.

As you will see, the manual contains instructions for the care-givers of the groups of handicapped children, so they can plan the sessions in great detail beforehand, and know how to facilitate the children's movements from the excellent drawings accompanying each step of the tasks presented.

In Hong Kong we have for many years benefited from having care-givers meet and discuss their experiences in their daily work. Many ideas have grown out of such meetings. Sometimes they have been able to invite 'specialists' to speak to them. Often they have just shared their experiences and found answers from other people's experiences. Hong Kong is a small place — China is a vast place. Perhaps it would nevertheless be possible for some users of this manual occasionally to meet and discuss their work together.

Out of such discussions grew 'The Hong Kong Conductive Education Source Book', where you can find many answers as how to do things for the handicapped children. Perhaps other parts of China will be able to write other volumes like that, thereby hastening the spread of these well-tested ideas of how to help more and more care-givers of children with motor disorders.

Much of the original work on adapting Pëto's ideas took place in the Spastics Association of Hong Kong, with generous contributions from many sides. It has been a truly co-operative effort by institutions and care-givers, by parents and children. Continuing the tradition which started in Hong Kong some twenty years ago, we are still learning and we shall go on sharing what we have learnt with those who wish to share our experiences.

It is therefore with great pleasure that I welcome this initiative to reach out to many more children with motor disorders and their care-givers. I see much work growing out of this important step. I trust we shall be there to assist.

Dr. Marion Fang, MBE, LLD (Hons)

Erik Kvan
Chairman, The Spastics Association of Hong Kong

Many people have helped us with this manual. In particular, we have been priviledged to work with wonderful children, parents and grandparents here in Hong Kong and in the Mainland. We are grateful for all they have taught us about living, about meeting challenges and about helping themselves and others.

Our enthusiasm for Conductive Education (CE) has been inspired by the work of the Pëto Institute, Budapest, Hungary, and also by Ester Cotton, who gave us the courage to start CE in Hong Kong and invaluable initial support and motivation. Ester graciously made the long trek here more than once to share with us her vast knowledge and experience.

We were fortunate in Hong Kong to have Professor Sir Harry Fang, whose unerring instinct for seizing the opportune moment proved crucial in moving the process forward both in Hong Kong and China. Dr. Marion Fang as Chairperson of the "Hong Kong Working Group on Conductive Education" under the Joint Council for the Physically and Mentally Disabled, Hong Kong Council of Social Service, who guaranteed us the vital support we needed especially in the early days. She faciliated our on-going training, particularly in Budapest, and conducted exchanges with various institutes around the world. Dr. Erik Kvan and Mrs. Chong Wong Chor Sar, Chairman and General Secretary, the Spastics Association of Hong Kong, who in the early 1980s boldly committed the Association to introducing CE.

We are indebted to the occupational therapists, physiotherapists, speech therapists, child care workers, nurses, and teachers at the John F. Kennedy Centre, the Caritas Medical Centre and the Spastics Association of Hong Kong who spearheaded CE here and without whose enthusiasm, professionalism, and commitment the effort would surely have foundered. We would like especially to give thanks to Mrs. Anita Tatlow for her guidance and suggestions during the early stages of writing this manual and for the indispensable role she has played in the development of CE in Hong Kong. Anita turned from being a physiotherapist piloting CE groups to become our mentor and scribe, and saw to it that theory kept pace with practice.

Very special thanks to the superintendents, staff, parents, and children of the Jockey Club Conductive Learning Centre and the Apleichau Pre-School Centre of the Spastics Association of Hong Kong for their time and patience, and for allowing us to take photographs of the practice. We also want to thank Edith Yuk Shan Yeung, Chan Siu Pik, and Clare Cheng for reading the main script and for their useful suggestions and comments.

We thank Miss Emily Li Kit Yiu and Miss Yasmin Li for their help in typing the musical notes.

In China, we would like to thank Mr. Yan Minfu who was Vice-Minister of the Ministry of Civil Affairs during our first years and who gave us invaluable support. We would also like to thank Professor Nan Dengkun, Professor Liu Sui, Professor Guo Zhengcheng at the Tongji Hospital, Wuhan, for providing space, staff, and support for a demonstration group of children for the first national training course on CE; Mr. Chen Sanding and the Hubei Centre for Deaf Children who wholeheartedly welcomed us to set up an all-day programme in their centre; the China Disabled Persons Federation who insured cerebral palsy was included in their national rehabilitation plan and have encouraged training and provision of services in the community. We are most grateful to the directors and staff of the welfare homes in Beijing, Ningbo, Guangzhou, Chengdu, and Nanjing where CE is now practised and where we gained experience which influenced every part of this manual.

Finally, sincere thanks to Miss Mabel Chau and the staff of the Hong Kong Society for Rehabilitation, especially our colleagues of the WHO Collaborating Centre for Rehabilitation who supported and encouraged us at every turn. Thanks also to the staff at Elite Business Services Limited, and the Vocational Rehabilitation and Retraining Centre for typing the manual. We owe a debt of gratitude to the staff of Springer-Verlag, Asia for their patience and understanding. We thank Misereor, Germany who have provided the major financial support for our work with disabled children in China.

To our families and extended families, and to our friends who have supported, encouraged, and kept us working, our deepest thanks.

Vast numbers of children in China with motor disorders have no access to rehabilitation. In response to the expressed needs of their care-givers, we have addressed the situation by compiling this manual in English and Chinese. It comes complete with a CD-ROM of songs in both languages. It is a practical, step-by-step guide of the activities of the daily programme/routine for different levels of functional ability. We hope to highlight the importance of the daily programme/routine in providing the children with the optimum opportunity for training, practice, and reinforcement when learning daily life skills.

Our approach is inspired by Conductive Education as originated and developed by Professor Andras Pëto and practised at the Institute for the Motor Disabled in Budapest, Hungary. In addition, many concepts are based on Ester Cotton's publication *The Basic Motor Pattern* (Cotton 1980). Anita Tatlow has the following to say about the usefulness of this publication (Tatlow 1993):

> *"This little booklet has been most valuable both to the neurologically impaired and to rehabilitation staff, as anyone who knows about recent developments in rehabilitation will acknowledge. The booklet uses a diction as simple as Pëto's; it reduces professional jargon to words which can be understood and accepted by all rehabilitation workers; it broke with the notion that normal child development can be followed at all times and instead aimed at essential function; and it gives confidence to large groups of rehabilitation workers to attempt using the Pëto-System."*

However, the main content is drawn from the practice of Conductive Education as it has evolved in the centres of the Spastics Association of Hong Kong since its introduction in the early 1980s.

The manual is in five parts. **Part A** discusses cerebral palsy and how it affects the whole development of the child. This should equip the care-giver with the knowledge and appreciation of the difficulties the child has to overcome in order to adapt to his immediate environment and learn to cope with the demands made upon him.

It also describes the early development of the normal child. In particular, it stresses the inter-relationship of all aspects of the child's development and should be seen by the care-giver as a unified holistic progression. It highlights play within loving, secure relationships as one of the main ingredients in the process.

In order to master the skills necessary for function, the first precondition is a structured learning environment wherein the child will be facilitated to learn all the skills he needs to function in life. The introduction to the Conductive Education system in **Part B** explains how this can be achieved and sets the groundwork for the actual implementation. The essence of Conductive Education is love and respect for the dignity of the child as a human being with his own unique personality, needs, and desires. In practice this is translated into a positive approach when assessing and observing the child. He is seen not as a list of problems to be dissected and treated one by one but, rather, the emphasis is on setting realistic goals for the child to succeed in achieving.

Having set the goals, **Part C** takes the child step by step through the implementation process. It also spells out how the care-giver can structure the day for the child. Hopefully, she can turn any part of the day into a learning situation for him. Every task the child needs to learn during the day is included in this part, for example, getting out of bed in the morning, walking to the toilet, putting on shoes and socks. We have divided the abilities of the children into four levels. For certain tasks with more advanced children, we have included a fifth level of ability.

Part D deals with the task series. The task series presented here are basic, and on the whole are common to most children with motor disorder. They are designed to teach the children the skills they need at different levels and in the following positions: the lying position, the sitting position on stool, a mat, and at a table, the standing position, and walking.

What we present here is an intensive daily programme. We recognise that circumstances of time, place, and manpower will largely dictate the quantity of input at any given time. In particular, we recommend the care-giver is mindful of the child's level of tolerance in accepting the programme. Nevertheless, a consistent, structured but flexible timetable is important for learning.

The need for a discussion on how to tackle certain problems which may arise has been apparent from the beginning. No two children are the same, but as a general rule the demands of function are common to most children. However, each child will have problems which require specific adaptations. This we have attempted to deal with in **Part E**.

The **Appendix** includes some of the special furniture and other teaching aids which has been found useful when implementing the programme. The songs and games are suggestions only; we very much hope that those working with children will draw on their own ideas and creativity, and develop a repertoire of songs and rhymes to suit their own cultural milieu.

It is not within the scope of this manual to detail the overall cognitive input of the developing child. In recent years in China, adequate material is available for this purpose. Hopefully, you the care-givers will make full use of what is available to enhance and enrich the quality of the programme.

The manual is primarily directed towards middle-level rehabilitation workers, but doctors, nurses, therapists, childcare workers, teachers, and parents will find it a useful guide in their daily practice. We hope that all who use this manual will make useful suggestions which will undoubtedly improve the quality of future editions.

For ease of reference, children will be referred to throughout as male and care-givers as female. The term care-giver is used to stand for child care workers, therapists, nurses, parents, grandparents, doctors, teachers, in short, all those who are involved in the development of children with motor disorders. In parts A, B and C we have used the singular for child. In Part D for ease of expression we interchange singular and plural.

Chapter 1

Cerebral Palsy

WHAT IS CEREBRAL PALSY?

Cerebral Palsy refers to a broad range of motor disorders which includes lifelong disturbance of tone, movement, posture, and balance. There is damage to the immature brain which can occur before, during, or after birth. The resultant motor disorder may not be apparent at birth; however, as the child develops and grows, the diagnosis is usually made when he presents with poor or no control of his motor movements.

CAUSES

Pre-natal (Before birth)
a. Maternal infection during the early stages of pregnancy.
b. Maternal drug abuse.
c. Severe iodine deficiency before conception or during early gestation.
d. Multiple births.
e. Intra-uterine growth retardation.
f. Pre-term birth.
g. Genetic defects.

Peri-natal (During birth)
a. Difficult birth with anoxia.
b. Birth injury trauma to the skull with resultant compression of the brain.

Post-natal (After birth)
a. Excessive jaundice.
b. Infections of the brain during the first years of life, e.g., meningitis, encephalitis.
c. Brain tumours.
d. Brain haemorrhage.
e. Head injuries.

DIAGNOSTIC TYPES OF CEREBRAL PALSY

As the damage can occur in different parts of the brain the clinical manifestations differ from one another.

Spastic
The limbs of a spastic child appear stiff. As a result, the child has poor or no control of his movements. He suffers what is commonly known as high muscle tone.

The body distribution is classified as follows:

a. Spastic hemiplegia — one side of the body is affected. (See Fig. 1.1.)

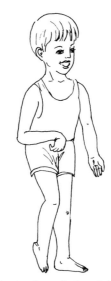

Fig. 1.1 Spastic hemiplegia

b. Spastic diplegia — the four limbs are affected with the lower limbs more affected than the upper limbs. (See Fig. 1.2.)

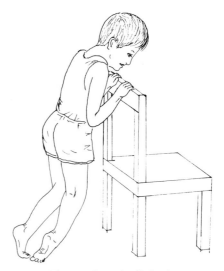

Fig. 1.2 Spastic diplegia

c. Spastic quadriplegia — the four limbs are affected with the upper limbs more affected than the lower limbs. (See Fig. 1.3.)

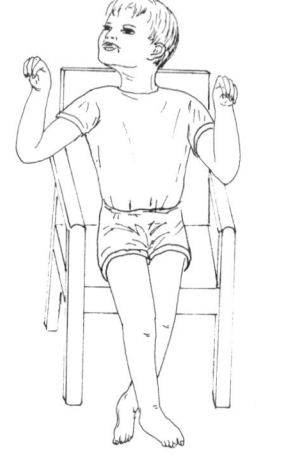

Fig. 1.3 Spastic quadriplegia

In rare cases, there may be an incidence of spastic "monoplegia" where one limb is affected or "triplegia" where three limbs are affected.

Hypotonic
"Hypo" means below. The child's muscle tone is below normal. It can be transient and is more commonly seen in babies under two years of age. As the child grows, the muscle tone may change and becomes the dyskinetic type. The term "floppy child" is commonly used to describe this group of children. The muscle appears weak and floppy. He is usually referred to as a good baby as he rarely moves about. He sleeps most of the time and does not cry or make much sound. Because of his severe weakness and loss of strength, he has great difficulty carrying out even the slightest movement, for example, turning the head to one side or as shown in Fig. 1.4, the child has difficulty straightening his back and keeping his head in the mid-line.

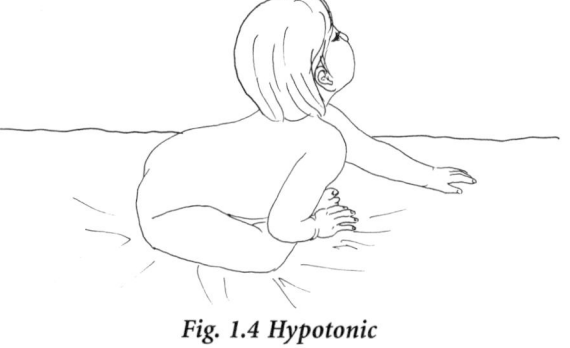

Fig. 1.4 Hypotonic

Dyskinetic
"Dyskinetic" — changes in the muscle tone. This group includes the "athetoid" and the "ataxic".

a. Athetoid. The child with athetosis has fluctuating muscle tone. He can appear very floppy and then suddenly become very stiff and tense. His movements are often exaggerated. Involuntary movements occur in the upper and lower limbs and are likened to movements performed by a ballet dancer. Involuntary movements may also occur in the tongue and cause slurring of speech. (see Fig. 1.5.)

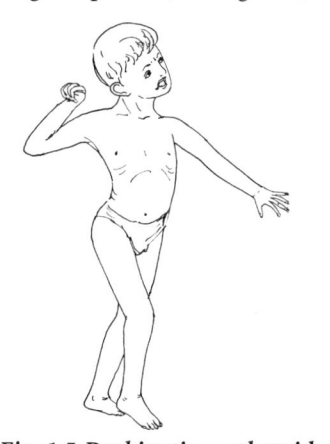

Fig. 1.5 Dyskinetic – athetoid

b. Ataxic. The child with ataxia has great difficulty with balance. Tremor is dominant in the head and trunk and appears in the limbs when he starts to move. The tremor increases when the child attempts to carry out a motor act. Because of his poor sense of balance the child is in constant fear of falling over. The speech is often soft and jerky.

Mixed type
As the damage to the brain is diffuse, quite a number of children present a mixed picture of the signs just discussed. A child may present as a spastic cerebral palsy with athetosis or a spastic cerebral palsy with ataxia.

ASSOCIATED DISORDERS AND COMPLICATIONS

The damage to the brain is often diffuse. As Phelps (1949, p. 106) states, "Cerebral Palsy differs from all other handicapping conditions because it includes all functions of the brain. It does not represent a motor handicap, such as poliomyelitis, but because of its origin in the brain it may include sensory and mental derivations as well."

The insult may or may not affect the child's intelligence. Some children may have average or above average intelligence, while others may suffer from mild, moderate, or severe degrees of intellectual deficiency. Moreover, the degree of motor disorder does not reflect the child's level of intelligence. A child with severe motor disorder may have a high intelligence quotient, however, because of his limited movement, he may be unable to express himself. Many children may have problems with vision, hearing, speech, visual perception, and sensation. Some children may suffer from epilepsy. Other problems which may also occur:

- Difficulty controlling body temperature;
- sleeplessness;
- constipation;
- dental problems;
- contractures and deformities.

SIGNS AND SYMPTOMS OF A CHILD WITH CEREBRAL PALSY

The clinical signs may not be obvious at birth but are observed as the child develops. He has difficulty controlling movement. The degree of severity varies. Some children may have problems with fine motor movements such as handwriting, while others have great difficulty moving different parts of the body. The motor disorder can vary from mild to severe involvement.

The child with cerebral palsy may have some or all of the following signs and symptoms:

- Difficulty in carrying out movements which can be jerky, stiff, writhing, and awkward.
- Difficulty in the timing of movements which can be delayed, sudden, uncoordinated, and slow.
- Poor balance including difficulty maintaining balance in certain positions, such as sitting, standing, walking.
- "Involuntary movements", movements the child is unable to control. For example, if the child wants to reach for a sweet or toy, his arm may first move backwards, then upwards before he can reach forward for the object.
- "Associated movements", movements that occur when the child tries to move one part of the body, the other parts also move. If the child wants to grasp a toy with his right hand, his left hand will also open and close imitating the movement of the right hand.

REFLEXES/MOTOR REACTIONS

Movements are needed for survival and for adapting to the environment. The movements of a newborn infant are limited and are dominated by a range of automatic reactions or stereotyped motor responses known as reflexes or motor reactions. These primitive motor reactions are strongest in the first days of life. As the infant develops and matures, they are modified within structures which incorporates the child's activities and experiences.

Because of the damage to the immature brain, some "primitive motor reactions" can persist unmodified in the child with cerebral palsy. Many children make use of these motor reactions for movement, resulting in stereotyped and inadequate movements which hinders them from acquiring normal movement patterns.

More Common "Primitive Reflexes or Motor Reactions"
Moro Reaction
This is evoked by a sudden sensory stimuli, e.g., a loud noise or bang. If the infant's head in the supine position is allowed to drop backwards, the arms will fly up and out in a backward direction in what is called the "embrace". This response can cause him to lose balance. (See Fig. 1.6.)

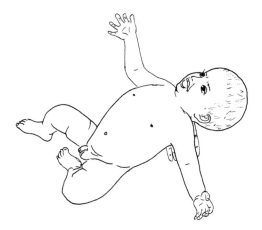

Fig. 1.6 Moro reaction

Palmar motor reaction
Strong pressure on the palm of the hand will cause the fingers to close and grasp the object. The persistence of this reaction can interfere with and prevent the infant from opening his hand. (See Fig. 1.7.)

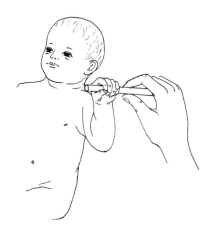

Fig. 1.7 Palmar motor reaction

Positive supporting reaction

When the infants's feet are in contact with a hard surface, the lower limbs will extend and he will be unable to bend at the hips, knees, and ankles. This will interfere with initiating steps for walking. (See Fig. 1.8.)

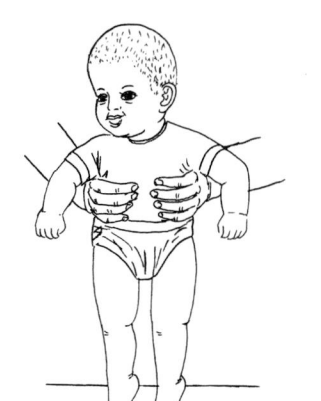

Fig. 1.8 Positive supporting reaction

Common "Pathological Tonic Reflexes or Motor Reactions"

The abnormal motor reactions, also known as pathological reflexes seen as a result of the brain damage include:

Tonic labyrinthine reflex or motor reaction (TLR)

This is elicited by changes in the position of the head in space. Clearly seen when the child lies on his back, the neck and back hyper-extend forcing the trunk to arch backwards. This position can prevent and interfere with the child lifting his head to initiate getting up from the supine lying position. When lying on his tummy, the child adopts a total flexion pattern preventing him from lifting his head and pushing up on his forearms. (See Figs. 1.9, 1.10)

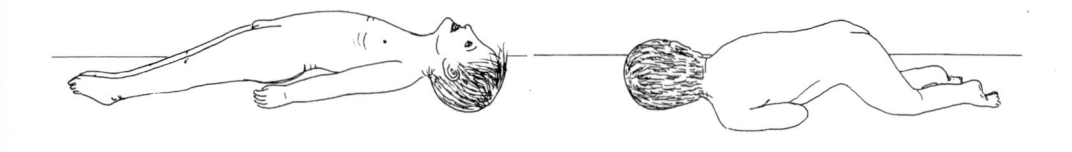

Fig. 1.9   *Fig. 1.10*
Tonic labyrinthine reflex/motor reaction

Symmetrical tonic neck reflex or motor reaction (STNR)

If the child bends his head in the crawling position, the elbows will also bend and the hips and knees will extend; this will hinder any attempts at crawling. Conversely, when the child lifts his head, the elbows will extend and the hips and knees flex. (See Fig. 1.11.)

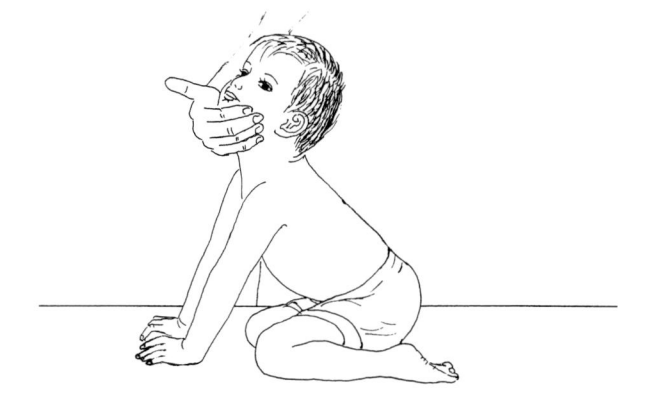

Fig. 1.11 Symmetrical tonic neck reflex/motor reaction

Asymmetrical tonic neck reflex or motor reaction (ATNR)

This is present in children with severe motor disorder. The position of the head determines the position of the limbs. When the head is turned towards the right side, the muscle tone on that side increases, causing the right arm and leg to extend. In severe cases, this can prevent the child bringing both hands together in the midline. Midline orientation is a precursor for function in activities of daily living. (See Fig. 1.12.)

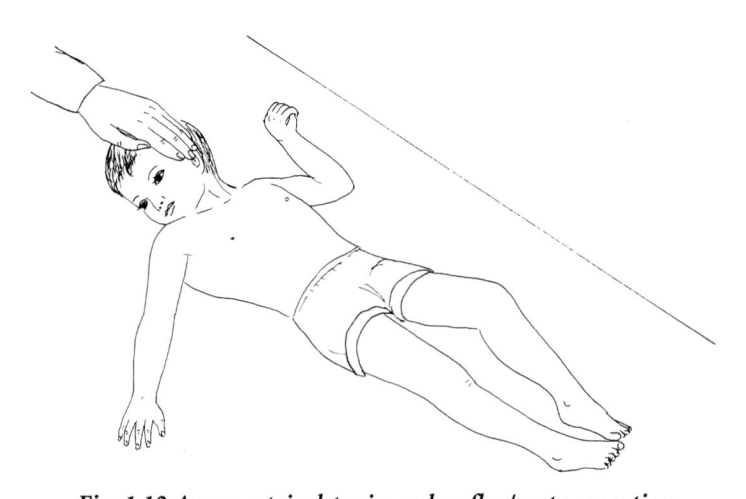

Fig. 1.12 Asymmetrical tonic neck reflex/motor reaction

SOME RECOMMENDATIONS FOR PARENTS ON HOW TO INTERACT WITH A CHILD WITH CEREBRAL PALSY

A child with cerebral palsy will demand a lot of attention especially from the mother. If the mother already has had children, she will have found it easy and natural to develop a relationship with them. However, it may be different with a child with cerebral palsy. The mother may experience many difficulties as it may not be easy understand the child's many needs. This may arise from the fact the child may not communicate through bodily or facial movements as the normal child. He may not be able to turn his head to look at and enjoy the toys the mother gives him. Because he cannot control his neck and facial muscles, he may not be able to smile at her or show how pleased he is to see her. This calls for great understanding. The mother should not stop communicating with the child despite the fact that he may not respond fully. Allow him experience what a normal baby would, such as touching, hugging, tickling, bouncing, taking him out shopping; in short, all the mothering and bonding as with a normal child.

Treat him as a normal baby and in time, this will encourage other members of the family, relatives, and friends to follow suit.

NEGATIVE FEELINGS

As a parent, it is natural to experience feelings of worry, fear, loneliness, and alienation. There are also times when there may be feelings of guilt and the need to compensate. These feelings are natural, and it is important to have an outlet for them — sharing with trusted friends, family members, parents who also have a child with cerebral palsy. Always remember, one is not alone with these feelings and problems.

POSITIVE ACTION

Worries, anxiety, and fears use up much energy and can leave one feeling exhausted. Conserve this energy and focus it on the child. Give priority to the many ways the child can be helped. As mentioned earlier, the child has difficulty with movement control. Focus on how he can be taught simple daily activities, i.e, to roll over in bed, to lift his bottom when changing his nappy, to sit properly, to learn to feed himself. This can be the beginning of positive experiences which will gradually lead the child to greater independence.

DAILY CHALLENGES FOR THE CHILD AND HIS FAMILY

Psychological
Relationship with parents
A new born baby is a helpless creature. He depends solely on others for survival. The mother becomes the mediator between the environment and the baby. She has to become familiar with his daily needs. This task of understanding and making sense of his many requirements can tax to the fullest her capacity, and in many cases, can lead to a breakdown in communication. This inevitably can interfere with the development of a close intimate relationship between mother and baby.

Dependent behaviour
Because of the difficulty in understanding the dynamics of building a secure relationship with the baby, the mother tends to become over-protective, or conversely, can neglect him. An over-protected child will demand everything to be done for him. This will prevent the child learning gradually to cope with his own life. The child is encouraged to adopt a "sick role". He quickly learns to become dependent on others because he is "sick" and demands to be cared for by others. On the other hand, frustration and lack of understanding of the child's needs can result in rejection by the mother. This rejection and human isolation takes its toll on the child and he becomes apathetic and passive.

Decreased motivation
Children easily learn to adapt to the demands of their particular environment. A child who is neglected and has few demands made upon him quickly learns to become passive and lacks the motivation to interact with his environment.

Unpleasant behaviour
As the child's needs, desires, and personality are suppressed, his disappointment may be expressed in unpleasant behaviour, e.g., temper tantrums, aggressive behaviour, and other expressions of attention-seeking.

Any or all of these affect the growing child's personality. Over dependence on adults, reluctance to take on responsibility, and an over-demanding attitude can become major obstacles for future learning.

Medical
Poor health
Due to weakness of the respiratory muscles, the child with cerebral palsy suffers from frequent upper respiratory tract infections.

Prone to injuries
Because of his problems with movement control, the child can suffer joint dislocation, especially of the hip. He may also suffer torn tendons and inflammation. Usually these problems necessitate frequent hospitalisation.

Contractures and deformities
Contractures develop as a result of irreversible shortening of the muscles due to muscle imbalance or faulty positioning. This can lead to a decrease in the range of movement of the joints. A child who spends most of his days sitting in a wheelchair will quickly develop contractures at the hips and knees; consequently, he will have great difficulty stretching the muscles of the hip and knee joints.

"Muscle Imbalance" occurs when one side of the muscle is stronger than the other. In a child with cerebral palsy, the muscles which flex the wrist are often stronger than those which extend it. The stronger group of muscles will pull the wrist joint into flexion resulting in the condition known as "dropped wrist". If this condition persists, the flexor muscles of the wrist will shorten, preventing active and passive movement of the wrist joint. The pull of the flexor muscles can be so strong it can cause a fixed deformity of the wrist. This condition deteriorates with time.

Epilepsy

Quite a number of children with cerebral palsy suffer from epilepsy. Fits can occur at a very young age or later in life. The duration of a fit can last from one to two seconds or sometimes up to 20 minutes. It varies with different children. It may present as a blinking of the eyelid, staring of the eyes, or a lapse into unconsciousness. In a severe fit, there may be drooling of saliva and loss of bladder control. Severe and frequent fits can cause further damage to the brain. Some children need medication.

Poor bowel and bladder control

A great majority of children suffer from this problem. This can be caused by poor control of the abdominal muscles. This problem causes many children to become distressed and agitated.

Poor attention span

A child with cerebral palsy is easily distracted. He may have great difficulty concentrating on a target for a reasonable length of time. This may be further complicated by other sensory problems such as visual, auditory, and tactile. The ability to concentrate depends on the ability to collect and integrate all sensory input in a systematic manner.

Poor sleeping pattern

The child with cerebral palsy may also have problems adjusting to daily routine patterns. This may be due to deficits in sensory perception or to the child's lack of activity during the day. It is important the child learns to develop a regular sleeping pattern.

Physical

Poor movement control

"A human being is designed to move." (Tatlow, 1994) Movement keeps a person healthy and promotes a normal sense of well-being. Because of the presence of abnormal muscle tone, the child with cerebral palsy has difficulty controlling his movements. This is the greatest single factor in preventing him from learning to explore his environment, also from developing feelings of accomplishment and success, and the inborn desire to be autonomous.

Poor balance control

Poor movement control leads to a poor sense of balance. The child develops feelings of insecurity and a fear of falling. This aggravates his inability to control his body.

Pain

The abnormal muscle tone and poor movement control can lead to contractures and deformity. Prolonged periods of immobility in bad positioning can hasten this problem.

Eventually the child may complain of pain. This will affect him both physically and psychologically.

Poor communication

Speech, language, facial expression, and gestures are the basis of communication. Children with cerebral palsy can be affected in any of these aspects. The inability to express himself leads to frustration and misunderstanding on both sides. This can be one of the greatest challenges the child has to deal with.

Sensory Perception

As the damage to the brain is diffuse, the child may also suffer various degrees of sensory perception deficits. The clinical signs may be manifested as:
a. inability to select a target for focus and differentiate it from its background, for example, the child cannot focus on his mother when she is talking to him face to face.
b. inability to feel and recognise one's own body parts, for example, a child with hemiplegia usually neglects his affected side.
c. inability to orientate and integrate all the sensory input of a highly stimulated environment, for example, a child on a visit to the market may feel uncomfortable and agitated, he can become upset and express this by crying.

Cognitive

Intelligence deficits may be caused by the damage to the brain or due to the lack of opportunities for normal childhood learning experiences. Every opportunity must be given to the child with cerebral palsy to experience and learn what a normal child of the same age experiences.

PRECAUTIONS WHEN HANDLING AND CARRYING A CHILD WITH CEREBRAL PALSY

Before handling the child,
a. always approach him from the front.
b. make contact with the child and give him sufficient time to understand the instructions. Many children cannot verbalise their needs. Develop a sensitivity to their needs, desires, likes, and dislikes. Explore different methods of communicating, e.g., body gestures, signs, facial expressions. Give one message at a time.
c. never move him suddenly, it can increase his anxiety.
d. do not force against tight muscles as this increases resistance. Hold him gently but firmly and give him time to relax.
e. when lifting, do not lift by the arm only as this may cause injury to the shoulder joint.
f. change the child's position every half hour to prevent the development of contractures and deformities which can occur if the child is left in a static position for too long.

Figure 1.13 shows a child with a typical spastic pattern. The child with quadriplegia has problems with head control. His shoulders are retracted with the arms turning outwards, the elbows flexed, and the hands fisted with the thumb inside. The trunk can be flexed or extended backwards, the hips, knees, and ankles are extended with the legs crossed.

When carrying a floppy child with poor head control, he will need full support. Depending on the ability of the child decrease the support. (See Fig. 1.16)

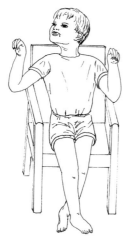

Fig. 1.13 Child with typical spastic pattern

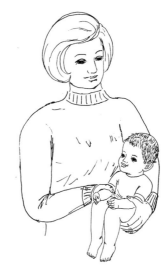

Fig. 1.16 Ensuring full support for the child's head

Bend his knees and hips, separate his legs, and support him at the trunk when carrying him. If carrying him from the front, encourage him to put his arms around the care-giver's neck. If required, support the head. If his head control is good he can be carried at the side or on the back. (See Figs. 1.14 and 1.15)

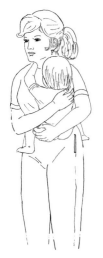

*Fig. 1.14 Carrying spastic child
at the side*

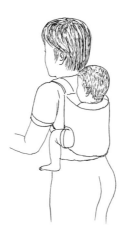

*Fig. 1.15 Carrying spastic child
on the back*

Chapter 2

How Children Learn and Develop

As children develop and grow, they are simultaneously learning. Growing and learning interweave and are never-ending processes, one facilitating the other. Crucial changes occur during the first three years of life. If, for medical reasons, the motor development of the child is interrupted during these vital years, the child's learning process will be hindered. To understand the impact this interference can have on the child, we need to look closely at normal child development and appreciate the importance of the inter-relationship between all the different aspects. We present normal child development under five different headings: motor and vision, hearing and communication, play, intellectual and psycho-social. However, we stress from the beginning the total integration of this developmental process and, in reality there is no division. Hopefully, through an understanding of the inter-relatedness of all facets of development, we can recognise, understand, and appreciate the difficulties and frustrations, at times expressed in terms of anger or aggressive behaviour in a child with cerebral palsy trapped in his body because of the interruption of his motor development, and how this can profoundly affect the whole process of development.

Table 2.1 Normal Child Development

Age	Motor and Vision	Hearing and Communication	Play	Intellectual	Psycho-social	Developmental Health Watch
0–1 month	*Lies on back* • With head more to one or the other side • Large jerky movements of arms • Hands usually fisted with thumbs inside palm *Lies on tummy* • With arms bent under body • Legs bent • Buttocks pushed up • Lifts head slowly and slightly, then turns to one side (see Fig. 2.1.) *Fig. 2.1 Baby in prone* *Vision* • Stares at large brightly coloured objects, large patterned pictures especially of black and white colours • Watches care-giver's face when being fed • Follows light briefly with eyes	*Hearing* • Startled by sudden loud noise • Soothed by soft human voice *Expression* • Cries when uncomfortable or hungry *Oral-motor control* • Sucks well	• Experiences different sensations as play — sucking, patting, gentle swinging, etc. • Enjoys listening to soft human voice or music • Stares at care-giver's face/light (see Fig. 2.2.) *Fig. 2.2 Care-giver rocking a baby.* **Give him** • some music to listen to • a clown's face to look at • a mobile over his bed	• Depends on sensation — tactile, vestibular, visual, and auditory senses • Very sensitive to touch and the way he is being handled • Able to feel and understand moods and feelings from the way he is being touched	• Sleeps most of the time, wakes for short periods only • Stops crying when comforted and when picked up • Cries in response to physiological needs • A time for developing trust and a sense of security between the baby and the environment (the care-giver) (see Fig. 2.3.) *Fig. 2.3 Care-giver feeding a baby — looking & rocking* **Remember to** • cuddle him • rock him in your arms • pat him on his shoulders and back • talk to him face-to-face • talk to him when you feed him • hum a song to him	If the baby shows the following sign(s), seek advice from a doctor • Sucks poorly and feeds very slowly • No response to a bright light shining in front • Does not attempt to follow a moving object when placed about 6 – 8 inches from him • No response to sounds • Arms and legs are stiff and show no movement • The whole body is floppy and the limbs appear very loose

Table 2.1 Cont'd

Age	Motor and Vision	Hearing and Communication	Play	Intellectual	Psycho-social	Developmental Health Watch
3 months	*Lies on back* • With head in midline and symmetrical • Waves arms • *Midline orientation.* Brings two hands to midline over chest • Directs hands to mouth accidentally • Kicks alternately *Lies on tummy* • Lifts head high and turns to explore environment • Supports weight on forearms • Buttocks lie flat *Supported sitting* • Holds head up momentarily • Back straight *Hands* • Holds rattle but cannot grasp • More open (see Fig. 2.4.) **Fig. 2.4 Baby in supine playing with the hands** *Vision* • Alert, follows care-givers movements • Follows a brightly coloured toy at 6–10 inches through 120° • Watches own hands in midline	*Hearing* • Still startled by sudden loud noise but to a lesser extent • Soothed by care-giver's voice when screaming • When an interesting sound is heard, may blink his eyes, stare, or move head from side-to-side to look for sound *Expression* • Vocalises and smiles when care-giver talks to him • Grows quiet when hears sounds of milk being prepared • Cries when uncomfortable *Oral-motor control* • More active sucking, swallowing, lip and jaw movement when feeding • Better lip closure	*Active body discovery* • Two hands meet together in midline • Directs hands to mouth and discovers own mouth • Sensation of touching own body • looks at own hands and their movements **Give him** • a rattle to hold in his hands • a dangling toy hanging near his chest **Time to Spend with him** • hold and clap his hands • hold his hands and show him how to touch your face, mouth, and eyes • guide him to look at rattle in his hand (see Fig. 2.5.) **Fig. 2.5 Baby in supine — a dangling toy in front of him**	• Begins to explore environment visually and physically by turning his head • Starts to collect information from environment visually, auditorily, and tactile • Starts to become aware of his own body parts through touching • Recognises feeding bottle (See Fig. 2.6.) **Fig. 2.6 Care-giver holding the baby's hands to touch her face**	• A time for developing trust and a sense of security between baby and care-giver • Eager/Begins to show interest in the environment **Remember to** • cuddle him • rock him • pat him • talk to him face-to-face • talk to him when feeding him • respond to his physiological needs • play with and talk to him at the same time (see Fig. 2.7.) **Fig. 2.7 Care-giver holds a baby and talks to him, cuddles him, rocks him and pats him**	If the baby shows the following sign(s), seek advice from a doctor • No response to sounds • Does not smile at the sound of the care-giver's voice • Does not follow a moving object when placed about 6 – 8 inches distance from him • Does not move one or both eyes in all directions • Shows no awareness of his hands • Does not grasp and hold objects when placed in his hands • Does not smile at people • Cannot lift his head in the prone position • Arms and legs are stiff and show no movement • No babbling • Does not push down with the legs when placed on a hard supporting surface

Table 2.1 Cont'd

Age	Motor and Vision	Hearing and Communication	Play	Intellectual	Psycho-social	Developmental Health Watch
6 months	**Lies on back** • Lifts head from pillow • **Hip mobility.** (BMP) Plays with toes and may pull them to mouth (see Fig. 2.9.) • Holds arms up to be lifted • Kicks strongly with alternating legs • Rolls to side **Lies on tummy** • **Elbow extension.** (BMP) Pushes up on straight arms (see Fig. 2.8.) • **Develop points of fixation.** (BMP) Pivots on extended arms • Rolls from prone to supine **Sitting** • When pulled to sit he actively helps by using arms for pull • Sits on floor and may still use hands for propping up • Back is straight and able to turn head to either side **Supported standing** • When held standing on floor, feet bounce up and down actively **Hands** • **Grasp and release.** (BMP) Begins to transfer toys from one hand to the other • Grasps using the whole hand (palmar grasp). • Lots of grasping but without good release **Vision** • Begins to move eyes independent of head movement • Very visually orientated • Fixates on interesting objects within a distance of a foot and directs arms to grasp them	**Hearing** • Turns immediately to care-giver's voice across the room • Responds to different emotional tones of care-giver • Responds to the sound of milk being prepared **Expression** • Imitates sounds, e.g. da – da – da, goo – goo – goo • Laughs, grunts, chuckles during play • Screams with annoyance **Oral-motor control** • Handles some semi-solid food; munches • Moves food in mouth to both sides • Does not have good lip control, therefore, messy when drinking from a cup. Good lip closure around the bottle **Fig. 2.8 Baby prone on extended arms looking at teddy bear.**	• Enjoys manipulating objects with both hands • Has better elbow control, therefore is able to shake rattle to make sound • Pats on milk bottle when feeding • Plays with toes • Takes everything to mouth, even toes • Occasionally may show shyness or anxiety towards strangers; otherwise, friendly • Smiles and vocalises at own mirror image **Give him** • a rattle • an appropriate-sized object that his hands can hold, e.g., cubes, bells, spoon • mouthing toys • toys of different textures, e.g., a small sponge ball, a small cloth ball, a hard plstic rattle, a soft cloth rattle, etc. • a mirror (unbreakable) • household objects, e.g., cups, spoons, small towels, plates, etc. • a squeaky toy **Fig. 2.9 Baby plays with his toes.**	• Begins to understand object permanence. If something is taken away from him, he protests because he realises it still exists (see Fig. 2.10.) • Continues to manipulate objects around him as he realises he can make things happen. He understands the relationship between hitting a mobile and causing it to move **Fig. 2.10 Care-giver takes away the toy, baby protests**	• Sleeps throughout the night and takes two naps a day • Smiles at familiar people and at own mirror image • From playing with his toes, he realises his body is separate from his mother, from the environment and this may increase his anxiety • Realisation of the social situation — the difference between familiar faces and strangers may make his behaviour seem more aggressive. He may pull hair, grab glasses, or other people's clothing (see Fig. 2.11.) **Fig. 2.11 Baby grabs the hair of the care-giver**	If the baby shows the following sign(s), seek advice from a doctor • Very stiff with tight muscles • Whole body is floppy • Head drops backwards in supported sitting • Uses one hand only • Takes no weight when supported in standing • Refuses to be cuddled and cries incessantly when touched • Shows no signs of affection towards care-giver • One or both eyes consistently turns upwards or outwards • Does not follow an object when placed at a distance of a foot • No response to sounds around him • Does not turn to source of sound • Does not laugh or make any sound

Note

The Basic Motor Pattern (BMP) is present at six months:

1. grasp and release
2. elbow extension
3. midline orientation
4. hip mobility
5. fixing one part of his body while moving another noted to be well coordinated in a baby of six months.

11

Table 2.1 Cont'd

Age	Motor and Vision	Hearing and Communication	Play	Intellectual	Psycho-social	Developmental Health Watch
9 months	**Sitting** • Variety of sitting positions — sits on floor, stool, chair (see Fig. 2.12.) • When sittings on floor, baby can rotate body sideways to reach out and grasp toys ***Fig. 2.12 Baby sits on floor*** **Standing** • Pulls to stand by holding onto furniture or care-giver's hands May pull himself up to half — kneeling, then squatting, then standing • Lots of movements with hips bending and stretching (hip mobility) **Mobility** • Creeps on floor, some may start crawling • Enjoys pulling himself up to stand and lowering himself down onto floor • Cruises along furniture **Hands** • Pokes at small objects with index finger • Uses thumb when grasping (radial grasp) • Grasps small objects between thumb and index finger • Releases toys against hard surface **Vision** • Watches activities of others for several seconds • Watches and follows a ball rolling towards him or across the room	**Receptive language** • Understands "no, no" and "bye bye" **Expressive language** • More vocalisation — ma ma, da da, la la • Imitates and babbles sounds accurately • Begins to attract attention • Tries to imitate adult's playful sound, e.g., cough **Oral-motor control** • Begins drinking from cup • Good downward lip control • Able to transfer food from middle to sides of mouth • Bites and chews biscuits (See Fig. 2.13.) ***Fig. 2.13 Baby holds a biscuit and bites***	• Takes objects to mouth • Shakes rattle, waves it, or bangs it on table • Enjoys peek-o-boo • Shows toys to adult but cannot give • Moves body to get objects out of reach • Brings object in each hand together for comparison (see Fig. 2.14.) ***Fig. 2.14 Baby holds a cube in each hand and compares*** **Give him** • a small and safe corner of the room to explore • some safe furniture where his hands can hold on to and pull himself up to stand and down onto the floor again • time to actively participate in feeding and dressing, e.g., allow him to hold a spoon, to pull out sleeves by himself	**Perceptual** • He shows excitement when he sees food he likes • Depth perception begins to develop — he often peers inside of tins/boxes/cups. Enjoys putting things into and taking them out of boxes • Approaches a ball with both hands — eyes and hands co-ordinate • Searches for an object which is hidden from view, e.g., a toy covered by a towel (object permanence) • Shows great persistence in getting objects • Explores different means to an end and cause and effect relationship, e.g., moves his body to get a toy which is our of reach	• As his mobility improves, child begins to move away from care-giver and becomes more assertive. This is important for development of self-esteem • Although he is able to play by himself for an hour he likes to have familiar persons around him • With strangers around, he clings to familiar adults and needs reassurance before accepting their advances. This is the beginning of separation anxiety • Begins to respond to other people's expressions of emotion	If the baby shows the following sign(s), seek advice from a doctor • Does not sit on the floor independently • Rolls to one side only • Reaches with one hand only • Cannot stand when supported • No babbling • Does not use gestures such as waving hands • Does not point to objects

Table 2.1 Cont'd

Age	Motor and Vision	Hearing and Communication	Play	Intellectual	Psycho-social	Developmental Health Watch
1 year	*Sitting* • Sits on floor, pivots, and shuffles • Enjoys getting in and out of sitting position, crawling, or pulling onto furniture to stand *Standing* • Enjoys standing and walking • Stands on his own grasping or pulling onto furniture • Cruises around furniture • Walks with one hand or both hands held (see Figs. 2.16a & b.) • May stand independently for a few seconds *Hands* • Neat pincer • Controlled release with wrist extension. • May show hand preference • Immitates scribbling and holds crayon in fist (See Fig. 2.15.) *Fig. 2.15 Picks up small object with neat pincer* *Vision* • Aware of familiar faces approaching him from 20 or more feet away • Watches movements of animals or cars intently *Figs. 2.16a & Fig. 2.16b A child walking with one hand held*	*Receptive language* • Knows own name and responds by turning around • Understands several words within the daily context, e.g., meal, family names • Understands simple commands accompanied by gestures, e.g., bye bye, give, hug hug • Responds to "no" *Expressive language* • Begins to communicate his desires by pointing, crawling, or gesturing towards his target • Imitates gestures of adults • Babbles loudly and tunefully • Recognises syllables like "ba", "da", "ga", and "ma" • Begins to use head shaking for "no" *Oral-motor control* • Chews solid food • Uses spoon for feeding and plays with it • More tongue control • Chews and moves food to either side of mouth	• Play centers around interaction with his space world by manipulating toys in various ways — dropping objects — watching movement of objects — stacking cubes — pushing a cart forwards and backwards — putting objects into and taking them out of a container — looking at the inside of container — pulling strings to grasp objects out of reach • Enjoys looking at own body movement in mirror (See Fig. 2.17.) *Fig. 2.17 Child looks into container* *Give him* • stacking toys of different sizes, shapes, and colours • cups, empty boxes, or any other unbreakable container • bath toys which float, sponges, containers which hold water • large dolls and puppets • plastic cars • balls of different sizes • musical toys • push and pull toys • large picture cards	• Explores different properties of objects • Finds hidden objects easily. (See Fig. 2.18.) • Identifies some common objects when named • Begins to use objects correctly, e.g., spoon for eating, cup for drinking, telephone for talking, etc. • Lots of imitation especially body movements • Relates objects, e.g., uses spoon to stir in a cup • May begin taking turns with the help of adults *Fig. 2.18 Child searches for a toy covered with a towel*	• Can at times be open, affectionate, and outgoing with care-giver, but at other times, anxious, clingy, and easily frightened by strangers (see Fig. 2.19.) • As his separation anxiety increases, he may resist going to bed and has difficulty with sleep. Much patience with child is needed at this stage • May begin testing parental responses to his actions such as refusing food, crying when parents leave the room • Has a strong sense of identity and is conscious of care-giver as a separate person *Fig. 2.19 Child clings to care-giver*	If the baby shows the following sign(s), seek advice from a doctor • Does not stand when held with both hands • Always sits on floor, does not know how to move in and out of sitting position • No single words, e.g., ma ma, da da, etc. • Does not look for toys being hidden while still watching • No grasp and release

Table 2.1 Cont'd

Age	Motor and Vision	Hearing and Communication	Play	Intellectual	Psycho-social	Developmental Health Watch
1½ years	**Sitting** • Sits on small chair and pivots • Climbs onto adult-chair and sits on it **Standing** • Walks independently • Pulls toys as he walks • Stands on tiptoe • Walks upstairs holding rail or unaided with both feet on each step • Runs awkwardly **Hands** • Scribbles spontaneously • Imitates vertical strokes • Turns container over and pours out contents (see Fig. 2.20.) • Picks up a rolling ball • Puts small objects into bottles • Takes toys apart and puts them together again • Picks up toys from floor without falling **Fig. 2.20 Child pours out contents** **Vision** • Points to distant objects out of doors • Recognises tiny interesting objects 10 feet away	**Receptive language** • Follows everyday simple commands • Enjoys nursery rhymes and wants to join in **Expressive language** • Begins to express himself in short phrases • Points to picture when named (see Fig. 2.21.) • Recognizes names of familiar people, objects, and some body parts • Repeats words overheard in adults' conversation • Vocabulary of about 10 – 20 words • Attempts to sing **Fig. 2.21 Child points to familiar picture when named** **Daily Living Skills** • Takes off socks and shoes • Drinks from a cup and uses straws independently • Holds cup and puts it down without spilling • Holds spoon and feeds self but messy • Bites and eats solids • Some rotatory movements when chewing • May indicate toilet needs by showing restlessness	• Explores and gathers information about the way different things work • Shows special interest with mechanical devices such as wind-up toys, switches, buttons, doorknobs • Imitates adult activities such as brushing hair, cleaning furniture, talking on the telephone (see Fig. 2.22.) • Enjoys taking turns in play • Directs others to play with him • Imitates new facial expressions or gestures **Fig. 2.22 Immitates adult activites** **Children like to** • say 'no' • get what they want immediately • climb up stairs	• Finds objects even when hidden under two covers • Begins make-believe play • Begins to use extended reach e.g., a long stick to obtain an object out of reach • Matches objects with pictures • Begins to sort shapes and objects **Give him** • Picture books (with large pictures of children) • nesting toys • kitchen sets, dolls • cars, trains • bath toys • balls • outdoor play, e.g., slides, swings, sandplay • Musical instruments • toy telephone • large crayons • shape sorting box (See Fig 2.23.) **Fig. 2.23 Child begins to play with dolls, imitating the actions of adults**	• Has acquired better understanding of separation from care-giver • Begins to play alone contentedly but still likes to have adults around • Shows concern about things in relation to himself but has no idea of the thoughts or feelings of others • Plays along side other children and competes for toys, but does not know how to play with others • No concept of sharing (see Fig. 2.24.) • May show possessiveness • Because they have little awareness of others' feelings, they may hit or slap others unaware that it hurts **Fig. 2.24 Child refuses to share toys with others**	If the baby shows the following sign(s), seek advice from a doctor • cannot put feet flat on the floor while standing or walking • does not walk independently • does not speak more than five words • does not know the use of some common objects, e.g., spoon, cup, etc.

Table 2.1 Cont'd

Age	Motor and Vision	Hearing and Communication	Play	Intellectual	Psycho-social	Developmental Health Watch
2 years	*Mobility* • Walks with a heel-toe gait • Runs in a hurried manner and avoids obstacles • Walks up and down steps, holding handrail with one hand, with both feet on each step • While walking, he can stop suddenly, squat down, pick up objects from floor and stand up independently (see Fig. 2.25.) • Jumps with one foot first • Kicks a ball *Fig. 2.25 Child squats down and picks up a toy* *Hands* • Screws lids • Definite hand preference • Turns pages of a book one at a time • Throws a ball forward • Copies horizontal lines • Imitates a closed circle with crayon • Removes sweet wrappings	*Communication* • Uses 50 or more words • Composes simple sentences • Uses own name to indicate self • Talks to himself while playing • Always repeats words said to him (echolalia) • Constantly asking names of different objects • Enjoys nursery rhymes and songs (See Fig. 2.26.) *Fig. 2.26 Child enjoys scribling* *Daily living skills* • Puts on pants, socks and shoes (see Fig. 2.27.) • Washes own hands • Spoon feeds himself without too much of a mess. Chews with slight rotatory movement • Requests food and drink • Discriminates food from inedible objects • Verbalises toilet needs occasionally *Fig. 2.27 Child puts on own socks and shoes*	• Follows adults around the house and imitates domestic work during play • Enjoys listening to stories • Observes older children at play and wants to take part but does not know how • Looks at details in picture books • Enjoys throwing objects, bouncing • Enjoys playground play such as crawling through tunnels, slides, etc. • Sequence appears in make-believe play, e.g., bathing a doll	• Awareness of spatial dimension increases as he moves around and climbs • Begins to observe surrounding details and asks "why" incessantly of himself. He is developing elementary reasoning and symbolic knowledge • Recognizes family faces in photos • Remembers the whereabouts and is aware of the absence of certain people or objects *Give him* • picture books (see Fig. 2.28.) • domestic play sets • simple shape sorters • beginners tricycles • dressing up clothes • baskets, old magazines, boxes, tubes, pots, wooden spoons, etc. *Fig. 2.28 Child turns pages of a picture book one by one*	• Constantly demands attention • Clinging when tired, frustrated, or sick • May have temper tantrums especially when frustrated but can be easily distracted • Enthusiastic with the company of other children • Jealous of attention shown towards other children • Imitates behaviour of other children and adults *Remember that* • each child moves at his own pace. Some children may be naturally shy. Give him time to adapt to adults and new situations • a child can build up frustration. He may express it with temper tantrums or aggressive behaviour. Give him positive outlets to release his energy, e.g., playground activities	If the baby shows the following sign(s), seek advice from a doctor • does not have a heel-toe gait • does not speak a two-word sentence • does not imitate actions or words • does not follow simple instructions • does not point to pictures when object is named

Table 2.1 Cont'd

Age	Motor and Vision	Hearing and Communication	Play	Intellectual	Psycho-social	Developmental Health Watch
2½ years	**Mobility** • Walks upstairs with both feet on each step • Walks downstairs holding rail, both feet on each step • Walks on tip toes • Runs • Pushes toys but has difficulty steering them around obstacles • Jumps with both feet together **Hands** • Strings beads of one inch • Imitates horizontal lines • Begins to use scissors to cut • Holds a cup with one hand	**Communication** • Verbalises past experiences and holds simple conversations with adults and playmates • Asks lots of question on "what", "where", and "who" • Gives full name and sex when asked **Daily living skills** **Dressing** • Takes off clothing • Puts on pants, socks and shoes but cannot differentiate left and right • Opens zips, unbuttons large buttons, unties shoe laces • Manages zips • Begins to manage large buttons **Feeding and drinking** • Pours water from a jug into a cup • Eats tidily with a spoon **Toileting** • No need for diapers at night when reminded to go to toilet just before bedtime **Grooming** • Washes face • Assisted showering • Uses soap when washing hands • Blows nose with handkerchief • Brushes teeth and gargles	• Attention span is longer • Enjoys drawing, building, and manipulating objects • Runs around • Enjoys looking at coloured books/magazines • Enjoys imitating and pretend play • Takes turns in games • Understands concept of "mine" and "yours" **Give him** • paper and crayons • picture books • thread and beads • tea set, beauty sets, medical sets for make-believe play (see Fig. 2.29.) **Fig. 2.29 Child enjoys make-believe play** **Fig. 2.30 A child dances to music**	• Less easily distracted • Recognises and identifies most common objects and pictures • Begins to understand simple time concepts • Begins to understand relationship between objects • Increased understanding of cause and effect with greater interest in switches, wind up toys, etc **Fig. 2.31**	• Appears to be selfish and self-centered as he refuses to share things that interests him • Does not know how to interact with other children • Cannot understand others' feelings and thinks that everyone else thinks and feels as he does • Imitates playmates and adults • Emotional changes occur frequently (see Fig. 2.32.) • May throw violent temper tantrums when thwarted **Fig. 2.32 Emotional changes occur frequently** **Fig. 2.33 Plays and interacts with other children**	If the baby shows the following sign(s), seek advice from a doctor • no heel-toe gait • difficulty in manipulating small objects • persistent drooling and unclear speech • failure to understand simple instructions

Table 2.1 Cont'd

Age	Motor and Vision	Hearing and Communication	Play	Intellectual	Psycho-social	Developmental Health Watch
3 years	*Mobility* • Walks upstairs independently with alternating steps • Walks downstairs alone with two feet on each step • Jumps from low step • Runs around corners and obstacles • Rides bicycles and turns at corners • Stands on one foot momentarily • Catches a large ball • Throws a small ball *Eye-hand coordination* • Picks up thread and pins with neat pincer • Wiggles thumb in imitation • Copies a closed circle • Does simple drawings • Cuts with scissors • Has more control in using tools and utensils to perform certain tasks such as using spoon, pen, comb, cup, etc.	*Communication* • Uses 200 or more recognisable words • Knows own name • Talks continuously with lots of infantilisms • Enjoys asking "what" • Starts using pronouns "I" and "you" • Says a few nursery rhymes • Enjoys listening to stories • Follows a two-step command *Daily living skills* • Rotatory chewing • Eats skilfully with spoon • Enjoys using chopsticks though clumsy • Verbalises toilet needs during the day • Dry throughout the night with occasional accidents • Pulls off loose T-shirts (see Fig. 2.34.) *Fig. 2.34 Child pulls off his loose T-shirt*	• Sings and dances to music • Imitates others and follows simple rules • Follows rules of games led by adults • Begins to ask for permission from other children before taking their toys • Enjoys listening to stories and asks questions • Retells part of stories already heard	• Begins to acquire the concept of sizes, weights, and shapes • Begins to classify objects into different categories, e.g., socks and shoes, edible objects, etc • Begins to match and name primary colours • Shows more sensitivity to spatial relationships between objects • Knows own and others' daily routine, e.g., will wait eagerly for father's return from work in the evening • Understands the concepts of same and different	• Greets others without being reminded • Begins to say "thank you" • Begins to answer phone calls • Appears to be less self-centred than at two years old • Plays and interacts with other children • Recognises that not everyone thinks as he does • Recognizes he is a whole person, with a body, mind, and feelings • Begins to fantasize and cannot distinguish between fantasy and reality • Cannot express feelings fully and may feel frustrated • Has difficulty making decisions when several choices are presented	If the baby shows the following sign(s), seek advice from a doctor • frequent falling and has difficulty with stairs • unable to copy lines or circle • unable to communicate in short phrases • no involvement in pretend play • no interest in other children

Chapter 3

Introduction to Conductive Education

Conductive Education is an integrated system which has as its ultimate goal the task of preparing the child with motor disorder to function in life. This presupposes the child will acquire during the process the capacity and the wherewithal to deal with the challenges he will meet daily in society. It was developed in Hungary in the 1940s by Professor Andras Petö (1893–1967). He founded the State Institute for The Motor Disabled and Conductors Training College in Budapest. As well as cerebral palsy, the Institute also deals with children with spina bifida and adults suffering from strokes and head injuries, Parkinson's disease and multiple sclerosis. Dr. Maria Hari took over the running of the Institute after Petö. The impressive results which they have achieved over the years has generated international interest in the system.

Petö saw the child with motor disorder as being persistently unable to engage constructively with the demands of his immediate environment during his developing years. For example, a child seeing an attractive toy within reach automatically moves towards it to explore it and play with it. The child with motor disorder has the same spontaneous reaction, but because of his inability to move and stretch his arms he cannot grasp and play with the toy. Consequently, repeated incidents such as these during the crucial early years causes the child to miss out on significant areas of normal childhood experiences and development. This failure to interact, adapt, and adjust affects the child not only physically, but also leaves him with deep feelings of confusion, alienation, dependence, and diminished self esteem.

Believing that brain-damaged children are usually left with a considerable residual capacity, Petö set out to utilise this asset to its fullest. Basing his practice on the theory of the brain's plasticity, he sought ways and means to forge new motor pathways for function. In particular though, he set out to create an approach which would develop the child's personality and promote their capacity to adapt to their environment. He made no claims of a cure, but he held that even profoundly handicapped children can master tasks provided they are given the correct goals, and are motivated to work and learn within the appropriate environment.

Familiar with and drawing on the vast heritage of Russian psychology, particularly the works of Pavlov, Vygotskii, Luriya and Bernstein, Petö combined the background theories of Neurophysiology and Neuropsychology when formulating his system. He made use of the existing knowledge available regarding the acquisition of motor skills and the regulation of behaviour. Departing from the traditional "treatment" approach, Petö from the outset used educational principles to help the children achieve their goals and function in life. His favourite dictum was *"the child must learn everything from sitting on the pot to the A.B.C."*.

The Institute's motto is *"Not because of but in order to"*. *"It is future or goal-oriented not focusing on the past or on the aetiology of the problem."* (Hari and Tillemans 1984)

The characteristic of the work can be defined as the direction of all resources and energies on reaching the goals and not on pinpointing the symptoms. The goals are shaped by the demands of society.

Petö lived with the children and spent long hours working with them developing and evaluating his system. Broad-based, it encompasses the needs of the whole child, i.e., physical, functional, social, emotional, and cognitive. Within the framework for guiding the children, it aims to promote active and self-initiated learning through goal-directed, carefully designated activities. Ideally, it puts the child at the centre and maps out for him a direction, where he has to learn to find his own solution to his problems.

The facilitations Petö used to mediate his system and promote the child's personality development and learning are for the most part unique to Conductive Education. In the Conductive milieu facilitations include everything that fosters and encourages the child to take an active part in his own learning. Anita Tatlow (1993) has the following to say about the child's active learning:

> *"With activity is meant the child wants to move. Facilitations must therefore be used in such a way that the child has the impression he is the active one, he himself found the movement, and that any progress was his achievement. This is what will motivate the child to find his own solutions and to persevere with his tasks."*

At the Institute in Budapest, the following *facilitations* have proved to be a foolproof recipe for the remarkable success of the work:

- **The Role of the Conductor.**
- **The Structure and Dynamics of the Group.**
- **Rhythmical Intention.**
- **Task Series and the Acquisition of Skills.**
- **The Daily Programme/Routine.**
- **The Learning Environment (Physical and Psychological).**
- **Manual/Hands on Facilitation.**

THE ROLE OF THE CONDUCTOR

The key professional in the Petö System is called the conductor. It is often asked why the word conductor is used in this context. Dr. Hari (1968) gives the following answer to the question:

> *"Like the Conductor of an orchestra, the Conductor regulates the activities of her group; occasionally practising individually with one child to bring his performance into tune with the rest of the group but normally leading the group which works collectively as a social unit in which one child's progress assists the performance of the others."*

The conductor is a state registered profession in Hungary. Trainees with A-level or equivalent qualifications undergo four years of intensive training in the Conductors College within the Institute complex in Budapest. On completion of training, they combine the roles of teacher, nursery nurse, and therapist for all with motor disorders. Ester Cotton has the following to say about the impact this holistic profession has on the overall outcome of the approach:

> "In Conductive Education there is no multi-disciplinary team, integration is complete within the person of the conductor and within the programme. There is an inter-connectedness which has a positive effect."

The conductor is first and foremost an educator. She is committed to using educational principles to help the children achieve their goals. To ensure that this is carried out in a consistent manner, the conductors work in shifts similiar to the nursing model. This guarantees the central tenet of the system which is an unbroken flow of conduction throughout the children's waking hours. It prevents confusion and fragmentation which can occur in the multi-disciplinary team approach.

In her practice, she is responsible for the following:

a. Establishing meaningful relationships with the children.
b. Careful assessment and observation of the children both individually and in daily life situations.
c. Setting long-term and short-term goals.
d. Organising the children into homogeneous groups.
e. Planning the daily/weekly programme/routine. This should embrace the whole child and ensure that all aspects of development are included i.e. the skills the child has to master. It also involves preparing task series, teaching aids, furniture, and the learning environment.
f. Implementing the daily/weekly programme/routine wherin she guides the children in a consistent pattern of learning.
g. Using her professional autonomy and familiarising herself with each child's strengths and weaknesses, modifying the programme as required.

Depending on the size of the group and the functional levels of the children, two to three conductors work together. They are expected to work harmoniously, their united goal being to create a secure, trusting, and at the same time, challenging environment for the children. Throughout the day, they guide the activities of the group. When carrying out the task series, one conductor runs the group assisted by the other conductors. The latter help the children under the direction of the leading conductor. From the beginning, the leading conductor will make contact with the children telling them what they are going to learn during the session. She takes care to speak in a slow and clear manner and at all times to ensure a smooth flow throughout the series.

The tasks the conductors set for the children should be geared to their level. They should be concrete and should motivate the children to actively participate. Above all, the conductors should strive to instill in the children a sense of personal effort.

Throughout the day, the conductors constantly seek ways and means to ensure the transfer of learning from one activity to another. For example, if a child is learning to grasp, they will make sure the child has the opportunity to grasp in all daily life situations, i.e.,

sitting grasping the plinth, grasping the spoon while eating, standing up grasping the ladderback chair.

They strive to foster a positive attitude and are constantly alert to the child's slightest effort and achievement. This, they highlight for praise. They ignore, on the whole, negative behaviour. Continuously challenging the children in a loving manner, they direct them to work for themselves and gradually learn to stand on their own two feet.

In places where teams of different professionals are available, it has proved possible to deliver the services to the children through an integration of all disciplines involved. The staff involved share their expertise on each child at the level of assessment, goal setting, and programme planning. In carrying out the work, professional boundaries are superseded in the common goal of creating the optimum learning environment. Thus, this programme also embodies Petö's dictum "he who pots must also teach".

THE STRUCTURE AND DYNAMICS OF THE GROUP

To facilitate the implementation of the daily/weekly programme/routine, the activities of the children takes place in a group situation. Group orientation is common in Eastern Europe and the East. In Chinese culture, the use of the group as a tool for learning is highly valued and developed.

The group offers the best opportunity for the children to interact with each other and with adults, and promotes interpersonal relationships which is basic for personality development. The children begin to look at, communicate with, and gradually become involved with each other. In the non-threatening environment of the group situation, they become familiar with their surroundings and develop feelings of belonging and security. They are stimulated to become actively involved and share activities. They learn to wait for one another, take turns, and gradually shoulder some responsibility. The group situation introduces a competitive spirit and provides them with opportunities for repetition and reinforcement. Success in the group energises and motivates all the children and makes them eager to achieve. It has been noted that the children's concentration in the conductive groups improves significantly.

Much effort and preparation goes into the selection of the children in the composition of a group. Dr. Hari has the following to say about this process (Hari and Tillemans 1983):

> "A group comes into being through a consideration of several characteristics of the children. Selection for group membership is a process of examining and re-examining children on diverse measures. The group must be large enough to permit individual differences and the formation of subgroups around similarities. It must create a favourable climate for teacher-student and student-student interaction. It must ensure success. Working in a group is more than merely training group spirit and a sense of responsibility for others: it sets the stage for activities in which members of the group learn to find ways to solve their problems."

The common demands for function makes it possible for children with different levels of motor disorder to be grouped together when carrying out the task series. However, each child can work at his own pace and at his own level of performance. For example, the child learning to stand up from a sitting position at Level 2 may need gaiters to straighten his elbows and manual help to sustain grasp of the ladderback chair as he stands up, whereas, the child at Level 4 may be learning to stand up independently. Each child's problem is different and the conductors must constantly seek ways and means to help solve it. Solutions will vary, however, it is important that the child reaches his goal and furthers his learning process.

Learning to attain goals and master skills should not be a grinding process of boring exercises. On the contrary, the conductors must see to it that all is done through age-appropriate activities, games and play. Optimum learning takes place when the children are enjoying and are actively participating in each task.

RHYTHMICAL INTENTION

Greatly influenced by the works of the Russian psychologists Vygotskii, Luriya, and Pavlov regarding the important influence speech has in regulating motor behaviour, Petö developed rhythmical intention. According to Luriya:

> "… any movement is aimed at a goal and carries out a certain motor task. At the level of instinctive behaviour, with its elementary structure these tasks are dictated by inborn programmes. At the level of complex conscious action during life they are dictated by intentions which are formed with the close participation of speech regulating behaviour."

Petö used rhythmical intention as a learning method by which the children use language to help them organise and carry out a movement.

Rhythmical Intention has two elements: intention and rhythm.

Intention

Before a movement is carried out the child must consciously want to achieve a certain goal. Through the use of vocalization, he expresses his intention and is mentally preparing to carry out the action. Movement and speech are linked together and facilitate the learning of movement and the attainment of the goal.

Rhythm

Rhythmical counting, the repetition of dynamic words or rhythmical songs gives the children a sense of timing which is vital in helping them to co-ordinate the movement. For example,

"I clasp my hands   1   2   3   4   5"

"I clasp my hands" is the intention. Counting one to five is the rhythm. When counting, use a slow even tempo. This is important when working with children who have spasticity. For children who constantly move, they should learn to fixate for the count of one, and hold from the count of two to five.

Dynamic speech may sometimes be used. This will depend on the level of the children and the goal to be achieved. For example,

"I grasp the stick   grasp   grasp   grasp"

The word "grasp" highlights the intention, thus giving the word "grasp" extra impetus in the situation.

When using Rhythmical Intention, it is important the child uses language he understands and is meaningful to him. It should be stressed that the child should also succeed in carrying out the goal set for him.

Children who cannot speak will benefit from the repitition of rhythmical intention. They can imitate the movements and actions of the conductor and the other children in the group and gradually link these experiences with language.

Rhythmical Intention

a. Emphasises 'I' thus highlighting from the outset the necessity for the child to take responsibility and become actively involved.
b. Focuses on the goal and helps eliminate all other distractions.
c. It helps them prepare mentally to learn a movement. When they are taught to express the intention, this helps form the internal speech pattern.
d. It helps them concentrate on the action and develops motor memory.
e. It equips them with an indispensable tool whereby they can gradually take over their own direction and thus phase out dependence on the conductor.
f. It harmonizes the group.
g. It regulates the timing and quality of the movement for both the athetoid and spastic child.
h. It predisposes the children to adopt a positive outlook in the way they want to live, solve problems, and strive to take control of their own lives.
i. It is the most effective way to impart to the parents the skills they need to help their children. In the normal relaxed atmosphere of the programme, the focus is off the parents and they gradually imbibe and learn every step their child needs to take. Following the rhythmical instructions, they in fact are learning along with their children.

TASK SERIES AND THE ACQUISITION OF SKILLS

The ability to master a task which can be either physical or mental is called a skill. The task may be a motor action, motor movement, intellectual process, or a combination of these. Skills can be specific or can be grouped together. In order to adapt to the environment and the demands of daily life, children have to learn many skills such as motor, functional, concentration, problem-solving, communication, social, creative, and imaginative. While normal children learn the foundation of these skills for the most part by assimilation, they have to be taught to children with motor disorders.

In the long process of acquiring daily-life skills, Petö used the *task analysis* approach. Each task is broken down into steps and the child is taken through these steps one at a time in order to reach the goal. Rhythmical Intention focuses the child's attention on the particular step and insures the correct timing of the movement. In this process, every opportunity must be given to the child to practise and transfer the skill he is learning.

Task analysis is based on knowledge and understanding of the child's abilities and needs, and an analysis of the movements and concepts involved in all functional activities. For example, the child at Level 2 — learning to drink from a two handled mug — must learn the following:

a. to recognise the mug, its characteristics, use, and position in space.
b. look at the mug and direct his hands towards it to grasp the handles.
c. coordinate the movement of bringing the mug to his mouth and adjusting the angle to enable the lips to seal the edge of the mug.
d. oral-motor coordination when swallowing.

At the initial stages of learning, this can prove to be a complex task for the child. However, if he has the opportunity to practise the task every time he takes a drink, he will gradually learn to master it. The number of steps in any given task depends on the functional and mental level of the children.

Essential tasks the child must learn will be found in Parts C and D of this manual. These tasks are based on the "*Basic Motor Pattern*" by Ester Cotton, who, working closely with Dorothy Seglow (Senior Physiotherapist, Watford Spastics Centre), realised there were fundamental movements that underlie all motor skills. These movements can be clearly observed in normal child development, however, they are missing or inadequately developed in the child with cerebral palsy. They include the ability to:

a. grasp and release
b. extend the elbows
c. develop fixation, i.e., fixing one part of the body while moving another part
d. acquire midline orientation
e. develop hip mobility

These fundamental movements will be practised within the essential tasks of the task series in various positions. When tasks are linked together and planned in a meaningful sequence this process is called task series. Built around the child's existing abilities it focuses on his immediate goals and gradually helps him at his pace master the skills he needs for independent living. Tasks to be learnt must be practised in different positions

e.g. in the lying position   — Lying Task Series
    in the sitting position — Sitting to Standing/Hand Task Series
    in standing   — Sitting to Standing/Transfer/Walking Task Series
    in walking   — Walking Task Series

The conductor plans and organises the task series and determines the·number of tasks she needs to teach the children in any one session. She should take into consideration the number of children, the level of their ability, the nature of the task series, and the number of staff available.

To encourage and motivate the children to actively engage in the task demands, the steps are taught within play and game situations. For example, giving the child a sweet, and giving him time to take off the wrapper before he eats it enables him learn the movement and master the "pincer grasp". Motivating activities and play makes everything meaningful and relevant for the children.

The tasks the children learn to master in the task series should be practised and reinforced consistently within the daily programme/routine. For example,

a. babies learning "bridging" in the lying task series have many opportunities throughout the day for practice and reinforcement every time the mother changes the nappy.
b. likewise, children at Level 1 learning the same task "bridging" in the lying task series have the opportunity for practice and reinforcement when pulling up and pushing down the pants in the supine lying position.

Task analysis and Rhythmical Intention interwine in the learning process for the child. This combination is a powerful facilitator in the hands of the conductor when teaching daily-life skills in the group situation. The conductor's yardstick for repeating a motor task in a series is the quality of enjoyment and lively participation on the part of the children.

THE DAILY PROGRAMME/ROUTINE

Practice makes perfect — with the exception of athletes training for sports events, no where has this axiom been adopted and utilised to its maximum as in the Petö Institute for Conductive Education. It is fair to say it is the greatest contributor to the excellence and overall success of the system in Budapest. In effect, it can be said the system revolves around the daily programme/routine wherein the children have the time and opportunity to practise and reinforce the skills they need to master. Indeed, so fundamental is it in Conductive Education that Petö demanded his professional, the conductor, work shift duty in order to implement the principle. It certainly underlines one of his favourite dictums: *No part of the day is better for learning than another.* It guarantees unity, prevents episodic training, and fully and consistently supports the children in their efforts.

All children need a regular routine to help them adjust to their environment, and learn to adapt to the demands made on them. Believing the child with cerebral palsy suffers a learning problem, the daily programme/routine was Petö's way of providing a learning environment for the child. Within this programme, the child has the opportunity to practise and repeat the skills he is learning or has learnt. When the child wakes in the morning, the conductor is on hand to make sure he learns to roll over as he has been taught in the task series, push off the bed, learn to sit down on the potty, or walk to the toilet using a ladderback chair, quadripods or walking stick. In the morning session, the child is guided by the conductor to transfer the skills he has learnt in the task series to activities of daily living. However tedious and time consuming it may appear, this first effort in the morning is for him a big step towards being able to take control of his life at a later stage in the conductive process.

Within the system, great emphasis is given to the planning of the programme/routine. All aspects of the child's development is included — physical, functional, psychological, social, cognitive. The automatic movements which we take for granted in our daily lives do not exist in the child with cerebral palsy. These movement patterns have to be learnt. For example, for the functional movement "raising the arms above the head to put on a sweater", the child with motor impairment must practise it in many different situations, i.e., in supine lying, in sitting, in standing, before he can do it automatically. The well-planned, comprehensive programme will provide and create situations where this can be learned and implemented daily.

However, despite the best planned programme, the most committed and skilled conductors, the most cooperative children, if time is not allowed for them to carry out the tasks and reach the goals at their pace, all effort is in vain. The uniqueness of the system in Budapest is the manner in which time is used in the learning process.

"Time is a very important ingredient in the process of learning: It is needed for locomotion, communication and motor activities, to be practised throughout the day. Time must be made available for the acquisition of such self-care functions as locomotion and toilet training in an unhurried fashion".

(Hari and Tillemans 1984)

From this, it is abundantly evident that the timetable is planned with the child at its centre. As the system revolves around the programme/routine, time should revolve around the child.

Tables 3.1 and 3.2 show a sample of a curriculum and a daily programme/routine in a pre-school centre of The Spastics Association of Hong Kong. The children in this centre range between two and six years of age.

Table 3.1 Curriculum

Task series
- Hand task series
- Sitting to standing/Transfer/ walking task series
- Lying task series (Cognitive, speech, and social skills training are integrated into the task series)

Lessons
- Play skills (object recognition)
- Pre-school concepts
- Social games
- Symbolic play
- Cooperative play
- Language activities
- Story telling
- Speech activities
- Music and games
- Fun and food
- Outdoor/Gross motor activities
- Arts and crafts
- Sensory stimulation
- Sensory motor training
- Oral motor training
- Self care
- Computer training

Other activities
- Outings
- Picnics
- Field trips
- Birthday parties
- Festival celebrations

Table 3.2 Timetable in a conductive education system

Time	Activity
7:00–8:00 a.m.	Getting up Toileting at the bedside Walking to the plinth for dressing and stretching Dressing
8:00–8:50 a.m.	**Breakfast, toileting**
8:50–9:10 a.m.	Walking to the classroom
9:10–9.20 a.m.	Prepare for classes
9:20–10:10 a.m.	1st group session/task series
10:10–10:45 a.m.	**Snacks, toileting**
10:45–11:30 a.m.	2nd group session
11:30–12:40 p.m.	**Toileting, lunch, toileting**
12:40–1:00 p.m.	Walking to the bedroom
1:00–2:15 p.m.	**Nap**
2:15–2:40 p.m.	Walking to the classroom, toileting
2:40–3:20 p.m.	3rd group session/task series
3:20–3:45 p.m.	**Toileting, snacks**
3:45–4:00 p.m.	Prepare for bathing
4:00–5:00 p.m.	Bathing/dressing
5:00–6:00 p.m.	**Toileting, dinner, toileting**
6:00–6:45 p.m.	4th group session: Group activity
6:45–7:00 p.m.	Toileting
7:00–7:45 p.m.	Homework/Positioning/TV
7:45–8:30 p.m.	**Snacks, toileting, brushing teeth, washing face**
8:30–8:45 p.m.	Walking to the bedroom
8:45 p.m.	Bed time

THE LEARNING ENVIRONMENT

The learning environment is a crucial facilitator within the system. Taking account of the child's motor, conceptual, and functional abilities, the careful organisation of the environment promotes learning, ensures the implementation of the programme, and assists the child in achieving his goals. However, much of the success depends on the combined efforts and organisation of the staff.

The room where the children work should be safe, well-ventilated, and attractively decorated. Unnecessary stimuli should be kept to a minimum. The furniture and teaching aids necessary for different sessions should be prepared and arranged beforehand. This gives the children the assurance they are expected, are important and will reinforce their sense of self-value and help them adopt a positive attitude towards learning. Furthermore, it minimises the level of distractions and helps them to focus on what they are doing.

The special Petö furniture (see Appendix) is an important facilitator as it promotes increasing independence physically and psychologically. The arrangement of the furniture should at all times encourage the children to be as active as possible. For example, if a child is learning to part his legs, the plinth should be placed in such a manner the child will have to cruise along the side of it in order to reach the stool where he sits for his meals.

Toys and teaching aids (see Appendix) should be placed at the child's level and space should be made available to facilitate and encourage their active exploration. Children should never be picked up and carried from one point to another, instead they should be taught how to move from one place to another in a manner which is appropriate for them at their functional level.

The conductors are responsible for generating a positive, supportive attitude both amongst themselves and with the children. They should unceasingly create an atmosphere which encourages the child's development of self-confidence and a realistic perception of his community and of the world. This demands hard work and total concentration on their part and on the task at hand. The following Fellowship Report by Marion Marx and Judy Ferren, United Cerebral Palsy of NYC, Inc. (1989) aptly describes the environment in a pre-school centre of The Spastics Association of Hong Kong:

> *"The staff worked incredibly hard, and with full concentration on the children. The atmosphere was not at all stern, however, but very cheerful and upbeat. Children were praised enthusiastically for good performances, and everyone in each group was made aware of each child's success. Songs were sung frequently to accompany the tasks. The games and activities were creative and age-appropriate, and the props and wall decorations were colorful and attractive."*

MANUAL FACILITATION

Manual facilitation is necessary to give the child the experience of a movement/position which he needs when learning functional activities. In this training manual, manual facilitations are needed for children at the mother and baby level and children at levels 1 and 2. They should be phased out as soon as possible at levels 3 and 4. Throughout this training manual where manual facilitation is used, it is clearly explained and illustrated.

When using manual facilitation, the care-giver should keep in mind the Basic Motor Pattern, especially the necessity for the child to learn to fixate one part of his body while moving another part. Priority should be given to helping the child learn to fixate the non-moving part, leaving him free to use the moving part.

Chapter 4

Observation of the Child with Cerebral Palsy and Goal-Setting in Conductive Education

The care-giver will need to have a clear understanding of the abilities of the child and the demands of the functional task in order to set realistic goals. A systematic and thorough observation of the child is required. This enables the care-giver to understand the child's abilities and helps her when setting goals for him. The functional record form is used to record the child's progress and reflect his abilities. It records the functional abilities of the child in the following daily activities:

a. feeding and drinking.
b. toileting.
c. dressing and undressing.
d. grooming.
e. showering/bathing.
f. sitting.
g. transferring.
h. getting in and out of bed.
i. standing and walking.
j. advanced hand skills.
k. advanced motor skills.

GUIDELINES FOR COMPLETING THE FUNCTIONAL SKILLS RECORD FORM

1. All care-givers should learn to complete the functional skills record form.
2. The record form should be completed once every 4–6 months.
3. The record form should be completed within the first month of the child's admission into the programme.
4. It is preferable to observe the child's daily activities to ensure that the functional abilities of the child are recorded.
5. For each record, the maximum functional level of the child should be recorded. Only gross estimation is required for items involving a time element.
6. Scoring system:
   ✔— the child's performance matches the description.
   ✗— the child's performance does not match the description.

7. If available, we recommend the use of a different coloured pen/pencil for each recording to indicate the child's progress during the given period of time.

   1st recording (date): _____
   2nd recording (date): _____
   3rd recording (date): _____
   4th recording (date): _____

HOW TO RELATE THE FUNCTIONAL SKILLS RECORD FORM TO GOAL SETTING AND PROGRAMME PLANNING

1. After completing the Functional Skills Record Form, the column with the most number of "✔"is the *maximum* functional level of the child and should be the base line for training.
2. The child may be at different levels in different functional tasks.
3. The training goals for the child should be those as stated in the description of the *next* functional level.
4. The child should be given the opportunity to participate in the activities of the daily routine as described in the next functional level in *Part C* of the manual — *The task analysis of activities of the daily routine.*
5. Furthermore, the child should be given the opportunity to participate in the task series as described at the next functional level in *Part D* of the manual — *The Task Series.*
6. For particular problems, the care-giver can refer to *Part E* of the manual — *Problem Solving.*
7. For information concerning equipment, furniture, teaching aids, please refer to the *Appendix.*

Feeding and Drinking Functional Record Form

1st record   (date): _____

2nd record   (date): _____

3rd record   (date): _____

4th record   (date): _____

a. *Finger Feeding*

Aims

1. Self-feeding.
2. Active reaching of upper limbs.
3. Eye-hand coordination.
4. Grasp and release.
5. Hand-mouth coordination.
6. Bite-off.
7. Lip closure.
8. Chewing.
9. Swallow.

b. *Spoon Feeding*

Aims

1. Self-feeding.
2. Active reaching of upper limbs.
3. Eye-hand coordination.
4. Grasp and release.
5. Hand-mouth coordination.
6. Lip closure.
7. Chewing.
8. Swallow.

c. *Using Chopsticks*

Aims

1. Self-feeding.
2. Fine-finger coordination.
3. Supination/pronation.

d. *Drinking*

Aims

1. Independent drinking.
2. Grasp and release.
3. Eye-hand coordination.
4. Hand-mouth coordination.
5. Elbow fixation.
6. Lip closure.
7. Swallow.

Feeding and Drinking Functional Record Form

Oral-Motor Control

	Yes	No			Yes	No
1. Dislikes others touching the mouth area.	☐	☐	6. Bites on spoon and unable to let go.		☐	☐
2. Drools copiously.	☐	☐	7. Chokes easily.		☐	☐
3. Unable to close lips.	☐	☐	8. Tongue thrust.		☐	☐
4. Unable to open mouth for food.	☐	☐	9. Unable to chew.		☐	☐
5. Unable to suck from milk bottle.	☐	☐	10. Unable to swallow.		☐	☐

Level 0	Goals = Level 1	Goals = Level 2	Goals = Level 3	Goals = Level 4
a. Finger Feeding				
1. Unable to focus on food. ☐	1. Looks at food. ☐	1. Looks at food. ☐	1. Looks at food. ☐	1. Finger feeds independently for all types of food. ☐
2. Unable to reach for food. ☐	2. Reaches for food. ☐	2. Reaches for food. ☐	2. Reaches for food. ☐	2. Eats tidily. ☐
3. Unable to grasp food and sustain grasp. ☐	3. Unable to grasp food and sustain grasp. ☐	3. Grasps and holds food. ☐	3. Grasps and holds food. ☐	
4. Unable to bring food to mouth. ☐	4. Brings food to mouth. ☐	4. Brings food to mouth. ☐	4. Brings food to mouth. ☐	
5. Unable to bite off food. ☐	5. Bites off food. ☐	5. Bites off food. ☐	5. Bites off food. ☐	
6. Unable to sustain grasp of food. ☐	6. Unable to sustain grasp of food. ☐	6. Sustains grasp of food. ☐	6. Sustains grasp of food. ☐	
7. Unable to finish last bit of food in hand. ☐	7. Unable to finish last bit of food in hand. ☐	7. Unable to finish last bit of food in hand. ☐	7. Finishes last bit of food in hand. ☐	
			8. Unable to finger feed tidily. ☐	

Level 0	Goals = Level 1	Goals = Level 2	Goals = Level 3	Goals = Level 4
b. Spoon Feeding				
1. Unable to focus on spoon. ☐	1. Looks at spoon. ☐	1. Looks at spoon. ☐	1. Looks at spoon. ☐	1. Spoon feeds independently. ☐
2. Unable to reach for spoon. ☐	2. Reaches for spoon. ☐	2. Reaches for spoon. ☐	2. Reaches for spoon. ☐	2. Spoon feeds tidily. ☐
3. Unable to grasp and hold spoon. ☐	3. Grasps and holds spoon. ☐	3. Grasps and holds spoon. ☐	3. Grasps and holds spoon. ☐	
4. Unable to scoop food onto spoon. ☐	4. Unable to scoop food onto spoon. ☐	4. Unable to scoop food onto spoon. ☐	4. Scoops food onto spoon. ☐	
5. Unable to bring spoon towards mouth. ☐	5. Unable to bring spoon towards mouth. ☐	5. Brings spoon to mouth. ☐	5. Brings spoon to mouth. ☐	
6. Unable to remove food from spoon with lips. ☐	6. Unable to remove food from spoon with lips. ☐	6. Unable to remove food from spoon with lips. ☐	6. Removes food from spoon with lips. ☐	
7. Unable to remove spoon from mouth and return it to bowl/plate. ☐	7. Removes spoon from mouth and returns it to bowl/plate. ☐	7. Removes spoon from mouth and returns it to bowl/plate. ☐	7. Removes spoon from mouth and returns it to bowl/plate. ☐	
			8. Unable to spoon feed tidily. ☐	
c. Using Chopsticks				
			1. Reaches for chopsticks. ☐	1. Reaches for chopsticks. ☐
			2. Holds chopsticks properly. ☐	2. Holds chopsticks properly. ☐
			3. Uses chopsticks to scoop rice to mouth. ☐	3. Uses chopsticks to scoop rice to mouth. ☐
			4. Unable to use chopsticks to pick up food. ☐	4. Uses chopsticks to pick up food. ☐

Level 0	Goals = Level 1	Goals = Level 2	Goals = Level 3	Goals = Level 4
d. Drinking				
1. Unable to focus on mug. ☐	1. Looks at mug. ☐	1. Looks at mug. ☐	1. Looks at mug. ☐	1. Looks at cup. ☐
2. Unable to reach for mug. ☐	2. Reaches for mug. ☐	2. Reaches for mug. ☐	2. Reaches for mug. ☐	2. Reaches for cup. ☐
3. Unable to grasp and hold mug. ☐	3. Unable to sustain grasp of mug. ☐	3. Grasps mug. ☐	3. Grasps mug. ☐	3. Grasps cup. ☐
4. Unable to bring mug to mouth. ☐	4. Initiates bringing mug to mouth. ☐	4. Brings mug to mouth. ☐	4. Brings mug to mouth. ☐	4. Brings cup to mouth. ☐
5. Unable to seal lips over rim of mug. ☐	5. Unable to seal lips over rim of mug. ☐	5. Unable to seal lips over rim of mug. ☐	5. Seals lips over rim of mug. ☐	5. Seals lips over rim of cup. ☐
6. Unable to drink from mug. ☐	6. Drinks from mug. ☐	6. Drinks from mug. ☐	6. Drinks from mug. ☐	6. Drinks from cup. ☐
7. Unable to drink from mug continuously. ☐	7. Unable to drink from mug continuously. ☐	7. Unable to drink from mug continuously. ☐	7. Drinks from mug continuously. ☐	7. Drinks from cup continuously. ☐
8. Unable to return mug to table. ☐	8. Unable to return mug to table. ☐	8. Returns mug to table. ☐	8. Returns mug to table. ☐	8. Returns cup to table. ☐
			9. Unable to sip from straw. ☐	9. Sips from straw. ☐

Toileting Functional Record Form

1ˢᵗ record (date): _____

2ⁿᵈ record (date): _____

3ʳᵈ record (date): _____

4ᵗʰ record (date): _____

a. *Sitting Down on Potty using ladderback chair (LBC)*

Aims

1. Standing balance.
2. Head control.
3. Body symmetry.
4. Grasp and release.
5. Hip mobility.
6. Knee flexion and extension.
7. Ankle dorsiflexion.
8. Stretching of hamstrings.
9. Transfer from standing to squatting.
10. Weight shifting.
11. Pulling down pants.
12. Learn body parts — hand, head, trunk, knee, hip, foot, bottom.
13. Learn concept "apart".

b. *Sitting on Potty*

Aims

1. Sitting balance.
2. Head control.
3. Body symmetry.
4. Elbow extension.
5. Sustained grasp.
6. Trunk extension.
7. Hip flexion.
8. Ankle dorsiflexion.
9. Lower limb abduction.
10. Learn body parts — head, trunk, elbow, hand, hip, knee, ankle, foot.
11. Learn concept "apart".

c. *Standing up from Potty*

Aims

1. Transfer — sitting on potty to standing.
2. Head control.
3. Body symmetry.
4. Grasp and release.
5. Elbow extension.
6. Trunk extension.
7. Hip mobility.
8. Knee extension.
9. Weight bearing through lower limbs.
10. Weight shifting.
11. Learn body parts — head, trunk, elbow, hand, knee, hip, bottom, foot.
12. Pull up pants.

d. *Bladder and Bowel control*

Aims

1. Bowel and bladder control.
2. Clean self after using toilet.

Toileting Functional Record Form

Level 0	Goals = Level 1	Goals = Level 2	Goals = Level 3	Goals = Level 4
a. Sitting Down on Potty Using Ladderback Chair (LBC)				*Sitting Down on Potty/Toilet without Aids*
1. Unable to stand grasping LBC in front. ☐	1. Unable to stand grasping LBC in front. ☐	1. Stands grasping LBC in front. ☐	1. Stands grasping LBC/handrails/plinth in front. ☐	1. Stands independently. ☐
2. Unable to release hand from rung of LBC. ☐	2. Releases hand from rung of LBC. ☐	2. Releases hand from rung of LBC. ☐	2. Pushes down pants. ☐	2. Pushes down pants. ☐
3. Unable to grasp rung. ☐	3. Grasps rung. ☐	3. Grasps rung. ☐	3. Squats down. ☐	3. Squats down. ☐
4. Unable to use alternate hands to climb down LBC. ☐	4. Unable to use alternate hands to climb down LBC. ☐	4. Uses alternate hands to climb down LBC. ☐	4. Sits on potty independently. ☐	4. Sits on potty/toilet independently. ☐
5. Unable to push down pants. ☐	5. Unable to push down pants. ☐	5. Unable to push down pants. ☐		
6. Unable to squat. ☐	6. Squats down. ☐	6. Squats down. ☐		
7. Unable to sit on potty grasping LBC in front. ☐	7. Sits on potty grasping LBC in front. ☐	7. Sits on potty grasping LBC in front. ☐		

Level 0	Goals = Level 1	Goals = Level 2	Goals = Level 3	Goals = Level 4
b. Sitting on Potty				*Sitting on toilet*
1. Unable to maintain head in midline. ☐	1. Maintains head in midline. ☐	1. Maintains head in midline. ☐	1. Maintains head in midline. ☐	1. Maintains head in midline. ☐
2. Unable to keep back straight. ☐	2. Unable to keep back straight. ☐	2. Keeps back straight. ☐	2. Keeps back straight. ☐	2. Keeps back straight. ☐
3. Unable to sustain grasp of LBC in front. ☐	3. Grasps LBC. ☐	3. Grasps LBC. ☐	3. Stretches elbows. ☐	3. Flexes hips. ☐
4. Unable to keep elbows straight. ☐	4. Unable to keep elbows straight. ☐	4. Stretches elbows. ☐	4. Flexes hips. ☐	4. Parts knees. ☐
5. Unable to keep hips well flexed. ☐	5. Flexes hips. ☐	5. Flexes hips. ☐	5. Parts knees. ☐	5. Keeps feet flat on floor. ☐
6. Unable to part knees. ☐	6. Parts knees. ☐	6. Parts knees. ☐	6. Keeps feet flat on floor. ☐	6. Sits independently. ☐
7. Unable to keep feet flat on floor. ☐	7. Keeps feet flat on floor. ☐	7. Keeps feet flat on floor. ☐	7. Sits independently for 10 mins. ☐	
8. Unable to maintain sitting position for 5 mins. ☐	8. Unable to maintain sitting position for 5 mins. ☐	8. Sits for 10 mins. ☐		

Level 0	Goals = Level 1	Goals = Level 2	Goals = Level 3	Goals = Level 4
c. Standing Up from Potty				
1. Unable to sit on potty grasping LBC in front. ☐	1. Sits on potty grasping LBC in front. ☐	1. Sits on potty grasping LBC in front. ☐	1. Sits on potty independently. ☐	1. Sits on toilet independently. ☐
2. Unable to push LBC forward. ☐	2. Unable to push LBC forward. ☐	2. Pushes LBC forward. ☐	2. Grasps and pushes LBC forward. ☐	2. Stands up independently. ☐
3. Unable to release hands from rung of LBC. ☐	3. Releases hand from rung. ☐	3. Releases hand from rung. ☐	3. Uses alternate hands to climb up LBC. ☐	3. Stands independently. ☐
4. Unable to grasp rung. ☐	4. Grasps rung. ☐	4. Grasps rung. ☐	4. Takes weight over feet. ☐	4. Pulls up pants. ☐
5. Unable to use alternate hands to climb up LBC. ☐	5. Unable to use alternate hands to climb up LBC. ☐	5. Uses alternate hands to climb up LBC. ☐	5. Stands up. ☐	
6. Unable to bend forward and take weight over feet. ☐	6. Bends forward and takes some weight over feet. ☐	6. Bends forward and takes weight over feet. ☐	6. Stands straight grasping LBC. ☐	
7. Unable to lift up bottom. ☐	7. Unable to lift up bottom. ☐	7. Lifts up bottom. ☐	7. Releases one hand to pull up pants. ☐	
8. Unable to stretch knees. ☐	8. Stretches knees. ☐	8. Stretches knees. ☐		
9. Unable to use alternate hands to climb up LBC. ☐	9. Unable to use alternate hands to climb up LBC. ☐	9. Uses alternate hands to climb up LBC. ☐		
10. Unable to extend hips. ☐	10. Extends hips. ☐	10. Extends hips. ☐		
11. Unable to stretch elbows. ☐	11. Stretches elbows. ☐	11. Stretches elbows. ☐		
12. Unable to stand grasping LBC in front. ☐	12. Stands grasping LBC in front. ☐	12. Stands grasping LBC in front. ☐		
13. Unable to pull up pants. ☐	13. Unable to pull up pants. ☐	13. Pulls up pants with assistance. ☐		

Level 0	Goals = Level 1	Goals = Level 2	Goals = Level 3	Goals = Level 4
d. Bladder and Bowel Control				
1. Unable to respond to potty during the day. ☐	1. Uses potty occasionally. ☐	1. Uses potty regularly. ☐	1. Uses potty. ☐	1. Indicates toilet needs. ☐
2. Unable to keep dry during the day. ☐	2. Unable to keep dry during the day. ☐	2. Dry during the day. ☐	2. Dry during the day. ☐	2. Dry during the day. ☐
3. Unable to keep dry at night. ☐	3. Unable to keep dry at night. ☐	3. Unable to keep dry at night. ☐	3. Dry at night. ☐	3. Dry at night. ☐
4. Unable to empty bowel while sitting on potty. ☐	4. Unable to empty bowel while sitting on potty. ☐	4. Empties bowel while sitting on potty. ☐	4. Empties bowel. ☐	4. Cleans self after toileting. ☐
5. Unable to clean self after toileting. ☐	5. Unable to clean self after toileting. ☐	5. Unable to clean self after toileting. ☐	5. Indicates toilet needs when asked. ☐	
			6. Unable to clean self after toileting. ☐	

Dressing Functional Record Form

1st record   (date): _____
2nd record   (date): _____
3rd record   (date): _____
4th record   (date): _____

a. *Putting on Socks*
  Aims
1. Sitting balance on bed/plinth/floor/stool.
2. Grasp and release.
3. Elbow extension.
4. Bilateral hand coordination.
5. Abduction and extension of thumb in grasp and pull.
6. Concentrate on task.
7. Learn body parts — toe, foot, ankle.
8. Learn the concept of sock.
9. Putting on socks.

b. *Putting on Shoes*
  Aims
1. Sitting balance on bed/plinth/floor/stool.
2. Grasp and release.
3. Elbow extension.
4. Abduction and extension of thumb.
5. Concentrate on task.
6. Learn body parts — toe, foot, ankle.
7. Learn concept of left and right.
8. Identify the left and right shoe.
9. Putting on shoes.

c. *Putting on Tops*
  Aims
1. Sitting balance.
2. Bilateral hand coordination.
3. Grasp and release.
4. Head control.
5. Elbow extension.
6. Abduction and extension of thumb in grasp and pull.
7. Concentrate on task.
8. Learn body parts — arm, elbow, shoulder, trunk, head.
9. Learn different parts of garments, sleeve, collar, front/back, top/bottom, inside/outside.
10. Learn garments suitable for different weather conditions.
11. Putting on garment.

d. *Putting on Pants*
  Aims
1. Sitting/standing balance.
2. Basic transfer skills — side lying ↔ supine lying sit ↔ stand.
3. Bilateral hand coordination.
4. Grasp and release.
5. Elbow extension.
6. Abduction and extension of the thumb in grasp and pull.
7. Concentrate on task.
8. Learn body parts — foot, leg, knee, bottom, waist.
9. Learn inside/outside, front/back of pants.
10. Learn garments suitable for different weather conditions.
11. Putting on pants.

Dressing Functional Record Form

Level 0	Goals = Level 1	Goals = Level 2	Goals = Level 3	Goals = Level 4
a. Putting on Socks				
1. Unable to sit well on care-giver's lap for 1 min.	1. Unable to tailor sit on bed/plinth/floor with support.	1. Tailor sits/Long sits on bed/plinth/floor with support.	1. Tailor sits/Long sits on bed/plinth/floor.	1. Long sits on bed/plinth/floor/sits on stool.
2. Unable to maintain looking at sock/foot for 1 min.	2. Looks at sock and foot.	2. Looks at sock and foot.	2. Looks at sock and foot.	2. Puts on sock.
3. Unable to put sock on toes.	3. Unable to put sock on toes.	3. Puts sock on toes.	3. Puts sock on toes.	3. Puts on sock, aware of inside/outside of sock.
4. Unable to grasp sock and pull.	4. Grasps sock and pulls.	4. Grasps sock and pulls up with thumb inserted inside sock.	4. Grasps sock and pulls with thumb inserted inside sock.	4. Puts on sock independently.
5. Unable to pull sock over heel.	5. Unable to pull sock over heel.	5. Unable to pull sock over heel.	5. Pulls sock over heel.	
6. Unable to pull up sock.	6. Pulls up sock with thumb inserted inside sock.	6. Pulls up sock with thumb inserted inside sock.	6. Pulls up sock with thumb inserted inside sock.	
b. Putting on Shoes				
1. Unable to sit well on care-giver's lap for 1 min.	1. Unable to tailor sit on bed/plinth/floor with support.	1. Tailor sits/Long sits on bed/plinth/floor with support.	1. Tailor sits/Long sits on bed/plinth/floor.	1. Long sits on bed/plinth/floor/sits on stool.
2. Unable to maintain looking at shoe/foot for 1 min.	2. Looks at shoe/foot.	2. Looks at shoe/foot.	2. Looks at shoe/foot.	2. Puts on left/right shoe correctly.
3. Unable to grasp shoe.	3. Grasps shoe.	3. Grasps shoe.	3. Grasps shoe.	3. Puts on shoes independently.
4. Unable to pull shoe over toes.	4. Puts shoe on toes.	4. Puts shoe on toes.	4. Puts shoe on toes.	
5. Unable to pull shoe over heel.	5. Unable to pull shoe over heel.	5. Unable to pull shoe over heel.	5. Pulls shoe over heel.	
6. Unable to adjust shoe on foot.	6. Unable to adjust shoe on foot.	6. Adjusts shoe on foot.	6. Adjusts shoe on foot.	
7. Unable to affix straps.	7. Unable to affix straps.	7. Begins to affix straps.	7. Affixes straps.	

Level 0	Goals = Level 1	Goals = Level 2	Goals = Level 3	Goals = Level 4
c. Putting on Tops				
1. Unable to sit well on care-giver's lap for 1 min. ☐	1. Sits well on care-giver's lap for 1 min. ☐	1. Sits at plinth/bed with support. ☐	1. Sits at plinth/bed. ☐	1. Sits at plinth/bed. ☐
2. Unable to maintain look at top x 1 min. ☐	2. Looks at top. ☐	2. Looks at top. ☐	2. Looks at top. ☐	2. Arranges top. ☐
3. Unable to grasp top. ☐	3. Grasps top with one hand. ☐	3. Grasps top with both hands. ☐	3. Unable to arrange top. ☐	3. Puts on top independently. ☐
4. Unable to put arms into sleeves. ☐	4. Unable to put arms into sleeves. ☐	4. Puts arms into sleeves. ☐	4. Grasps top with both hands. ☐	4. Chooses appropriate top for different weather conditions. ☐
5. Unable to bend head. ☐	5. Bends head. ☐	5. Bends head. ☐	5. Puts arms into sleeves. ☐	
6. Unable to pull top over head. ☐	6. Unable to pull top over head. ☐	6. Unable to pull top over head. ☐	6. Bends head. ☐	
7. Unable to pull down top. ☐	7. Pulls down top. ☐	7. Pulls down top. ☐	7. Pulls top over head. ☐	
8. Unable to adjust top. ☐	8. Unable to adjust top. ☐	8. Adjusts top. ☐	8. Pulls down top. ☐	
			9. Adjusts top. ☐	

Level 0	Goals = Level 1	Goals = Level 2	Goals = Level 3	Goals = Level 4
d. Putting on Pants				
1. Unable to lie still on bed/plinth. ☐	1. Lies still on bed/plinth. ☐	1. Sits on stool at plinth. ☐	1. Sits on stool. ☐	1. Sits on stool. ☐
2. Unable to maintain looking at pants for 1 min. ☐	2. Looks at pants. ☐	2. Looks at pants. ☐	2. Unable to arrange pants on floor. ☐	2. Arranges pants. ☐
3. Unable to lift up leg to put on pants. ☐	3. Fixates one leg and lifts the other to put on pants. ☐	3. Attempts to put leg into pants. ☐	3. Puts legs into pants. ☐	3. Puts on pants independently. ☐
4. Unable to bend both knees and keep both feet flat in the bridging position. ☐	4. Bends both knees and keeps both feet flat in the bridging position. ☐	4. Unable to pull up pants from above ankle. ☐	4. Grasps and pulls pants up over knees. ☐	4. Chooses pants suitable for different weather conditions. ☐
5. Unable to lift up bottom. ☐	5. Lifts up bottom slightly. ☐	5. Pulls up pants from below knee. ☐	5. Grasps plinth/handrails in front. ☐	
6. Unable to stretch both knees and relax. ☐	6. Grasps pants and pulls with assistance. ☐	6. Unable to stand up without assistance. ☐	6. Stands up with hands grasping support in front. ☐	
	7. Stretches both knees and relaxes. ☐	7. Stands with one hand grasping plinth with assistance. ☐	7. Maintains standing position with one hand holding onto support in front. ☐	
		8. The other hand attempts to grasp and pull up pants. ☐	8. Pulls up pants with the other hand with assistance. ☐	

Undressing Functional Record Form

1st record (date): _____
2nd record (date): _____
3rd record (date): _____
4th record (date): _____

a. *Taking off Socks*
   Aims
   1. Sitting balance.
   2. Bilateral hand coordination.
   3. Grasp with thumb in abduction and extension and push.
   4. Grasp and release.
   5. Elbow extension.
   6. Concentrate on task.
   7. Learn body parts — heel, toe, foot.
   8. Learn concept of sock.
   9. Learn inside/outside of sock.
   10. Learn pairing of socks and shoes.
   11. Take off socks.

b. *Taking off Shoes*
   Aims
   1. Sitting balance.
   2. Bilateral hand coordination.
   3. Grasp with thumb in abduction and extension and push.
   4. Grasp and release.
   5. Elbow extension.
   6. Concentrate on task.
   7. Learn body parts — heel, toe, foot.
   8. Learn concept of shoe.
   9. Learn left/right shoe.
   10. Learn pairing of socks and shoes.
   11. Take off shoes.

c. *Taking off Tops*
   Aims
   1. Sitting balance.
   2. Bilateral hand coordination.
   3. Elbow extension.
   4. Head control.
   5. Grasp and release.
   6. Concentrate on task.
   7. Learn body parts — neck, head, trunk, arm, hand.
   8. Learn parts of garment — front, back, collar, sleeve, inside/outside, top, bottom.
   9. Take off tops.

d. *Taking off Pants*
   Aims
   1. Standing/sitting balance.
   2. Transfer from standing to sitting and sitting to standing.
   3. Grasp and release with thumb in abduction and extension.
   4. Elbow extension.
   5. Hip mobility.
   6. Stepping in sitting/standing position.
   7. Concentrate on task.
   8. Learn body parts — waist, bottom, knee, leg, left and right foot.
   9. Learn different parts of pants — waist, leg, inside/outside.
   10. Take off pants.

Undressing Functional Record Form

Level 0	Goals = Level 1	Goals = Level 2	Goals = Level 3	Goals = Level 4
a. Taking off Socks				
1. Unable to sit well on care-giver's lap for 1 min. ☐	1. Tailor sits on bed/ plinth/floor with support. ☐	1. Tailor sits/long sits on bed/plinth/floor. ☐	1. Tailor sits/long sits on bed/plinth/floor. ☐	1. Sits on stool independently. ☐
2. Unable to maintain looking at sock for 1 min. ☐	2. Looks at sock. ☐	2. Bends one knee to allow the hand to reach the foot. ☐	2. Bends one knee to allow the hand to reach the foot. ☐	2. Removes socks independently. ☐
3. Unable to reach for sock. ☐	3. Reaches for sock. ☐	3. Grasps sock with thumb out. ☐	3. Grasps sock with thumb out and pushes down. ☐	3. Puts socks away tidily. ☐
4. Unable to grasp sock. ☐	4. Unable to grasp sock properly. ☐	4. Pushes down sock. ☐	4. Pushes sock over heel. ☐	
5. Unable to insert thumb in sock and push down sock. ☐	5. Pushes down sock. ☐	5. Unable to push sock over heel. ☐	5. Removes sock. ☐	
6. Unable to push sock over heel. ☐	6. Unable to push sock over heel. ☐	6. Grasps and pulls off sock. ☐	6. Puts socks in shoe. ☐	
7. Unable to grasp and pull off sock. ☐	7. Grasps and pulls sock off the toes. ☐	7. Relaxes and stretches knees. ☐		
	8. Relaxes and stretches knees. ☐			

Level 0	Goals = Level 1	Goals = Level 2	Goals = Level 3	Goals = Level 4
b. Taking off Shoes				
1. Unable to sit well on care-giver's lap for 1 min. ☐	1. Tailor sits on bed/plinth/floor with support. ☐	1. Tailor sits/long sits on bed/plinth/floor. ☐	1. Tailor sits/long sits on bed/plinth/floor. ☐	1. Sits on stool. ☐
2. Unable to maintain look at shoe x 1 min. ☐	2. Looks at shoe. ☐	2. Bends one knee to allow the hand to reach the foot. ☐	2. Bends one knee to allow the hand to reach the foot. ☐	2. Removes shoes independently. ☐
3. Unable to grasp strap of shoe. ☐	3. Grasps strap of shoe. ☐	3. Looks at shoe. ☐	3. Looks at shoe. ☐	3. Puts shoes away tidily. ☐
4. Unable to pull out strap. ☐	4. Pulls strap. ☐	4. Grasps and pulls strap. ☐	4. Grasps and pulls strap. ☐	
5. Unable to push off shoe. ☐	5. Pushes off shoe. ☐	5. Unable to push shoe over heel. ☐	5. Grasps shoe with thumb out. ☐	
		6. Pulls off loosen shoe. ☐	6. Pulls off shoe. ☐	
c. Taking off Tops				
1. Unable to sit well on care-giver's lap for 1 min. ☐	1. Sits well on care-giver's lap for 1 min. ☐	1. Sits at plinth/bed. ☐	1. Sits at plinth/bed. ☐	1. Sits on stool independently. ☐
2. Unable to maintain looking at top for 1 min. ☐	2. Looks at top. ☐	2. Unable to pull up top at the back. ☐	2. Pulls up top. ☐	2. Removes top independently. ☐
3. Unable to pull up top at the back. ☐	3. Unable to pull up top at the back. ☐	3. Bends head. ☐	3. Pulls top over head. ☐	3. Turns top inside out. ☐
4. Unable to bend head. ☐	4. Bends head. ☐	4. Grasps and pulls top over head. ☐	4. Pulls off top. ☐	4. Puts top away tidily. ☐
5. Unable to pull top over head. ☐	5. Unable to grasp and pull top over head. ☐	5. Pulls off top. ☐		
6. Unable to pull off top. ☐	6. Pulls off top. ☐			

Level 0	Goals = Level 1	Goals = Level 2	Goals = Level 3	Goals = Level 4
d. Taking off Pants				
1. Unable to lie still on bed/plinth/mat on floor. ☐	1. Lies still on bed/plinth/mat on floor. ☐	1. Grasps plinth with both hands and stands up. ☐	1. Stands grasping plinth/handrails in front with one hand. ☐	1. Stands grasping plinth/handrails in front with one hand. ☐
2. Unable to maintain looking at pants. ☐	2. Looks at pants. ☐	2. Unable to grasp pants with one hand and push pants down to knees. ☐	2. Grasps pants with thumb out with one hand. ☐	2. Pushes pants down to ankles. ☐
3. Unable to bend knees and keep feet flat on bed/plinth/mat. ☐	3. Bends knees but unable to keep feet flat on bed/plinth/mat. ☐	3. Sits down at plinth. ☐	3. Pushes pants down to knees. ☐	3. Lifts one leg at a time to step out of pants. ☐
4. Unable to lift up bottom. ☐	4. Lifts up bottom with assistance. ☐	4. Frees one hand to grasp pants at knees. ☐	4. Sits down on stool. ☐	4. Picks up pants from floor. ☐
5. Unable to grasp pants with both hands. ☐	5. Grasps pants with both hands. ☐	5. Pushes pants down to ankles. ☐	5. Pushes pants down to ankles. ☐	5. Puts pants away tidily. ☐
6. Unable to push down pants. ☐	6. Pushes down pants with assistance. ☐	6. Kicks off pants. ☐	6. Removes pants by lifting one leg at a time and stepping out of pants. ☐	
7. Unable to straighten legs and relax. ☐	7. Straightens both legs and relaxes. ☐		7. Picks up pants from floor with one hand. ☐	
8. Unable to kick off pants. ☐	8. Kicks off pants. ☐			

Grooming Functional Record Form

1st record   (date): _____

2nd record   (date): _____

3rd record   (date): _____

4th record   (date): _____

a. *Washing Hands*

Aims

1. Washing hands.
2. Midline orientation.
3. Hands in midline.
4. Flat hands.
5. Awareness of hands and fingers.
6. Personal Hygiene.

b. *Washing Face*

Aims

1. Washing face.
2. Wringing flannel.
3. Midline orientation.
4. Hands in midline.
5. Hands-to-face movement.
6. Elbow flexion and extension.
7. Flat hands.
8. Awareness of hands, face, and facial features.
9. Personal Hygiene.

c. *Brushing Teeth*

Aims

1. Brushing teeth and gargling.
2. Midline orientation.
3. One hand fixing one hand moving.
4. Grasp and release.
5. Bilateral hand coordination.
6. Crossing the midline.
7. Wrist mobility.
8. Fine finger movement.
9. Lip closure.
10. Personal Hygiene.

d. *Brushing Hair*

Aims

1. Brushing hair.
2. Midline orientation.
3. One hand fixing one hand moving.
4. Grasp and release.
5. Crossing the midline.
6. Elbow extension and flexion.
7. Shoulder extension and flexion.
8. Eye-hand coordination.
9. Personal Hygiene.

Grooming Functional Record Form

Level 0	Goals = Level 1	Goals = Level 2	Goals = Level 3	Goals = Level 4
a. Washing Hands				
1. Unable to put hands into basin.	1. Unable to put hands into basin.	1. Puts hands into basin.	1. Unable to turn on tap.	1. Turns on tap.
2. Unable to open hands for washing.	2. Opens hands for washing.	2. Opens hands for washing.	2. Opens hands for washing under tap.	2. Opens hands for washing under tap.
3. Unable to rub hands together.	3. Unable to rub hands together.	3. Rubs hands together.	3. Rubs hands together.	3. Rubs hands together.
4. Unable to lift hands out of basin.	4. Lifts hands out of basin.	4. Unable to use soap.	4. Uses soap.	4. Uses soap.
5. Unable to dry hands with hand towel.	5. Unable to dry hands with hand towel.	5. Lifts hands out of basin.	5. Unable to turn off tap.	5. Turns off tap.
		6. Wipes hands with hand towel.	6. Dries hands with hand towel.	6. Dries hands with hand towel.
b. Washing Face				
1. Unable to squeeze flannel.	1. Unable to squeeze flannel.	1. Squeezes flannel.	1. Unable to turn on tap.	1. Turns on tap.
2. Unable to bring flannel to face.	2. Brings flannel to face.	2. Brings flannel to face.	2. Squeezes flannel.	2. Squeezes flannel.
3. Unable to wash face with flannel .	3. Unable to wash face with flannel.	3. Washes face with flannel.	3. Holds flannel in outstretched palms and brings to face.	3. Holds flannel in outstretched palms and brings to face.
			4. Washes face with flannel.	4. Washes face.
				5. Washes and wrings out flannel.

Level 0	Goals = Level 1	Goals = Level 2	Goals = Level 3	Goals = Level 4
c. Brushing Teeth				
1. Cannot tolerate having teeth brushed by care-giver. ☐	1. Tolerates teeth being brushed. ☐	1. Grasps toothbrush and brings it to mouth. ☐	1. Grasps toothbrush and brings it to mouth. ☐	1. Grasps toothbrush and brings it to mouth. ☐
2. Unable to open mouth. ☐	2. Opens mouth. ☐	2. Squeezes tooth paste but messy. ☐	2. Unscrews cap of toothpaste. ☐	2. Unscrews cap of toothpaste. ☐
3. Unable to grasp toothbrush. ☐	3. Grasps toothbrush. ☐	3. Imitates movement of brushing teeth. ☐	3. Squeezes toothpaste. ☐	3. Squeezes toothpaste. ☐
4. Unable to rinse mouth and spit out. ☐	4. Unable to squeeze toothpaste. ☐	4. Unable to brush teeth at the side of the mouth. ☐	4. Unable to screw on cap of toothpaste. ☐	4. Screws on cap of toothpaste. ☐
	5. Unable to bring toothbrush to the mouth. ☐	5. Unable to rinse mouth and spit out. ☐	5. Brushes teeth. ☐	5. Rinses mouth and spits out. ☐
	6. Imitates movement of teeth brushing. ☐		6. Rinses mouth and spits out. ☐	6. Brushes teeth independently. ☐
	7. Unable to brush teeth at the side of the mouth. ☐			
	8. Unable to rinse mouth and spit out. ☐			
d. Brushing Hair				
1. Unable to grasp brush. ☐	1. Holds brush. ☐	1. Holds brush. ☐	1. Holds brush. ☐	1. Holds brush. ☐
2. Unable to bring brush to hair. ☐	2. Unable to bring brush to hair. ☐	2. Brings brush to hair. ☐	2. Brings brush to hair. ☐	2. Brings brush to hair. ☐
3. Unable to brush hair. ☐	3. Unable to brush hair. ☐	3. Imitates movement of hair brushing. ☐	3. Brushes hair but untidy. ☐	3. Brushes hair neatly. ☐

Showering/Bathing Functional Record Form

1st record   (date): _____

2nd record   (date): _____

3rd record   (date): _____

4th record   (date): _____

a. *Showering/Bathing*

Aims

1. Showering Bathing.
2. Transfer in/out of bathing area.
3. Sitting balance.
4. Upper limb movement.
5. Eye-hand coordination.
6. Personal Hygiene.

Showering/Bathing Functional Record Form

Level 0	Goals = Level 1	Goals = Level 2	Goals = Level 3	Goals = Level 4	Goals = Level 5
a. Showing/Bathing					
1. Unable to tolerate bathing (shows discomfort, frightened, or cries). ☐	1. Accepts being bathed by care-giver. ☐	1. Accepts being bathed by care-giver. ☐	1. Accepts being bathed by care-giver. ☐	1. Grasps handrails. ☐	1. Sits well for showering/ bathing. ☐
2. Unable to grasp handrails. ☐	2. Unable to grasp handrails with assistance. ☐	2. Grasps handrails. ☐	2. Grasps handrails. ☐	2. Sits with support. ☐	2. Rubs different parts of the body. ☐
3. Unable to sit with support. ☐	3. Sits with support. ☐	3. Sits with support. ☐	3. Sits with support. ☐	3. Rubs different parts of the body. ☐	3. Grasps flannel/ sponge and bathes independently. ☐
4. Unable to cooperate when bathing. ☐	4. Cooperates when being bathed. ☐	4. Cooperates when being bathed. ☐	4. Cooperates when being bathed. ☐	4. Grasps flannel/ sponge with one hand and grasps handrails with the other. ☐	4. Grasps and uses soap. ☐
5. Unable to look at different parts of the body when being bathed. ☐	5. Looks at different parts of the body when being bathed. ☐	5. Looks at different parts of the body when being bathed. ☐	5. Looks at different parts of the body when being bathed. ☐	5. Grasps and uses soap. ☐	5. Uses shower head properly. ☐
6. Unable to rub different parts of the body. ☐	6. Unable to rub different parts of the body. ☐	6. Unable to rub different parts of the body. ☐	6. Imitates rubbing of different parts of the body with one hand. ☐	6. Unable to use shower head properly. ☐	6. Follows the steps in bathing under supervision. ☐
7. Unable to grasp flannel/sponge. ☐	7. Unable to grasp flannel/sponge. ☐	7. Unable to grasp flannel/sponge. ☐	7. Occasionally holds flannel/ sponge. ☐	7. Follows the steps in bathing when reminded. ☐	7. Turns on tap. ☐
8. Unable to grasp and use soap. ☐	8. Unable to grasp and use soap. ☐	8. Unable to grasp and use soap. ☐	8. Grasps and uses soap. ☐		8. Turns off tap. ☐
					9. Controls the flow of hot/ cold water. ☐
					10. Moves into/out of bathing area independently. ☐

Sitting Functional Record Form

1st record   (date): _____

2nd record (date): _____

3rd record   (date): _____

4th record   (date): _____

a. *Sitting on Stool at Plinth*

Aims

1. Sitting balance.
2. Head control.
3. Symmetry.
4. Midline orientation.
5. Elbow extension.
6. Wrist dorsiflexion.
7. Sustain grasp.
8. Hip flexion.
9. Trunk extension.
10. Abduction of lower limbs.
11. Ankles in neutral position.
12. Symmetrical weight bearing.
13. Visual perception of the environment in the upright position.
14. Learn body parts — head, trunk, bottom, elbow, hand, foot.

b. *Long Sitting on Floor*

Aims

1. Sitting balance.
2. Head control.
3. Symmetry.
4. Weight bearing through upper limbs.
5. Elbow extension.
6. Flat hands.
7. Hip flexion.
8. Abduction of lower limbs.
9. Knee extension.
10. Visual perception of the environment in the upright position.
11. Learn body parts — head, trunk, bottom, elbow, hand, knee, leg.

Sitting Functional Record Form

Level 0	Goals = Level 1	Goals = Level 2	Goals = Level 3	Goals = Level 4
a. Sitting on Stool at Plinth				*Free Sitting on Stool*
1. Unable to grasp plinth. ☐	1. Grasps plinth. ☐	1. Grasps plinth in front leaving one hand free for play. ☐	1. Grasps side of stool. ☐	1. Sits on stool and plays with both hands. ☐
2. Unable to keep elbows straight. ☐	2. Unable to keep elbows straight. ☐	2. Keeps elbows straight for a period of time. ☐	2. Keeps elbows straight. ☐	2. Maintains head in midline. ☐
3. Unable to maintain head in midline. ☐	3. Maintains head in midline. ☐	3. Maintains head in midline. ☐	3. Maintains head in midline. ☐	3. Flexes hips. ☐
4. Unable to flex hips. ☐	4. Flexes hips. ☐	4. Flexes hips. ☐	4. Flexes hips. ☐	4. Keeps back straight. ☐
5. Unable to keep back straight. ☐	5. Unable to keep back straight. ☐	5. Unable to keep back straight. ☐	5. Unable to keep back straight. ☐	5. Parts legs. ☐
6. Unable to part legs. ☐	6. Unable to part legs. ☐	6. Parts legs. ☐	6. Parts legs. ☐	6. Places feet flat on floor. ☐
7. Unable to place feet flat on floor. ☐	7. Unable to place feet flat on floor. ☐	7. Unable to place feet flat on floor. ☐	7. Places feet flat on floor. ☐	7. Sits independently while hands are engaged in play. ☐
b. Long sitting on floor				
1. Unable to use hands for support. ☐	1. Uses both hands for support. ☐	1. Uses both hands for support. ☐	1. Uses one hand for support. ☐	1. Frees both hands for play. ☐
2. Unable to keep elbows straight. ☐	2. Unable to keep elbows straight. ☐	2. Keeps elbows straight for a period of time. ☐	2. Keeps elbows straight. ☐	2. Maintains head in midline. ☐
3. Unable to maintain head in midline. ☐	3. Maintains head in midline. ☐	3. Maintains head in midline. ☐	3. Maintains head in midline. ☐	3. Keeps back straight. ☐
4. Unable to keep back straight. ☐	4. Unable to keep back straight. ☐	4. Unable to keep back straight. ☐	4. Keeps back straight. ☐	4. Flexes hips. ☐
5. Unable to flex hips. ☐	5. Unable to flex hips. ☐	5. Flexes hips. ☐	5. Flexes hips. ☐	5. Stretches knees. ☐
6. Unable to stretch knees. ☐	6. Unable to stretch knees. ☐	6. Unable to stretch knees. ☐	6. Stretches knees. ☐	6. Parts legs. ☐
7. Unable to part legs. ☐	7. Unable to part legs. ☐	7. Parts legs. ☐	7. Parts legs. ☐	

Transfer Functional Record Form

1st record (date): _____

2nd record (date): _____

3rd record (date): _____

4th record (date): _____

a. *Transfer from Sitting on Stool to Standing at Plinth*
   Aims
   1. Change of position from sitting on stool to standing up at plinth.
   2. Sustained grasp.
   3. Extension of elbows.
   4. Body symmetry.
   5. Weight shifting (posterior and anterior).
   6. Weight bearing through lower limbs.
   7. Extension of hips and knees.

b. *Transfer from Standing at Plinth to Sitting on Stool*
   Aims
   1. Change of position from standing at plinth to sitting on stool.
   2. Sustained grasp.
   3. Extension of elbows.
   4. Body symmetry.
   5. Weight shifting (posterior and anterior).
   6. Weight bearing through lower limbs.
   7. Flexion of hips, knees and ankles.

c. *Tranfer from Standing to Long Sitting on Floor Using LBC*
   Aims
   1. Transfer from standing at LBC to long sitting on floor.
   2. Transfer from standing to kneeling.
   3. Transfer from kneeling to long sitting on floor.
   4. Change from side sitting to long sitting.
   5. Grasp and release.
   6. Extension of elbows.
   7. Weight bearing on flat hands.
   8. Extension of the knees with flexion of hips.
   9. Weight shifting.

d. *Transfer from long sitting on the floor to standing using LBC*
   Aims
   1. Transfer from long sitting to kneeling.
   2. Transfer from kneeling to standing using LBC.
   3. Change from long sitting to side sitting.
   4. Grasp and release.
   5. Extension of elbows.
   6. Weight bearing on flat hands.
   7. Extension of knees with flexion of hips.
   8. Weight shifting.

Transfer Functional Record Form

Level 0	Goals = Level 1	Goals = Level 2	Goals = Level 3	Goals = Level 4
a. From Sitting on Stool to Standing at Plinth				*From Sitting on Stool to Free Standing*
1. Unable to sit on stool grasping plinth in front. ☐	1. Unable to sit on stool grasping plinth in front. ☐	1. Sits on stool grasping plinth in front momentarily. ☐	1. Sits on stool grasping plinth in front. ☐	1. Free sits on stool. ☐
2. Unable to lean forward to initiate standing. ☐	2. Leans forward to initiate standing. ☐	2. Leans forward to initiate standing. ☐	2. Leans forward to initiate standing. ☐	2. Leans forward to initiate standing. ☐
3. Unable to lift up bottom to stand. ☐	3. Attempts to lift up bottom to stand. ☐	3. Unable to shift body weight forward. ☐	3. Attempts to shift body weight forward. ☐	3. Shifts body weight forward before standing up. ☐
4. Unable to bend the head and look at feet while standing up. ☐	4. Bends head and looks at feet while standing up. ☐	4. Begins to lift up bottom to stand up. ☐	4. Bends head while standing up. ☐	4. Clasps hands and stands up. ☐
5. Unable to sustain grasp of plinth while standing up. ☐	5. Unable to sustain grasp of plinth while standing up. ☐	5. Bends head while standing up. ☐	5. Lifts up bottom to stand up. ☐	5. Straightens hips and knees in standing. ☐
6. Unable to take weight through legs. ☐	6. Some weight bearing through legs. ☐	6. Maintains grasp of plinth while standing up. ☐	6. Maintains grasp of plinth while standing up. ☐	6. Stands straight with feet flat and apart. ☐
7. Unable to straighten hips and knees in standing. ☐	7. Unable to straighten hips and knees in standing. ☐	7. Weight bears through legs. ☐	7. Weight bears through legs. ☐	
8. Unable to stretch elbows in standing. ☐	8. Unable to stretch elbows in standing. ☐	8. Unable to straighten hips and knees in standing. ☐	8. Straightens hips and knees in standing. ☐	
9. Unable to stand straight. ☐	9. Unable to stand straight. ☐	9. Unable to stretch elbows in standing. ☐	9. Stretches elbows in standing. ☐	
		10. Unable to stand straight. ☐	10. Stands straight. ☐	

Level 0	Goals = Level 1	Goals = Level 2	Goals = Level 3	Goals = Level 4
b. From Standing to Sitting on Stool at Plinth				
1. Unable to stand grasping plinth in front with two assistants. ☐	1. Unable to stand grasping plinth in front with one assistant. ☐	1. Stands grasping plinth with one assistant. ☐	1. Stands grasping plinth without assistance. ☐	1. Free standing with clasped hands. ☐
2. Unable to bend head and look at feet. ☐	2. Bends head and looks at feet. ☐	2. Bends head and looks at feet. ☐	2. Bends head when sitting down. ☐	2. Bends head when sitting down. ☐
3. Unable to bend hips and knees. ☐	3. Bends hips and knees with assistance when sitting down. ☐	3. Bends hips and knees with minimal assistance when sitting down. ☐	3. Bends hips and knees without assistance when sitting down. ☐	3. Bends hips and knees gradually when sitting down. ☐
4. Unable to sustain grasp of plinth when sitting down. ☐	4. Unable to sustain grasp of plinth when sitting down. ☐	4. Sustains grasp of plinth when sitting down. ☐	4. Sustains grasp of plinth when sitting down. ☐	4. Keeps hands clasped when sitting down. ☐
5. Unable to sit properly with one assistant. ☐	5. Unable to sit well momentarily without assistance. ☐	5. Sits on stool momentarily without assistance. ☐	5. Sits on stool without assistance. ☐	5. Free sits on stool. ☐
	6. Unable to keep elbows straight in sitting. ☐	6. Unable to keep elbows straight in sitting. ☐	6. Keeps elbows straight in sitting. ☐	

Level 0	Goals = Level 1	Goals = Level 2	Goals = Level 3	Goals = Level 4
c. Transfer from Standing to Long Sitting on Floor Using Ladderback Chair (LBC)	*i. Transfer from Standing to Kneeling Using LBC*	*i. Transfer from Standing to Kneeling Using LBC*		
	1. Unable to stand grasping LBC with one assistant. ☐	1. Stands grasping LBC with one assistant. ☐	1. Stands grasping LBC without assistance. ☐	1. Stands grasping handrails. ☐
	2. Releases one hand and grasps rung to climb down LBC with minimal assistance. ☐	2. Releases one hand and grasps rung to climb down LBC. ☐	2. Uses alternate hands to climb down LBC. ☐	2. Bends one leg and half-kneels. ☐
	3. Unable to bend one leg and half-kneel. ☐	3. Bends one leg and half-kneels with assistance. ☐	3. Bends one leg and half-kneels with minimal assistance. ☐	3. Bends the other leg and kneels. ☐
	4. Unable to bend the other leg and kneel. ☐	4. Bends the other leg and kneels with minimal assistance. ☐	4. Bends the other leg and kneels. ☐	4. Kneels with bottom tucked well in. ☐
	5. Unable to kneel with bottom tucked well in. ☐	5. Kneels with bottom tucked in with minimal assistance. ☐	5. Kneels with bottom tucked well in. ☐	5. Pushes LBC forward. ☐
	ii. Transfer from Kneeling Using LBC to Long Sitting	*ii. Transfer from Kneeling Using LBC to Long Sitting*	6. Pushes LBC forward. ☐	6. Puts both hands flat on floor. ☐
	1. Unable to push LBC forward. ☐	1. Pushes LBC forward with minimal assistance. ☐	7. Releases both hands and puts hands flat on floor. ☐	7. Side sits on floor. ☐
	2. Unable to release both hands and put hands flat on floor. ☐	2. Unable to release both hands and put hands flat on floor. ☐	8. Side sits on floor. ☐	8. Puts one hand on each side. ☐
	3. Unable to side sit on floor. ☐	3. Unable to side sit on floor. ☐	9. Put one hand on each side. ☐	9. Stretches both legs to assume long sitting position. ☐
	4. Unable to put one hand on each side. ☐	4. Puts one hand on each side. ☐	10. Stretches both legs in front to assume tailor sitting position. ☐	10. Pushes through hands and pushes bottom back. ☐
	5. Unable to stretch out both legs in front. ☐	5. Stretches both legs in front to assume tailor sitting position. ☐	11. Pushes through hands and pushes bottom back. ☐	11. Sits with back straight and hips well bent. ☐
	6. Unable to push through hands and push bottom back. ☐	6. Unable to push through hands and push bottom back. ☐	12. Sits with back straight. ☐	

Level 0	Goals = Level 1	Goals = Level 2	Goals = Level 3	Goals = Level 4
d. Transfer from Long Sitting on Floor to Standing Using Ladderback Chair (LBC)	*i. Transfer from Long Sitting on Floor to Kneeling Using LBC*	*i. Transfer from Long Sitting on Floor to Kneeling Using LBC*		.
	1. Unable to long sit on floor. ☐	1. Unable to long sit on floor. ☐	1. Tailor sits on floor. ☐	1. Long sits on floor. ☐
	2. Unable to put both hands to one side and take weight through them. ☐	2. Unable to put both hands to one side and take weight through them. ☐	2. Brings both hands to one side and takes weight through them. ☐	2. Moves in to side sitting on floor. ☐
	3. Unable to bend both legs and side sit. ☐	3. Attempts to bend both legs and side sits. ☐	3. Bends both legs and side sits. ☐	3. Grasps LBC/ handrails in front. ☐
	4. Unable to bring both hands forward to grasp LBC in front. ☐	4. Grasps LBC in front. ☐	4. Grasps LBC in front. ☐	4. Kneels up grasping LBC/handrails in front. ☐
	5. Unable to kneel up grasping LBC in front. ☐	5. Unable to kneel up grasping LBC in front. ☐	5. Kneels up grasping LBC in front. ☐	5. Brings one leg forward to half-kneeling. ☐
	ii. Transfer from Kneeling to Standing Using LBC	*ii. Transfer from Kneeling to Standing Using LBC*	6. Unable to bring one leg forward to half-kneeling. ☐	6. Pushes up with the other leg and stands. ☐
	1. Unable to bring one leg forward to half-kneeling. ☐	1. Unable to bring one leg forward to half-kneeling. ☐	7. Pushes LBC forward. ☐	7. Stands straight with clasped hands. ☐
	2. Unable to push LBC forward. ☐	2. Unable to push LBC forward. ☐	8. Attempts to push up with the other leg. ☐	Goals = Level 5
	3. Unable to push up with the other leg. ☐	3. Unable to push up with other leg. ☐	9. Uses alternate hands to climb up LBC. ☐	1. Long sits on floor. ☐
	4. Unable to use alternate hands to climb up LBC. ☐	4. Uses alternate hands to climb up LBC with minimal assistance. ☐	10. Stands up grasping LBC without assistance. ☐	2. Moves into side sitting on floor. ☐
	5. Unable to stand straight. ☐	5. Stands grasping LBC with one assistant. ☐		3. Kneels up with clasped hands. ☐
				4. Brings one leg forward to half kneeling. ☐
				5. Pushes up with the other leg and stands up. ☐
				6. Stands straight with clasped hands. ☐

Getting into Bed Functional Record Form

(Transfer from standing → lying on bed)
(Transfer in standing, pulling onto bed, pivoting, rolling)

1st record   (date): _____
2nd record (date): _____
3rd record   (date): _____
4th record (date): _____

a. *Standing at Ladderback Chair (LBC) → Standing at side of bed*
   Aims
   1. Transfer from LBC to standing at bed/plinth.
   2. Grasp and release.
   3. Weight shifting.
   4. Trunk rotation.
   5. Upper and lower limb abduction.
   6. Standing balance.
   7. Cruising.

b. *Getting onto Bed*
   Aims
   1. Getting into bed.
   2. Hip flexion with knees in extension and ankle dorsiflexion.
   3. Hip and knee extension with lower limb abduction.
   4. Neck and trunk extension.
   5. Upper limb elevation.
   6. Grasp and release.
   7. Elbow extension and flexion.

c. *Pivot in Prone*
   Aims
   1. Moving around in prone lying.
   2. Abduction of upper and lower limbs.
   3. Extension of neck and trunk.
   4. One part fixing, one part moving.
   5. Weight shifting.
   6. Grasp and release.

d. *Rolling from Prone → Supine*
   Aims
   1. Rolling from prone to supine.
   2. Independent head movement.
   3. Independent upper limb elevation.
   4. Trunk extension.
   5. Independent movement of lower limbs.
   6. Trunk rotation.

Getting into Bed Functional Record Form

(Transfer from standing → lying in bed)

(Transfer in standing, pulling up onto bed, pivoting, rolling)

Level 0	Goals = Level 1	Goals = Level 2	Goals = Level 3	Goals = Level 4
a. From Standing at Ladder-back Chair (LBC) → Standing at Side of Bed				
1. Unable to stand with both hands grasping LBC. ☐	1. Unable to stand with both hands grasping LBC. ☐	1. Stands with both hands grasping LBC. ☐	1. Stands with both hands grasping LBC. ☐	1. Walks to side of bed with quoits/sticks or clasped hands. ☐
2. Unable to release one hand. ☐	2. Releases one hand. ☐	2. Releases one hand. ☐	2. Releases one hand. ☐	2. Releases the aid. ☐
3. Unable to part the hand and rest hand on bed. ☐	3. Unable to part hand and rest it on bed. ☐	3. Parts hand and rests it on bed. ☐	3. Parts hand and rests it on bed. ☐	3. Stands independently at side of bed. ☐
4. Unable to lift foot. ☐	4. Unable to lift foot. ☐	4. Lifts foot. ☐	4. Lifts foot. ☐	
5. Unable to move the leg forward towards the bed. ☐	5. Unable to move leg foward towards bed. ☐	5. Moves leg fowards towards bed. ☐	5. Moves leg forward towards bed. ☐	
6. Unable to weight bear through the leg. ☐	6. Some weight bearing through the leg. ☐	6. Takes some weight through the leg. ☐	6. Bears weight through the leg. ☐	
7. Unable to release opposite hand. ☐	7. Releases opposite hand. ☐	7. Releases opposite hand. ☐	7. Releases opposite hand. ☐	
8. Unable to move opposite hand towards the other hand and rest it on bed. ☐	8. Unable to move opposite hand towards the other hand and rest it on bed. ☐	8. Unable to move opposite hand towards the other hand and rest it on bed. ☐	8. Brings opposite hand towards the other hand and rests it on bed. ☐	
9. Unable to lift opposite foot. ☐	9. Unable to lift opposite foot. ☐	9. Unable to lift up opposite foot. ☐	9. Lifts opposite foot. ☐	
10. Unable to move opposite leg towards the other leg. ☐	10. Unable to move opposite leg towards the other leg. ☐	10. Unable to move opposite leg towards the other leg. ☐	10. Moves opposite leg towards the other leg. ☐	
11. Unable to weight bear through opposite leg. ☐	11. Some weight bearing through opposite leg. ☐	11. Takes some weight through opposite leg. ☐	11. Bears weight through opposite leg. ☐	
12. Unable to stand leaning on bed. ☐	12. Stands with assistance using arm gaiters. ☐	12. Stands leaning on bed. ☐	12. Stands straight leaning on bed. ☐	

Level 0	Goals = Level 1	Goals = Level 2	Goals = Level 3	Goals = Level 4
b. Getting onto Bed				
1. Unable to stand at side of bed. ☐	1. Stands with assistance at side of bed using arm gaiters. ☐	1. Stands with assistance at side of bed. ☐	1. Stands straight at side of bed. ☐	1. Stands at side of bed. ☐
2. Unable to keep feet flat on floor with hips flexed and trunk extended across bed. ☐	2. Unable to keep feet flat on floor with hips flexed and trunk extended across bed. ☐	2. Keeps feet flat on floor with hips flexed and trunk extended across bed. ☐	2. Keeps feet flat on floor with hips flexed and trunk extended across bed. ☐	2. Gets onto bed with both arms stretched above head and both legs apart. ☐
3. Unable to stretch both arms above head. ☐	3. Unable to stretch both arms above head. ☐	3. Stretches both arms above head. ☐	3. Stretches both arms above head. ☐	3. Pulls up the bed with both hands. ☐
4. Unable to grasp bed clothes with both hands. ☐	4. Grasps bed clothes with both hands. ☐	4. Grasps bed clothes with both hands. ☐	4. Grasps bed clothes with both hands. ☐	
5. Unable to pull onto bed using both hands. ☐	5. Unable to pull onto bed with both hands. ☐	5. Attempts to pull onto bed using both hands. ☐	5. Pulls onto bed with both hands. ☐	
6. Unable to stretch both legs. ☐	6. Stretches both legs. ☐	6. Stretches and parts both legs . ☐	6. Stretches and parts both legs. ☐	
c. Pivoting on Stomach				
1. Unable to lie on stomach with arms stretched above head. ☐	1. Unable to lie on stomach with arms stretched above head. ☐	1. Lies on stomach with arms stretched above head. ☐	1. Lies on stomach with arms stretched above head. ☐	1. Lies on stomach with arms stretched above head. ☐
2. Unable to lift up head. ☐	2. Lifts head. ☐	2. Lifts head. ☐	2. Lifts head in midline. ☐	2. Pivots and lies straight in bed. ☐
3. Unable to part one arm. ☐	3. Parts one arm. ☐	3. Parts one arm. ☐	3. Parts one arm. ☐	
4. Unable to part opposite leg. ☐	4. Unable to part opposite leg. ☐	4. Unable to part opposite leg. ☐	4. Parts opposite leg. ☐	
5. Unable to bear weight on arm and move the other arm towards it. ☐	5. Unable to bear weight on arm and move the other arm towards it. ☐	5. Bears weight on arm and moves the other arm towards it. ☐	5. Bears weight on arm and moves the other arm towards it. ☐	
6. Unable to bear weight on leg and move the other leg towards it. ☐	6. Bears weight on leg and moves the other leg towards it. ☐	6. Bears weight on leg and moves the other leg towards it. ☐	6. Bears weight on leg and brings the other leg towards it. ☐	
7. Unable to complete a 90° turn. ☐	7. Unable to complete a 90° turn. ☐	7. Unable to complete a 90° turn. ☐	7. Completes a 90° turn slowly. ☐	

Level 0	Goals = Level 1	Goals = Level 2	Goals = Level 3	Goals = Level 4
d. Rolling from Lying on Stomach → Lying on Back				
1. Unable to stretch both arms above head. ☐	1. Unable to stretch both arms above head. ☐	1. Unable to stretch both arms above head. ☐	1. Stretches both arms above head. ☐	1. Rolls onto back independently. ☐
2. Unable to lift head. ☐	2. Lifts head. ☐	2. Lifts head. ☐	2. Lifts head to midline. ☐	2. Lies straight in bed. ☐
3. Unable to turn face to one side to look at toy. ☐	3. Turns face to one side to look at toy. ☐	3. Turns face to the side. ☐	3. Turns face to one side. ☐	
4. Unable to bend opposite leg. ☐	4. Bends opposite leg. ☐	4. Bends opposite leg. ☐	4. Bends opposite leg. ☐	
5. Unable to roll to the side. ☐	5. Unable to roll to the side. ☐	5. Rolls to the side. ☐	5. Rolls to the side. ☐	
6. Unable to roll onto back. ☐	6. Unable to roll onto back. ☐	6. Unable to roll onto back. ☐	6. Rolls onto back. ☐	

Getting Out of Bed Functional Record Form

(Transfer from bed → standing at end of bed)
(Rolling, pivoting, pushing down, cruising)

1st record (date): _____
2nd record (date): _____
3rd record (date): _____
4th record (date): _____

a. *Rolling From Supine to Prone*
   Aims
   1. Getting out of bed.
   2. Rolling from supine to prone.
   3. Independent head movement.
   4. Independent upper limb elevation.
   5. Elbow extension.
   6. Crossing midline.
   7. Independent lower limb movement.
   8. Trunk rotation.

b. *Pivot in Prone*
   Aims
   1. Moving around in prone lying.
   2. Abduction of upper and lower limbs.
   3. Neck extension.
   4. Trunk extension.
   5. One part fixing, one part moving.
   6. Weight shifting.
   7. Alternate upper and lower limb movement.

c. *Pushing Down From Bed*
   Aims
   1. Transfer from bed/plinth to standing on floor.
   2. Neck extension.
   3. Upper limb elevation.
   4. Elbow flexion and extension.
   5. Trunk extension.
   6. Knee extension with hip in abduction.
   7. Hip flexion with knee extension and ankle dorsiflexion.
   8. Grasp and release.

d. *Cruising to End of Bed*
   Aims
   1. Cruising.
   2. Transfer from one place to another.
   3. Grasp and release.
   4. Weight shifting.
   5. Upper and lower limb abduction.
   6. Standing balance.

Getting Out of Bed Functional Record Form

(Transfer from bed → standing at end of bed)

(Rolling, pivoting, pushing down, cruising)

Level 0	Goals = Level 1	Goals = Level 2	Goals = Level 3	Goals = Level 4
a. Lying on Back → Lying on Stomach				
1. Unable to lie still. ☐	1. Lies still. ☐	1. Lies still. ☐	1. Lies still. ☐	1. Lies still. ☐
2. Unable to stretch both arms above head. ☐	2. Unable to stretch both arms above head. ☐	2. Unable to stretch both arms above head. ☐	2. Stretches both arms above head. ☐	2. Rolls onto stomach independently. ☐
3. Unable to turn face to one side to look at toy. ☐	3. Turns face to one side to look at toy. ☐	3. Turns face to one side. ☐	3. Turns face to one side. ☐	3. Lies straight. ☐
4. Unable to bend the opposite leg. ☐	4. Bends opposite leg. ☐	4. Bends opposite leg. ☐	4. Bends opposite leg. ☐	
5. Unable to roll to the side. ☐	5. Unable to roll to the side. ☐	5. Roll to the side. ☐	5. Rolls to the side. ☐	
6. Unable to roll onto stomach. ☐	6. Unable to roll onto stomach. ☐	6. Unable to roll onto stomach. ☐	6. Rolls onto stomach. ☐	
b. Pivot on Stomach				
1. Unable to lie on stomach with arms stretched above head. ☐	1. Unable to lie on stomach with arms stretched above head. ☐	1. Lies on stomach with arms stretched above head. ☐	1. Lies on stomach with arms stretched above head. ☐	1. Lies on stomach with arms stretched above head. ☐
2. Unable to lift head. ☐	2. Lifts up head. ☐	2. Lifts head. ☐	2. Lifts head. ☐	2. Pivots until body lies across the bed. ☐
3. Unable to part one arm. ☐	3. Parts one arm. ☐	3. Parts one arm. ☐	3. Parts one arm. ☐	
4. Unable to part opposite leg. ☐	4. Unable to part opposite leg. ☐	4. Unable to part opposite leg. ☐	4. Parts opposite leg. ☐	
5. Unable to bear weight on arm and move the other arm towards it. ☐	5. Unable to bear weight on arm and move the other arm towards it. ☐	5. Bears weight on arm and moves the other arm towards it. ☐	5. Bears weight on arm and moves the other arm towards it. ☐	
6. Unable to bear weight on leg and move the other leg towards it. ☐	6. Bears weight on leg and moves the other leg towards it. ☐	6. Bears weight on leg and moves the other leg towards it. ☐	6. Bears weight on leg and moves the other leg towards it. ☐	
7. Unable to complete a 90° turn. ☐	7. Unable to complete a 90° turn. ☐	7. Unable to complete a 90° turn. ☐	7. Completes a 90° turn slowly. ☐	

Level 0	Goals = Level 1	Goals = Level 2	Goals = Level 3	Goals = Level 4
c. Pushing off the Bed				
1. Unable to lie on stomach with arms stretched above head. ☐	1. Unable to lie on stomach with arms stretched above head. ☐	1. Lies on stomach with arms stretched above head. ☐	1. Lies on stomach with arms stretched above head. ☐	1. Lies on stomach. ☐
2. Unable to lift head. ☐	2. Able to lift head. ☐	2. Able to lift head. ☐	2. Lifts up head. ☐	2. Pushes off bed using both hands. ☐
3. Unable to stretch hips and knees. ☐	3. Stretches hips and knees. ☐	3. Stretches both hips and knees. ☐	3. Stretches hips and knees. ☐	3. Weight bears with feet flat on floor. ☐
4. Unable to use both hands to push off bed. ☐	4. Unable to use both hands to push off bed. ☐	4. Attempts to push off bed using both hands. ☐	4. Uses both hands to push off bed. ☐	4. Stands straight with clasped hands. ☐
5. Unable to put both feet flat on floor with hips flexed and trunk extended across bed. ☐	5. Puts both feet flat on floor with hips flexed and trunk extended across bed. ☐	5. Puts both feet flat on floor with hips flexed and trunk extended across bed. ☐	5. Puts both feet flat on floor with hips flexed and trunk extended across bed. ☐	
6. Unable to bear weight through both legs. ☐	6. Some weight bearing through both legs. ☐	6. Some weight bearing through legs. ☐	6. Weight bears through both legs. ☐	
7. Unable to push up through hands into standing. ☐	7. Unable to push up through hands into standing. ☐	7. Pushes up through hands into standing. ☐	7. Pushes up to standing with straight elbows. ☐	
8. Unable to keep feet flat on floor in standing. ☐	8. Unable to keep feet flat on floor in standing. ☐	8. Keeps feet flat on floor in standing. ☐	8. Keeps feet flat on floor in standing. ☐	
9. Unable to stand straight. ☐	9. Stands with assistance using arm gaiters. ☐	9. Stands straight with assistance. ☐	9. Stands straight. ☐	

Level 0	Goals = Level 1	Goals = Level 2	Goals = Level 3	Goals = Level 4
d. Walking Sideways to End of Bed (Cruising)				*Walking from Bed to Toilet*
1. Unable to release one hand. ☐	1. Releases one hand. ☐	1. Releases one hand. ☐	1. Releases one hand. ☐	1. Walks to toilet using walking aids. ☐
2. Unable to part hand and grasp. ☐	2. Unable to part hand and grasp. ☐	2. Parts hand and grasps. ☐	2. Parts hand and grasps. ☐	2. Walks to toilet independently. ☐
3. Unable to lift foot. ☐	3. Lifts foot. ☐	3. Lifts foot. ☐	3. Lifts foot. ☐	
4. Unable to part leg and move it sideways. ☐	4. Unable to part leg and move it sideways. ☐	4. Unable to part leg and move it sideways. ☐	4. Parts leg and moves it sideways. ☐	
5. Unable to weight bear through leg. ☐	5. Some weight bearing through leg. ☐	5. Weight bears through leg. ☐	5. Weight bears through leg. ☐	
6. Unable to release opposite hand. ☐	6. Releases opposite hand. ☐	6. Releases opposite hand. ☐	6. Releases opposite hand. ☐	
7. Unable to move opposite hand towards the other hand and grasp. ☐	7. Unable to move opposite hand towards the other hand and grasp. ☐	7. Brings opposite hand towards the other hand and grasps. ☐	7. Moves opposite hand towards the other hand and grasps. ☐	
8. Unable to lift opposite foot. ☐	8. Lifts opposite foot. ☐	8. Lifts up the opposite foot. ☐	8. Lifts opposite foot. ☐	
9. Unable to move opposite leg towards the other. ☐	9. Unable to move opposite leg towards the other. ☐	9. Moves the opposite leg towards the other leg. ☐	9. Moves opposite leg towards the other. ☐	
10. Unable to weight bear through the opposite leg. ☐	10. Some weight bearing through the opposite leg. ☐	10. Weight bears through the opposite leg. ☐	10. Weight bears through the opposite leg. ☐	
11. Unable to stand. ☐	11. Stands with assistance using arm gaiters. ☐	11. Stands straight with assistance. ☐	11. Stands straight. ☐	

Standing and Walking Functional Record Form

1st record   (date): _____

2nd record   (date): _____

3rd record   (date): _____

4th record   (date): _____

a. *Standing at Ladderback Chair (LBC)*

Aims

1. Standing balance.
2. Body symmetry.
3. Head control.
4. Extension of trunk, hips, and knees.
5. Ankles in neutral.
6. Abduction of lower limbs.
7. Extension of elbows and wrists.
8. Sustained grasp.
9. Symmetrical weight bearing.
10. Visual perception of the environment in the upright position.
11. Relationship of body parts.
12. Learn body parts — head/trunk/hips/bottom/leg/knee/foot/arm/ elbow.
13. Spatial concept — forward.

b. *Walking*

Aims

1. A means of moving from one place to another.
2. Walking balance.
3. Body symmetry.
4. Head control.
5. Extension of trunk/hips/knees.
6. Hip mobility.
7. Ankle mobility.
8. Weight bearing through lower limbs.
9. Weight shifting.
10. Extension of elbows and dorsiflexion of wrists.
11. Sustained grasp.
12. Maintain functional range of lower limb joint mobility.
13. Visual perception of the environment in upright position.
14. Relationship of body parts.
15. Learn body parts — head/trunk/hip/knee/foot/arm/elbow/ hand.
16. Spatial relationship.
17. Spatial concept — forward/at the side/left/right.
18. Improve circulation.

Standing and Walking Functional Record Form

Level 0	Goals = Level 1	Goals = Level 2	Goals = Level 3	Goals = Level 4
a. Standing at Ladderback Chair (LBC)				
1. Unable to grasp LBC in front. ☐	1. Grasps LBC in front. ☐	1. Grasps LBC in front. ☐	1. Grasps a tripod/quadripod/walking stick. ☐	1. Grasps a horizontal stick/quoit/clasped hands. ☐
2. Unable to maintain head in midline. ☐	2. Maintains head in midline. ☐	2. Maintains head in midline. ☐	2. Maintains head in midline. ☐	2. Maintains head in midline. ☐
3. Unable to keep elbows straight. ☐	3. Unable to keep elbows straight. ☐	3. Keeps elbows straight. ☐	3. Keeps elbows straight. ☐	3. Keeps elbows straight. ☐
4. Unable to maintain back upright. ☐	4. Unable to maintain back straight. ☐	4. Keeps back straight. ☐	4. Keeps back straight. ☐	4. Keeps back straight. ☐
5. Unable to extend hips. ☐	5. Unable to fully extend hips. ☐	5. Extends hips. ☐	5. Extends hips. ☐	5. Extends hips. ☐
6. Unable to weight bear through legs. ☐	6. Some weight bearing through the legs. ☐	6. Weight bears through the legs. ☐	6. Weight bears through the legs. ☐	6. Weight bears through the legs. ☐
7. Unable to maintain straight legs. ☐	7. Unable to maintain straight legs. ☐	7. Keeps knees straight. ☐	7. Keeps legs straight. ☐	7. Keeps legs straight. ☐
8. Unable to keep knees apart. ☐	8. Unable to keep knees apart. ☐	8. Unable to keep knees apart. ☐	8. Keep knees apart. ☐	8. Keeps knees apart. ☐
9. Unable to keep feet flat on floor. ☐	9. Unable to keep feet flat on floor. ☐	9. Unable to keep feet flat on floor. ☐	9. Keeps feet flat on floor. ☐	9. Keeps feet flat on floor. ☐
10. Unable to tolerate this position for 10 seconds. ☐	10. Maintains this position for 10 seconds. ☐	10. Maintains this position for 10 seconds. ☐	10. Keeps this position for 10 seconds. ☐	10. Keeps this position for 10 seconds. ☐

Level 0	Goals = Level 1	Goals = Level 2	Goals = Level 3	Goals = Level 4
b. Walking — *Using Ladderback Chair*				*Using tripods/quadripods/sticks*
1. Unable to stand grasping LBC in front. ☐	1. Stands grasping LBC in front with two assistants. ☐	1. Stands grasping LBC in front with one assistant. ☐	1. Stands grasping LBC in front under supervision. ☐	1. Standing grasping tripods/quadripods/ walking sticks. ☐
2. Unable to push LBC forward. ☐	2. Unable to push LBC forward. ☐	2. Unable to push LBC forward. ☐	2. Pushes LBC forward. ☐	2. Moves Rt. stick forward. ☐
3. Unable to take weight through Rt. leg. ☐	3. Unable to take weight through Rt. leg. ☐	3. Takes some weight through Rt. leg. ☐	3. Takes weight through Rt. leg. ☐	3. Takes a step with Lt. foot. ☐
4. Unable to straighten Rt. leg. ☐	4. Unable to straighten Rt. leg. ☐	4. Unable to straighten Rt. leg. ☐	4. Straightens Rt. leg. ☐	4. Moves Lt. stick forward. ☐
5. Unable to lift up Lt. leg. ☐	5. Lifts up Lt. leg. ☐	5. Lifts up Lt. leg. ☐	5. Lifts up Lt. leg. ☐	5. Takes a step with Rt. foot. ☐
6. Unable to bring Lt. leg forward. ☐	6. Unable to bring Lt. leg forward. ☐	6. Brings Lt. leg forward. ☐	6. Brings Lt. leg forward. ☐	6. Stands straight. ☐
7. Unable to place Lt. foot flat on floor. ☐	7. Unable to place Lt. foot flat on floor. ☐	7. Places Lt. foot on floor. ☐	7. Places Lt. foot flat on floor. ☐	
8. Unable to take weight through Lt. leg. ☐	8. Unable to take weight through Lt. leg. ☐	8. Takes some weight through Lt. leg. ☐	8. Takes weight through Lt. leg. ☐	*Goals = Level 5*
9. Unable to straighten Lt. leg. ☐	9. Unable to straighten Lt. leg. ☐	9. Unable to straighten Lt. leg. ☐	9. Straightens Lt. leg. ☐	*Using quoits/clasped hands*
10. Unable to lift up Rt. leg. ☐	10. Lifts up Rt. leg. ☐	10. Lifts up Rt. leg. ☐	10. Lifts up Rt. leg. ☐	1. Stands with clasped hands. ☐
11. Unable to bring Rt. leg forward. ☐	11. Unable to bring Rt. leg forward. ☐	11. Brings Rt. leg forward. ☐	11. Brings Rt. leg forward. ☐	2. Steps with Lt. foot forward. ☐
12. Unable to bring Rt. foot flat on floor. ☐	12. Unable to place Rt. foot flat on floor. ☐	12. Places Rt. foot on floor. ☐	12. Places Rt. foot flat on floor. ☐	3. Steps with Rt. foot forward. ☐
13. Unable to straighten Rt. leg. ☐	13. Unable to straighten Rt. leg. ☐	13. Unable to straighten Rt. leg. ☐	13. Straightens Rt. leg. ☐	4. Stands straight. ☐
14. Unable to weight bear through the legs. ☐	14. Some weight bearing through the legs. ☐	14. Weight bears through the legs. ☐	14. Weight bears through the legs. ☐	
15. Unable to stand straight. ☐	15. Unable to stand straight. ☐	15. Unable to stand straight. ☐	15. Stands straight. ☐	
			16. Turns LBC at corner. ☐	

Advanced Hand Skills Functional Record Form

1st record   (date): _____
2nd record   (date): _____
3rd record   (date): _____
4th record   (date): _____

Hand Preference: _____

a. *Grasp and Release*
  1. Makes fist with thumb out — left hand.   ☐ ☐ ☐ ☐
                                        — right hand.   ☐ ☐ ☐ ☐
  2. Makes fist with thumb up — left hand.   ☐ ☐ ☐ ☐
                                        — right hand.   ☐ ☐ ☐ ☐
  3. Radial grasp   — left hand.   ☐ ☐ ☐ ☐
                                        — right hand.   ☐ ☐ ☐ ☐
  4. Pincer grip   — left hand.   ☐ ☐ ☐ ☐
                                        — right hand.   ☐ ☐ ☐ ☐
  5. Releases small pellets
     (1 cm) into a bottle   — left hand.   ☐ ☐ ☐ ☐
                                        — right hand.   ☐ ☐ ☐ ☐
  6. Turns pages of a book one by one.   ☐ ☐ ☐ ☐
  7. Builds a tower of 2 with 2.5 cm cubes.   ☐ ☐ ☐ ☐
  8. Builds a tower of 4 with 2.5 cm cubes.   ☐ ☐ ☐ ☐
  9. Builds a tower of 6–8 with 2.5 cm cubes.   ☐ ☐ ☐ ☐
10. Builds a tower of more than 9 with
     2.5 cm cubes.   ☐ ☐ ☐ ☐
11. Unscrews a bottle with 2 cm cap.   ☐ ☐ ☐ ☐
12. Screws a bottle with 2 cm cap.   ☐ ☐ ☐ ☐

b. *Bilateral eye-hand co-ordinated activities*
  1. Threads beads of 2.5 cm in diameter.   ☐ ☐ ☐ ☐
  2. Threads beads of 1 cm in diameter.   ☐ ☐ ☐ ☐
  3. Tears a piece of drawing paper using
     pincer grip.   ☐ ☐ ☐ ☐
  4. Folds a piece of paper in half.   ☐ ☐ ☐ ☐
  5. Folds a piece of paper in half and then
     half again.   ☐ ☐ ☐ ☐
  6. Uses a pair of scissors to make a cut.   ☐ ☐ ☐ ☐
  7. Uses a pair of scissors to make 2 cuts
     successively.   ☐ ☐ ☐ ☐
  8. Cuts along a straight line.   ☐ ☐ ☐ ☐
  9. Cuts along curvature.   ☐ ☐ ☐ ☐
10. Cuts out a single shape.   ☐ ☐ ☐ ☐
11. Rolls a ball towards partner.   ☐ ☐ ☐ ☐
12. Receives a rolling ball.   ☐ ☐ ☐ ☐
13. Throws a ball from above head.   ☐ ☐ ☐ ☐
14. Throws a ball from above head towards target.   ☐ ☐ ☐ ☐
15. Throws a ball upwards.   ☐ ☐ ☐ ☐
16. Catches a ball thrown towards him/her.   ☐ ☐ ☐ ☐
17. Catches a bouncing ball.   ☐ ☐ ☐ ☐
18. Bounces a ball.   ☐ ☐ ☐ ☐

c. *Writing*
1. Holds crayon with tripod grip. ☐ ☐ ☐ ☐
2. Imitates horizontal strokes with crayon. ☐ ☐ ☐ ☐
3. Imitates verticle strokes with crayon. ☐ ☐ ☐ ☐
4. Imitates circles with crayon. ☐ ☐ ☐ ☐
5. Imitates crosses with crayon. ☐ ☐ ☐ ☐
6. Imitates diagonal lines with crayon. ☐ ☐ ☐ ☐
7. Draws a line using a pencil. ☐ ☐ ☐ ☐
8. Draws a line through a 2 cm wide path (20 cm long). ☐ ☐ ☐ ☐
9. Imitates simple Chinese characters within a boundary of 5 cm x 5 cm. ☐ ☐ ☐ ☐
10. Fixes the paper with one hand while writing with the other. ☐ ☐ ☐ ☐

Advanced Motor Skills Functional Record Form

1st record   (date): _____
2nd record   (date): _____
3rd record   (date): _____
4th record   (date): _____

a. *Related to Walking*
   1. Walks sideways.   ☐ ☐ ☐ ☐
   2. Walks backwards.   ☐ ☐ ☐ ☐
   3. Walks on uneven ground.   ☐ ☐ ☐ ☐
   4. Walks over obstacle.   ☐ ☐ ☐ ☐
   5. Walks up slope.   ☐ ☐ ☐ ☐
   6. Walks down slope.   ☐ ☐ ☐ ☐
   7. Walks along narrow space (e.g. balance beam).   ☐ ☐ ☐ ☐
   8. Single leg standing (15 secs.) — left leg.   ☐ ☐ ☐ ☐
                                         — right leg.   ☐ ☐ ☐ ☐

b. *Related to Stairs Management*
   1. Upstairs
      1.1 With both hands holding, 2 feet/step.   ☐ ☐ ☐ ☐
      1.2 With both hands holding, 1 foot/step.   ☐ ☐ ☐ ☐
      1.3 With one hand holding, 2 feet/step.   ☐ ☐ ☐ ☐
      1.4 With one hand holding, 1 foot/step.   ☐ ☐ ☐ ☐
      1.5 Without holding, 2 feet/step.   ☐ ☐ ☐ ☐
      1.6 Without holding, 1 foot/step.   ☐ ☐ ☐ ☐
   2. Downstairs
      2.1 With both hands holding, 2 feet/step.   ☐ ☐ ☐ ☐
      2.2 With both hands holding, 1 foot/step.   ☐ ☐ ☐ ☐
      2.3 With one hand holding, 2 feet/step.   ☐ ☐ ☐ ☐
      2.4 With one hand holding, 1 foot/step.   ☐ ☐ ☐ ☐
      2.5 Without holding, 2 feet/step.   ☐ ☐ ☐ ☐
      2.6 Without holding, 1 foot/step.   ☐ ☐ ☐ ☐

c. *Jumping*
   1. Jumps from low step.   ☐ ☐ ☐ ☐
   2. Jumps on spot.   ☐ ☐ ☐ ☐
   3. Jumps forward.   ☐ ☐ ☐ ☐
   4. Jumps successively forward.   ☐ ☐ ☐ ☐
   5. Jumps over obstacle.   ☐ ☐ ☐ ☐
   6. Single leg jumping.   ☐ ☐ ☐ ☐

d. *Ball Activites*
   1. Kicking
      1.1 Kicks a ball   — left leg.   ☐ ☐ ☐ ☐
                                 — right leg.   ☐ ☐ ☐ ☐
      1.2 Kicks a ball towards
           a target 1m away   — left leg.   ☐ ☐ ☐ ☐
                                 — right leg.   ☐ ☐ ☐ ☐
      1.3 Follows a ball and kicks.   ☐ ☐ ☐ ☐

e. *Other Activities*
   1. Rides a bicycle in a straight line.   ☐ ☐ ☐ ☐
   2. Rides a bicycle and turns at corners.   ☐ ☐ ☐ ☐
   3. Runs.   ☐ ☐ ☐ ☐
   4. Skips with a rope.   ☐ ☐ ☐ ☐

Guidelines on how to use Part C — the task analysis of the activities of the daily routine

a. Part C of this manual deals with the activities of the child in his daily routine. After identifying the functional level of the child in the different activities, please refer to this part of the manual.

b. Choose the task analysis that corresponds to the functional level of the child.

c. Read the whole page especially the column on "guide-lines" carefully.

d. Follow the instructions on "analysis of motor task" with reference to the column on "guidelines". Use the "speech/songs/rhymes" suggested. Give the instruction clearly and request the child to repeat the words in the "speech/songs/rhymes" column.

e. Upgrade the child's ability as suggested in the column on "guidelines".

f. When the child can perform as described in the task analysis, repeat the observation of the child in Chapter 4 Functional Record Form. Complete the form of the particular task again and identify the child's new functional level.

g. Go to point (a) as described above and repeat the whole process again until the child is independent in the task.

Eating and Drinking

TASK 1: EATING WITH A SPOON
(LEVELS 1—4)

TASK 2: DRINKING
(LEVELS 1—4)

Eating and Drinking

The process of eating and drinking includes:

a. The ability to sit properly.
b. The ability to bring food to the mouth.
c. The ability to take food and swallow.

In this task analysis on eating and drinking, we highlight items a and b. For children who have specific difficulties in taking food, and swallowing, please seek a doctor's advice. Each child should be dealt with individually. Below are some guidelines to facilitate oral-motor control (see Table 5.1).

Table 5.1

Problems	Recommendations
Dislikes others touching mouth area.	a. Apply firm strokes to the mouth area. It is preferable to use the child's hands for the task.
Drools copiously or cannot close lips.	a. Apply firm, downward pressure on the upper lip, stroking from the center towards the sides. Repeat with the lower lip, starting from the centre, stroking firmly upwards and towards the sides. b. Use a straw for drinking. c. Encourage the child to pucker the lips as in kissing, blowing through the lips, or sucking an ice-pop. d. Wipe drooling by applying firm pressure around the lips, use upward pressure over the lower lip and downward pressure over the upper lip.
Cannot open mouth for food.	a. Apply firm, upward pressure on the lower jaw to initiate opening the mouth. b. Create an atmosphere which helps the child relax.

Table 5.1 cont'd

Problems	Recommendations
Cannot suck from milk bottle.	a. Carry out the above suggestions for lip closure. b. Use thin liquid at the beginning for sucking. c. Sucking can be stimulated by using a "squeeze" bottle.
Bites on spoon and cannot let go (bite reflex).	a. Avoid stimulating teeth, gums, or tongne when feeding the child. b. Child's head should be in midline with the chin slightly tucked in. c. When feeding, approach the child with the spoon in mid-position, unload the spoon towards the side. d. When child bites on the spoon, do not force the spoon from between the teeth, instead soothe the child to help him relax and open his mouth.
Chokes on food.	a. Scoop a small amount of food onto the spoon. Do not overload it. b. Be mindful of the temperature of the food, some children can be sensitive to hot/cold food. C. Be mindful of the texture of the food, some children are sensitive to food with a rough texture.
Tongue thrust.	a. When feeding, the child should sit well with the head in midline and the chin tucked in. b. When feeding, approach the child with the spoon in mid-position and unload the spoon towards the side to help him chew. c. Using the tip of the spoon, apply pressure on the inner half of the tongue when spoon feeding. d. Scoop a small amount of food onto the spoon. e. Desensitize the tongue by applying pressure on it and walk backwards about $^2/_3$ of the way along the tongue. Do this half an hour before feeding time.

Table 5.1 *cont'd*

Problems	Recommendations
Cannot chew.	a. Practise chewing on food such as a stem of vegetable or a long thick piece of cooked meat cut. The care-giver holds one end of the food while the other end is placed at the side of the child's mouth. The child is encouraged to chew on the food until it generates some juice. Care should be taken to prevent the child swallowing particles of the food to avoid choking. b. Wrap some meat, e.g., beef, in a sterilised gauze. The care-giver holds one end of it while the other end can be placed at the side of the child's mouth. Encourage the child to chew on the food but not swallow.
Cannot swallow.	a. Scoop a small amount of food onto the spoon at a time. b. Make sure the child is sitting well with the head in midline and the chin tucked slightly in. c. Help the child to swallow by stroking slowly and firmly downwards from under the chin to midway down along the neck. d. Help the child to swallow by applying firm pressure to the root of the tongue under the chin.

Analysis of Motor Task	*Speech/Songs/Rhymes*	*Guidelines*

1. Look at the spoon.

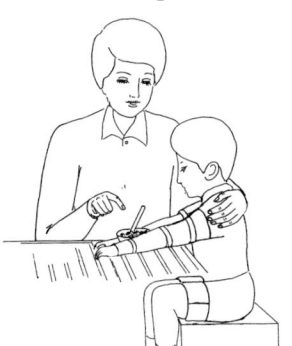

I look at spoon   look   look   look

2. Grasp the spoon.

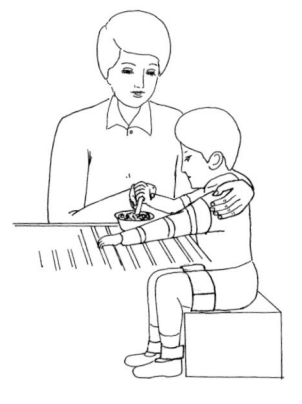

I grasp   grasp grasp grasp

3. Scoop the food.

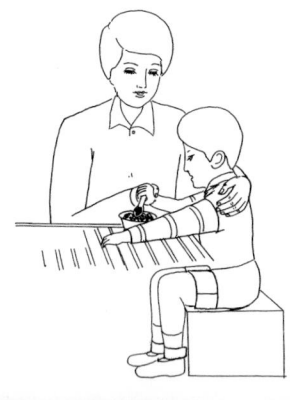

I scoop food   scoop scoop scoop

1. Make sure the child is sitting well for this task (see Chapter 10, Task 18, Level 1).

2. The child who cannot bring his head into the midline position may need gaiters on both arms and may also need flexion mitts to help him sustain grasp of the plinth/ horizontal hand bar (see Appendix) while being fed.

3. The care-giver should feed the child from the front to encourage him to bring his head into the midline position.

4. When the child can maintain his head in the midline position, he can begin to learn to grasp the spoon and the care-giver helps feed him while sitting by his side. If the child pushes his head and shoulders backwards, she should stabilise the opposite shoulder with her free hand.

5. The child may need a gaiter on the opposite hand to stretch his elbow and for security. He may also need a flexion mitt to help him sustain grasp of the plinth/ hand bar.

6. The care-giver says every step out loud and helps the child with each step.

7. Children who have difficulty in chewing and swallowing should be given small spoonfulls of food.

8. Give the child sufficient time to chew and swallow his food and do not rush him.

9. When finished eating, help him to grasp the flannel and wipe his mouth.

4. Bring the spoon to the mouth.   Spoon to mouth

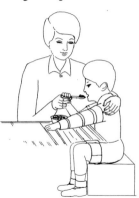

5. Remove the food from the spoon with the lips.

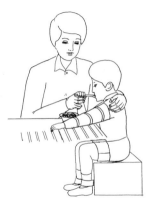

6. Return the spoon to the dish.   Spoon to dish   down   down   down

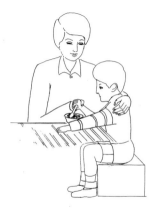

Analysis of Motor Task	*Speech/Songs/Rhymes*	*Guidelines*
1. Look at the spoon.	I look at the spoon look look look	1. Make sure the child is sitting well for this task (see Chapter 10, Tasks 18, Level 2).

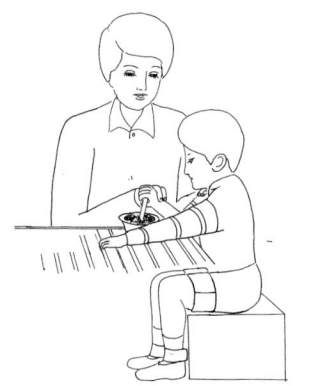

2. He may still need a gaiter on the opposite arm to stretch his elbow and grasp the plinth/hand bar.

3. The care-giver may still need to help the child to scoop the food and bring the spoon to the mouth.

4. Do not load the spoon with food and give the child sufficient time to chew and swallow the food.

5. As far as possible the care-giver should sit by the side of the child when helping him. Avoid sitting behind him. If the child pushes his head and shoulders backwards, she should stabilise the opposite shoulder with her free hand.

2. Grasp the spoon.

I grasp the spoon   grasp   grasp   grasp

6. Decrease assistance as soon as the child begins to feed himself independently.

7. Encourage the child to grasp the flannel and learn to wipe his mouth when finished.

8. This method may also be used for finger feeding.

3. Scoop the food.

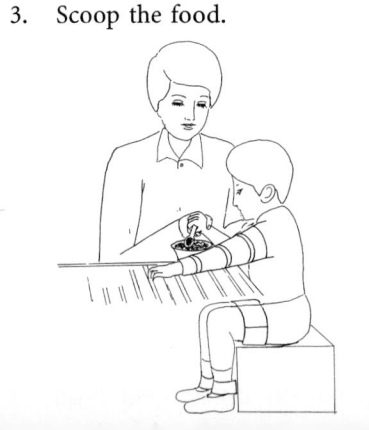

I scoop the food   1   2   3   4   5

4. Bring the spoon to the mouth.

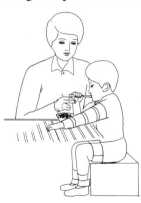

I bring the spoon to my mouth   1   2   3   4   5

5. Return the spoon to the dish.

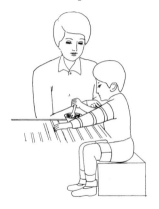

I return the spoon to the dish   1   2   3   4   5

6. Grasp the flannel and wipe the mouth.

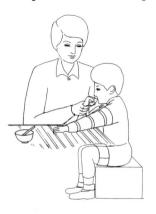

I grasp the flannel   1   2   3   4   5

Analysis of Motor Task	*Speech/Songs/Rhymes*	*Guidelines*

1. Look at the spoon.

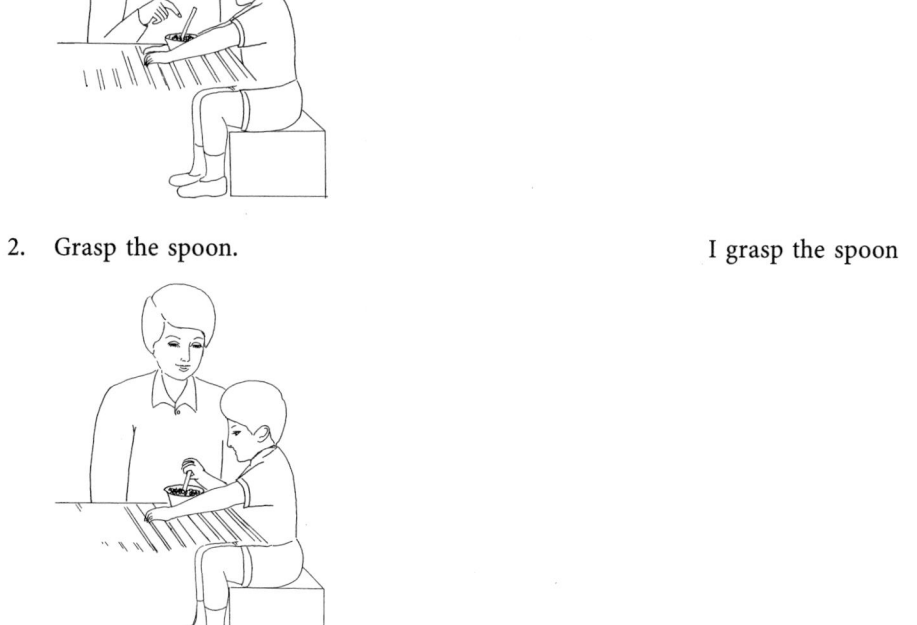

I look at the spoon   1 2 3 4 5

1. Make sure the child is sitting well before beginning the task.

2. Encourage the child to stretch his opposite arm and grasp the plinth.

3. The care-giver sits beside the child when assisting him.

4. The child should be able to grasp the spoon, scoop the food but may still need help to bring the spoon to his mouth.

5. Give him sufficient time to try and do each step.

6. If possible, the child with hemiplegia should be encouraged to use the affected hand. However, if he uses his unaffected hand, make sure he stretches the other hand and grasps the plinth/hand bar while eating.

7. Encourage the child to grasp the flannel and wipe his mouth when he finishes his meal.

2. Grasp the spoon.

I grasp the spoon   1 2 3 4 5

3. Scoop the food.

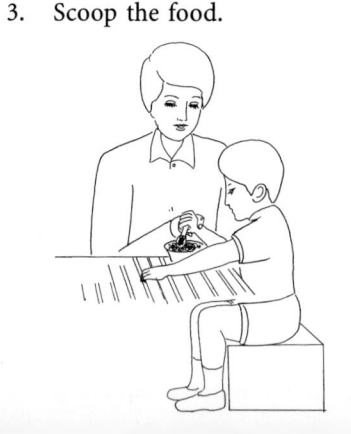

I scoop the food   1 2 3 4 5

4. Bring the spoon to the mouth.

I bring the spoon to my mouth   1   2   3   4   5

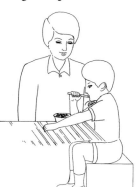

5. Return the spoon to the dish.

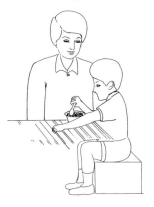

6. Wipe the mouth with the flannel.

I grasp the flannel and wipe my mouth

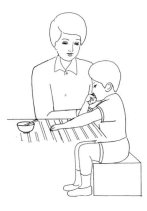

| | *Analysis of Motor Task* | *Guidelines* |

1. Grasp the spoon.

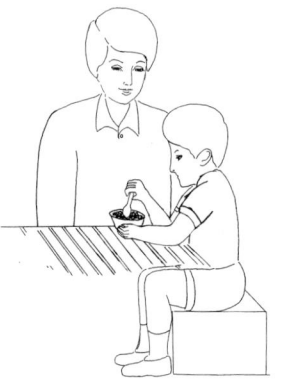

2. Scoop the food.

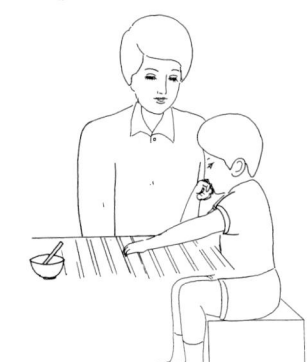

3. Bring the spoon to the mouth.

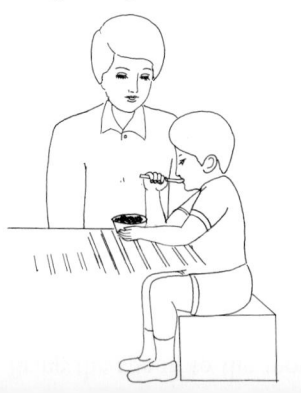

4. Return the spoon to the dish.

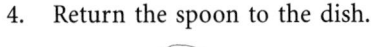

5. Wipe the mouth.

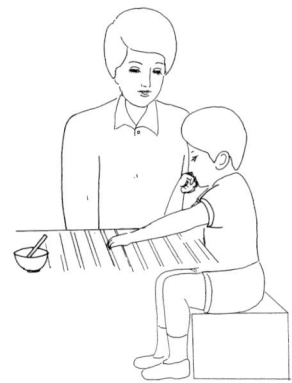

1. Make sure the child is sitting well.

2. Use speech to remind the child and preferably no manual assistance.

3. Encourage the child to eat tidily and wipe his mouth when he finishes his meal.

4. When the child has reached independence at this level, he should begin to learn to use chopsticks.

Analysis of Motor Task	*Speech/Songs/Rhymes*	*Guidelines*

1. Sitting task (Chapter 10, Task 18, Level 1)

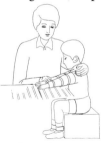

I Stretch my Hands and Hold on Tight

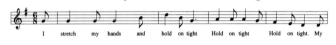

I   stretch   my   hands   and   hold   on   tight   Hold   on   tight   Hold   on   tight.   My

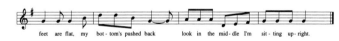

feet   are   flat,   my   bot - tom's   pushed   back   look   in   the   mid - dle   I'm   sit - ting   up - right.

1. Make sure the child is sitting well for this task (see Chapter 10, Task 18, Level 1).

2. Encourage the child to look at the fluid in the mug before he drinks. It is preferable to have the mug half filled for the task.

2. Look at the mug.

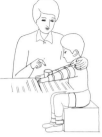

I look at mug   look   look   look

3. The care-giver sits beside the child and brings the mug to the child's mouth. However, in certain circumstances she may need to place herself behind the child for the task.

4. If the child has difficulty with lip closure, she uses her other hand to seal his lips over the mug.

3. Bring the mug to the mouth.

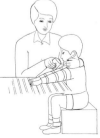

5. Do not give him too much fluid at any one time.

6. Give the child sufficient time to sip from the mug and swallow the fluid.

7. Encourage the child to look at the empty mug when it has been returned to the table.

4. Put the mug down on the table.

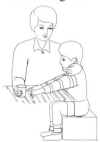

Analysis of Motor Task	*Speech/Songs/Rhymes*	*Guidelines*

1. Look at the mug.

I look at mug   look   look   look

2. Grasp the mug.

I grasp mug   grasp   grasp   grasp

3. Push the mug forward.

I push mug   push   push   push

1. This is an excellent task to teach the child with asymmetrical tonic neck reflex (ATNR) to bring his head into the midline.

2. Make sure the child is sitting well for the task (Chapter 10, Task 18, Level 1).

3. The care-giver should sit behind the child and will need to help him step by step.

4. Make sure the child pushes the mug well forward and looks at it before he attempts to bring it to his mouth.

5. While drinking, the care-giver should make sure the child is stabilised by fixating both elbows on the table.

6. If the child has difficulty with lip closure, the care-giver should help the child to seal his lips over the mug.

7. It is preferable to have a mug half-filled when teaching the child to drink.

8. The care-giver should say every step out loud and when possible encourage the child to speak.

4. Bend the elbows and bring the mug to the mouth (elbows have to be on the table).

I bend elbows  up   up   up

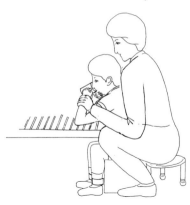

5. Return the mug to the table.

Mug down   down   down   down

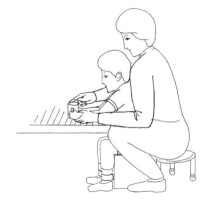

Analysis of Motor Task	*Speech/Songs/Rhymes*	*Guidelines*
1. Look at the mug. 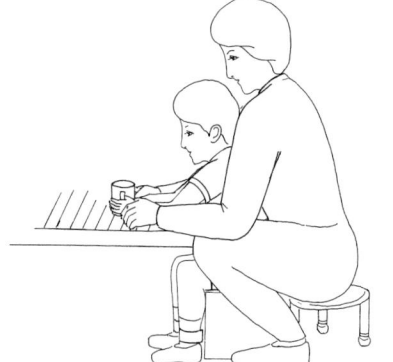	I look at the mug look look look	1. This is an excellent task to teach the child with asymmetrical tonic neck reflex (ATNR) to bring his head into the midline. 2. Make sure the child is sitting well for this task (see Chapter 10, Task 18, Level 2). 3. Whenever possible, give the child the opportunity to choose his drink. 4. If possible, the care-giver may sit/stand in front of the child and help him to fixate the elbows on the table while drinking. 5. The child may still need some help to seal his lips over the mug.
2. Grasp the mug.	I grasp the mug grasp grasp grasp	6. It is preferable to have a mug half-filled when teaching the child to drink. 7. The care-giver should say every step out loud and encourage the child to speak. 8. Encourage the child to grasp the flannel and wipe his mouth when finished.
3. Push the mug forward.	I push the mug push push push	

4. Look at the mug.

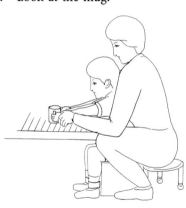

I look at the mug   look look look

5. Bring the mug to the mouth.

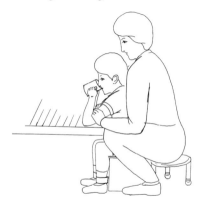

I bring the mug to mouth   1 2 3 4 5

6. Return the mug to the table and release hands.

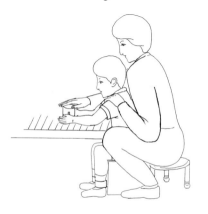

I put the mug down   1 2 3 4 5

Analysis of Motor Task	*Speech/Songs/Rhymes*	*Guidelines*

1. Look at the mug.

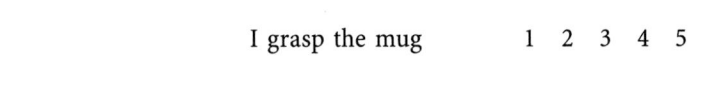

I look at mug   1 2 3 4 5

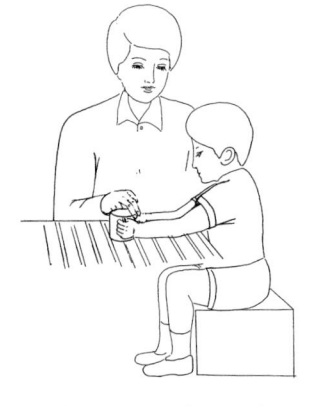

2. Grasp the mug.

I grasp the mug   1 2 3 4 5

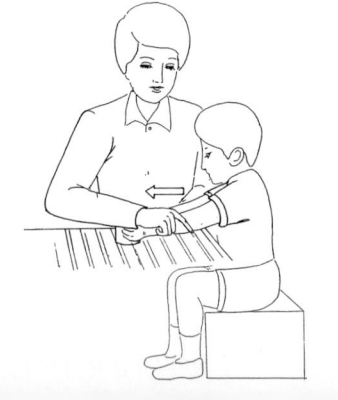

3. Push the mug forward.

I push the mug   1 2 3 4 5

1. Make sure the child is sitting well before he attempts this task (see Chapter 10, Task 18, Level 3).

2. Whenever possible, give the child the opportunity to choose his drink.

3. The child should be able to grasp the mug, push it forward and bring it to his mouth. However, he may still need help to fixate the elbows on the table.

4. Encourage the child to drink slowly and learn not to drool.

5. Encourage him to grasp the flannel and wipe his mouth when finished.

4. Bring the mug to the mouth.　　　　　　I bring mug to my mouth　　1　2　3　4　5

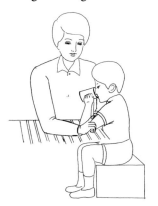

5. Return the mug to the table.　　　　　I put the mug down　　1　2　3　4　5

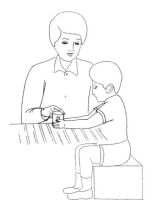

Analysis of Motor Task	*Speech/Songs/Rhymes*	*Guidelines*

1. Grasp the cup.

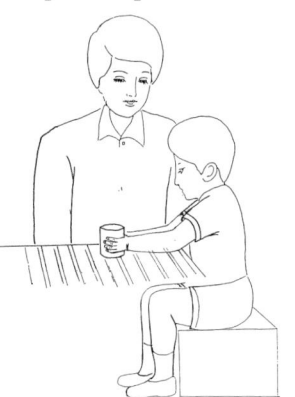

2. Bring the cup to the mouth.

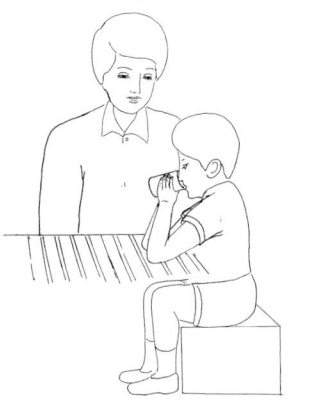

3. Return the cup to the table.

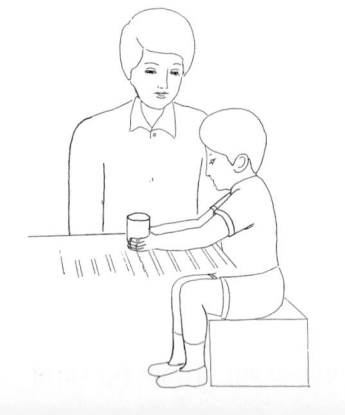

1. Make sure the child is sitting well for this task (see Chapter 10, Task 18, Level 4).

2. Give the child the opportunity to choose his drink.

3. Use speech to remind the child and preferably no manual assistance.

4. Encourage the child to drink tidily and wipe his mouth when finished.

Chapter 6

Toilet-Training

Task 3: Sitting Down on Potty/Toilet
(Levels 1 — 4)

Task 4: Standing Up from Potty/Toilet
(Levels 1 — 4)

Analysis of Motor Task	*Speech/Songs/Rhymes*	*Guidelines*

1. Release one hand and grasp the rung.

I release and grasp   grasp grasp grasp

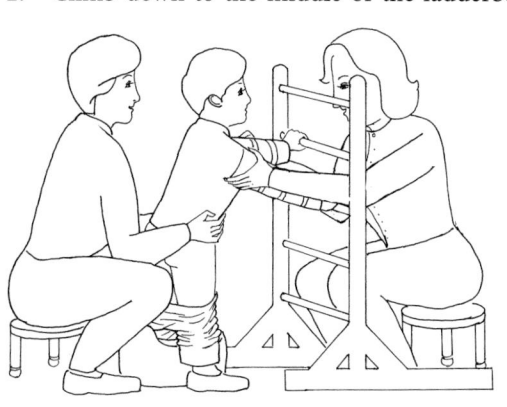

2. Climb down to the middle of the ladderback chair.

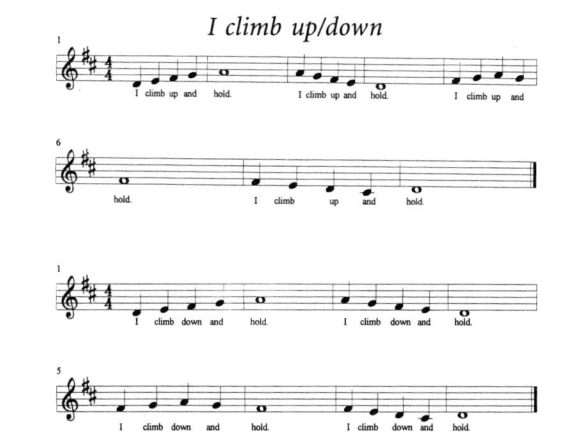

I climb up/down

I climb up and hold.   I climb up and hold.   I climb up and

hold.   I climb   up   and   hold.

I climb down and   hold.   I climb down and   hold.

I climb down   and   hold.   I climb down and   hold.

3. Bend the hips and knees and sit down.

I sit down   down down down

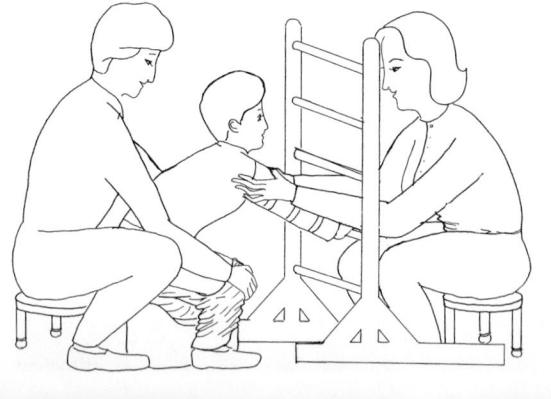

1. The age at which children begin toilet training depends to a large extent on the culture. The Chinese people look on independence in toileting as an important skill to acquire at an early age. Provided they are given a regular toileting routine (see Daily Timetable, Chap. 3, p. 23). Most 2–5 year-old motor disordered children can be toilet trained.

2. Children should not be picked up and put on potties/potty chairs/toilets. They should have the opportunity to learn to become actively involved in toilet-training.

3. Two care-givers need to assist the child. One supports the child from behind, the other helps the child grasp the rungs of the chair. At this level, the care-giver may have to facilitate the child at the shoulders or the elbows. Facilitating at the shoulders stabilises the shoulder girdle and helps the child with poor head control to lift his head and control its position.

4. The child may need gaiters on both arms to stretch the elbows and for stability. He may also need flexion mitts to help him maintain his grasp of the rung when he is sitting on the potty (see Appendix).

5. The care-giver assisting from behind should support the child at the trunk and knees and pull down the child's pants.

6. Help the child to climb down to approximately the middle of the ladderback chair. Encourage him to look at his feet. Then help him bend his hips and knees and sit down slowly on the potty.

7. Surround the child with cushions on the floor to prevent injury if he falls down. This is the best way for the child to begin to learn to take responsibility for himself and improve his trunk balance.

4. Feet flat.

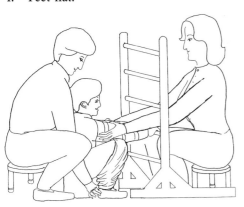

Feet flat flat flat flat

5. Feet apart.

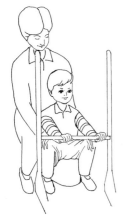

Feet apart apart apart apart

6. Push the ladderback chair forward and sit well.

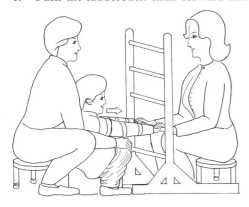

I push chair push push push

8. The care-giver should sit in front to help the child grasp the rungs. If the child keeps pushing backwards, grasp his shoulders firmly and hold him well forward.

9. If he cannot keep his feet flat on the floor, the care-giver should stabilise them by pressing down gently but firmly on his feet with her feet.

10. Talk/sing to the child to encourage him to sit in the midline position.

11. Avoid sitting behind the child as this encourages him to push backwards.

12. Praise him if he uses the potty and record it.

91

Analysis of Motor Task	*Speech/Songs/Rhymes*	*Guidelines*
1. Sit well.		1. Two care-givers need to assist the child. One supports the child from behind the other helps the child in front.
2. Feet flat and apart.	Feet apart apart apart apart	2. The child may need arm gaiters to stretch the elbows and for stability.
		3. Make sure child's feet are flat and apart.
		4. The care-giver in front should help the child release the hand and grasp the rung to climb up a little.
		5. Make sure the child pushes the chair well forward and his body weight is over his feet when preparing to stand up.
3. Push the ladderback chair forward.	I push chair push push push	6. The care-giver in front should stabilise the child by grasping his hands firmly on the rung or if he needs more stability, she may grasp him at the elbows or shoulders to prevent him from pulling backwards.
		7. The care-giver from behind may support the child at the waist with one hand and use the other to help him stand up.
		8. Encourage the child with poor head control to look at the care-giver.
4. Climb up the ladderback chair a little.	I release and grasp grasp grasp grasp	9. The care-giver pulls up the child's pants.

5. Lift up the bottom and stand up.

I stand up   1   2   3   4   5

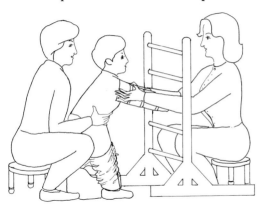

6. Climb up.

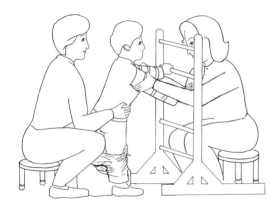

I climb up/down

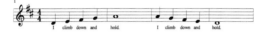
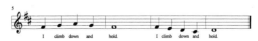

7. Standing straight (see Chapter 11, Task 19, Level 1)

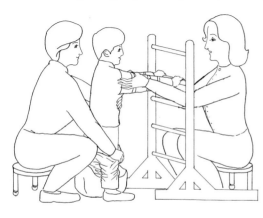

Look at me

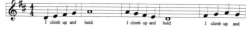
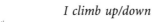
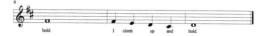

Analysis of Motor Task	*Speech/Songs/Rhymes*	*Guidelines*

1. Release one hand and grasp the rung.

    I relesase and grasp   grasp   grasp   grasp

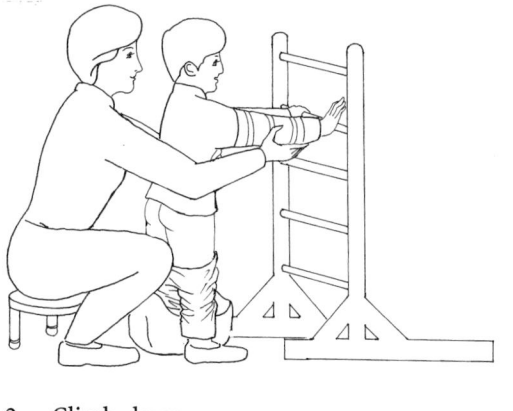

1. One care-giver facilitates the child from behind.

2. The child may still need gaiters to stretch the elbows and for stability.

3. The child should be able to grasp and release.

4. He climbs down to approximately the middle of the ladderback chair.

5. The care-giver helps the child to grasp his pants and learn to push it down to just above his knees.

6. The child may still need help to bend his hips and sit down slowly. Do not allow the child collapse when doing this movement.

2. Climb down.

I climb up/down

I climb up and hold.   I climb up and hold.   I climb up and

hold.   I climb up and hold.

I climb down and hold.   I climb down and hold.

I climb down and hold.   I climb down and hold.

7. Surround him with cushions for security.

8. Use song/toy to encourage the child to learn to maintain the midline position.

9. Remind him to sit well.

10. Praise the child if he uses the potty and record it.

3. Bend the hips and knees and sit down.

    I bend knees   1   2   3   4   5

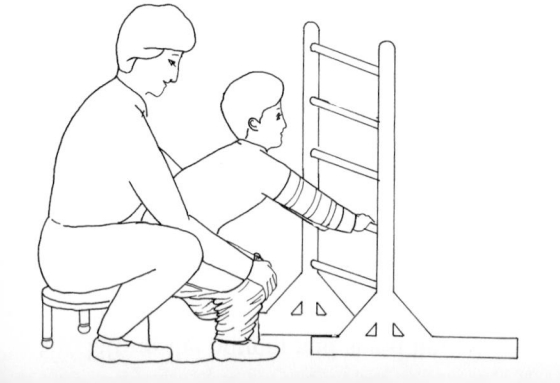

4. Sit down slowly.   I sit down   1   2   3   4   5

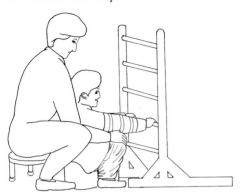

5. Push the ladderback chair forward.   I push chair   1   2   3   4   5

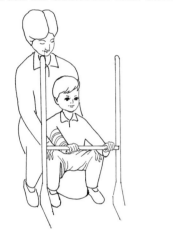

6. Sit well and look at the toy.   I look at toy   look   look   look

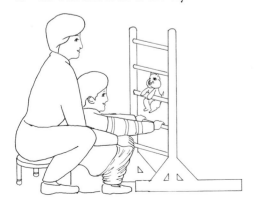

Analysis of Motor Task	*Speech/Songs/Rhymes*	*Guidelines*
1. Both feet flat.	My feet flat 1 2	1. One care-giver supports the child from behind.

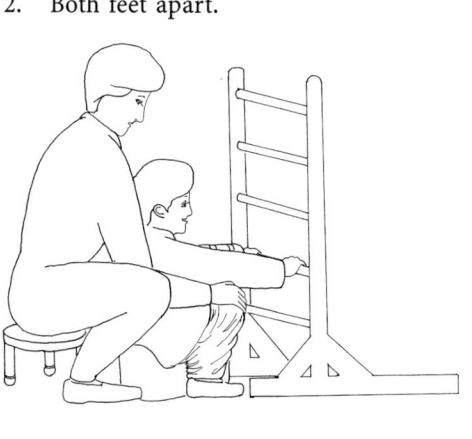

2. The child should be able to grasp and release.

3. The child may still need arm gaiters to stretch the elbows and for stability.

4. Make sure the child pushes the chair well forward and his weight is well over his feet when preparing to stand up.

5. The care-giver should help the child initiate standing up by pushing down firmly but gently on both knees.

6. Encourage him to climb up by singing.

2. Both feet apart.

My feet apart   apart   apart   apart

7. The care-giver pulls up the child's pants to above his knees and then encourages him to learn to grasp them and pull them up using alternate hands.

8. Give the child sufficient time to do the task and encourage him to use speech to guide his movements.

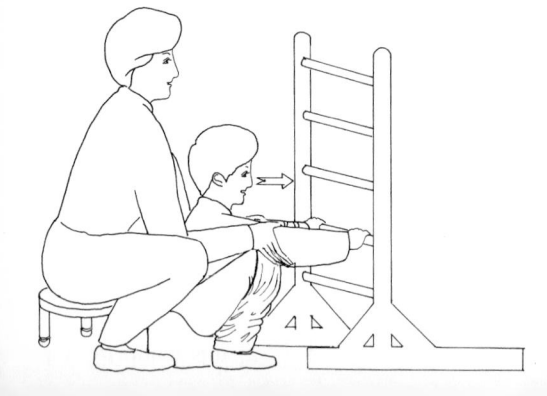

3. Push the ladderback chair forward.

I push chair   1   2   3   4   5

4. Climb up a little.

I release and grasp   grasp   grasp   grasp

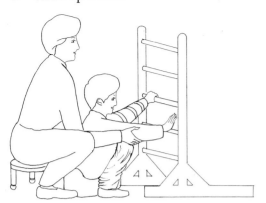

5. Lift up the bottom to stand and climb up.

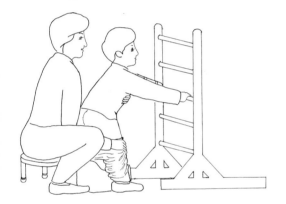

I climb up/down

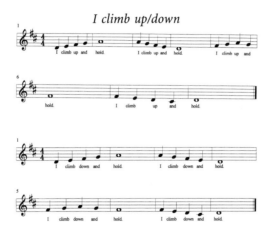

6. Standing straight (see Chapter 11, Task 19, Level 2).

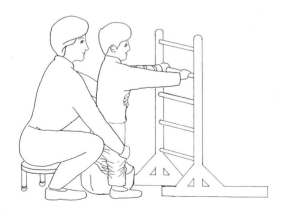

Look at me

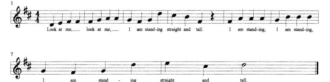

Analysis of Motor Task	*Speech/Songs/Rhymes*	*Guidelines*

1. Climb down.

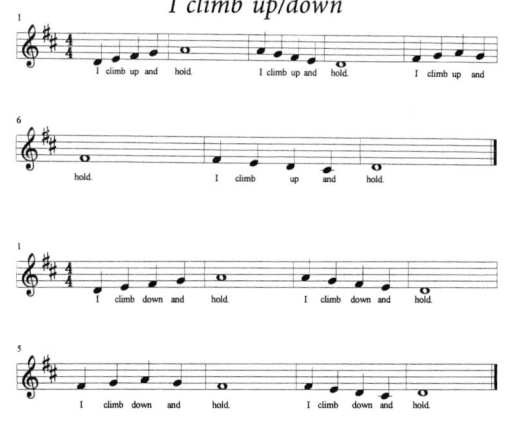

I climb up/down

1. The care-giver facilitates with speech and minimal manual facilitation.

2. Give the child sufficient time to learn to push down his pants.

3. At this level, the child does not need cushions as he should be able to maintain his balance on the potty.

4. While he is sitting on the potty, he may release his hands and play with a toy.

5. Remind him to sit well.

2. Grasp the rung with one hand.

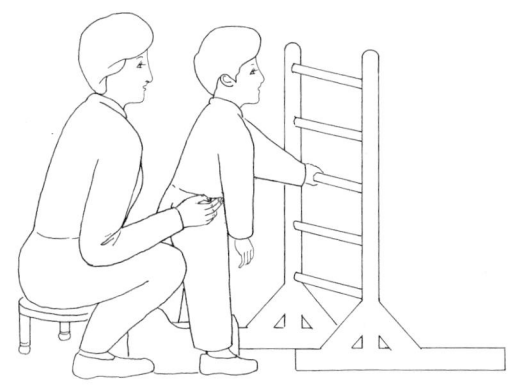

3. Grasp the pants with the other hand.

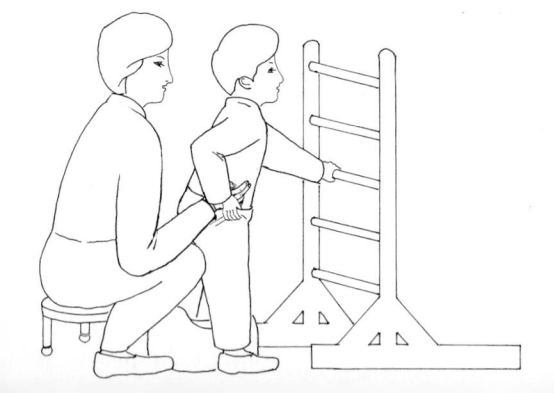

I grasp my pants   1   2   3   4   5

4. Push down the pants.

I push down my pants   push   push   push

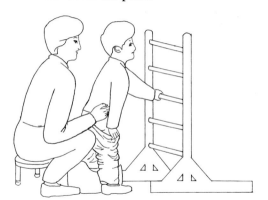

5. Bend the hips and sit down.

I sit down   1   2   3   4   5

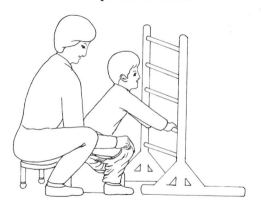

6. Release both hands and sit well.

I sit well

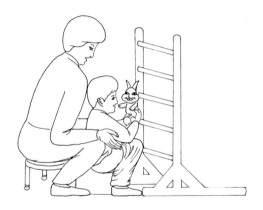

Analysis of Motor Task	*Speech/Songs/Rhymes*	*Guidelines*
1. Both feet flat and apart.	My feet are apart 1 2 3 4 5	1. Remind the child to stretch his elbows at all times to help him sit and stand straight.

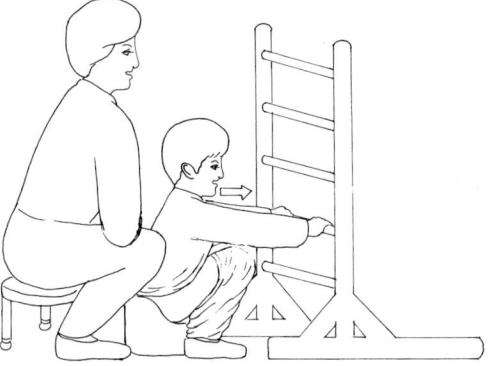

2. Facilitate with speech and minimal manual assistance.

3. Give the child sufficient time to learn to pull up his pants. Encourage the child to use alternate hands when doing this task. This is important for the child with hemiplegia as they prefer to use the unaffected hand.

4. Insist on good standing, i.e., feet flat and apart, knees straight, hips straight, back straight, head in the midline.

5. If the child feels insecure in the standing position while pulling up his pants he may stand against a wall/ ladderback chair/bed rail.

2. Push the ladderback chair forward.

I push the chair   1 2 3 4 5

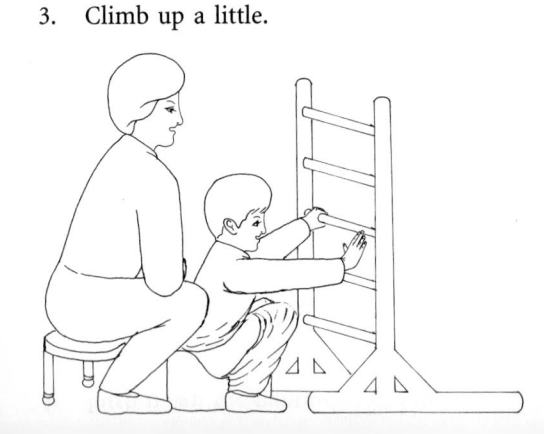

3. Climb up a little.

I climb up   1,2   1,2   1,2

4. Lift up the bottom and stand up.

I stand up   1   2   3   4   5

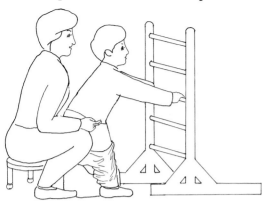

5. Climb up the ladderback chair.

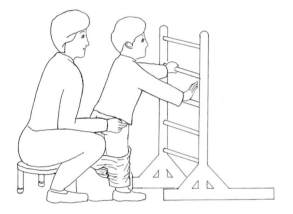

I climb up/down

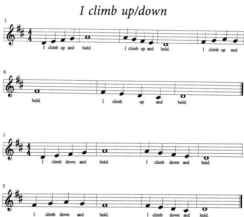

6. Pull up the pants.

I pull up pants   .   pull   pull   pull

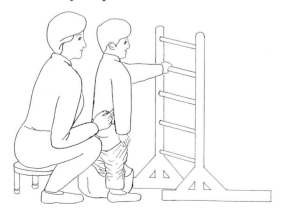

Analysis of Motor Task	_Speech/Songs/Rhymes_	_Guidelines_

1. Both feet flat and apart.

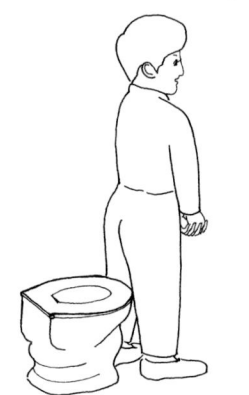

2. Push down the pants.

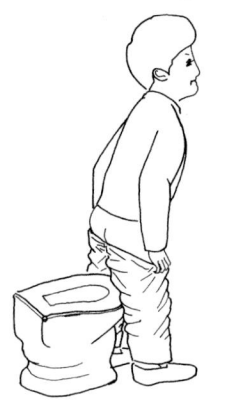

3. Sit down on the toilet.

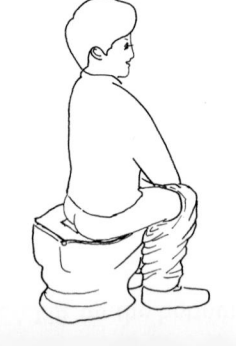

1. The child uses inner speech.

2. The care-giver supervises the child, preferably with no manual assistance.

3. The child should begin to learn to use toilet paper after using the toilet.

Analysis of Motor Task	Speech/Songs/Rhymes	Guidelines

1. Both feet flat and apart.

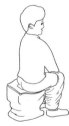

2. Stand up.

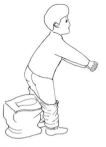

3. Pull up the pants.

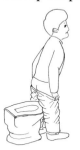

4. Stand tall.

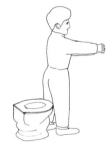

1. The child uses inner speech.

2. The care-giver supervises the child, preferably with no manual assistance.

3. The child should begin learn to use toilet paper and flush the toilet after use.

4. Give the child the opportunity to wash his hands after using the toilet.

Stand up Tall

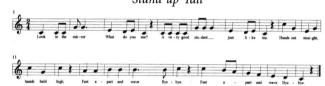

103

Chapter 7

Dressing and Undressing

TASK 5: PUTTING ON PYJAMA TOP
(LEVELS 1—4)

TASK 6: PUTTING ON PYJAMA LEGS
(LEVELS 1—4)

TASK 7: PUTTING ON SOCKS
(LEVELS 1—4)

TASK 8: PUTTING ON SHOES
(LEVELS 1—4)

TASK 9: TAKING OFF SHOES
(LEVELS 1—4)

TASK 10: TAKING OFF SOCKS
(LEVELS 1—4)

TASK 11: TAKING OFF PYJAMA TOP
(LEVELS 1—4)

TASK 12: TAKING OFF PYJAMA LEGS
(LEVELS 1—4)

Notes on Special Clothing

The following are some suggestions regarding suitable clothing for children with cerebral palsy. Hopefully, it will facilitate dressing/undressing. Always teach the children to dress/undress the more affected side first.

Underwear

a. Select garments x one size larger.
b. Pullover underwear with shoulder or a larger collar is preferred.
c. Pants with elastic waist.
d. Stretchable material such as polyester/cotton/jersey cotton.

Tops

a. Select garments x one size larger.
b. Polo or T-shirt.
c. Zipper fronts.
d. Front openings with large buttons.
e. Stretchable materials.

Pants

a. Select loose-fitting pants.
b. Pants with elastic waist.
c. Avoid jeans and garments with lining.

Skirts/Dress

a. Select loose-fitting.
b. Skirts with elastic waist.
c. Zipper closing in front or at the side opposite the good hand.
d. Front fastening.

Socks

a. Select stretchable material.
b. Easily identifiable ankle area.

Shoes

a. Select velcro attachment.
b. Elastic attachment.
c. Elastic shoelaces.

Outer Garments

a. Select coats or jackets x one size larger.
b. Large buttons and zips.
c. Raglan sleeves.
d. Light weight.
e. Attach a suitably sized ring or a piece of thick ribbon to the zip for ease of grasp.

Analysis of Motor Task	*Speech/Songs/Rhymes*	*Guidelines*
1. Long sitting on the floor (see Chapter 16, Task 18, Levels 2–4). 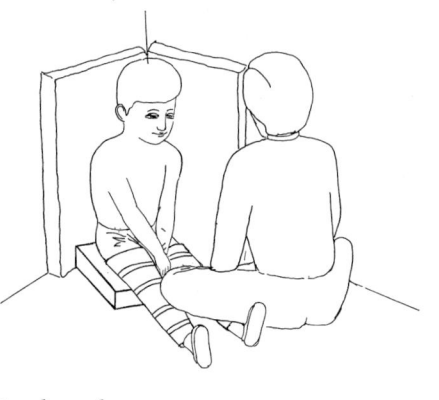	I sit well	1. The child may need to sit in a corner of the room for greater support for this task. His hips should be well flexed, his bottom pushed well back and his legs parted. If the child is unable to stretch his knees, he may need long leg gaiters (see Appendix).
2. Look at the top. 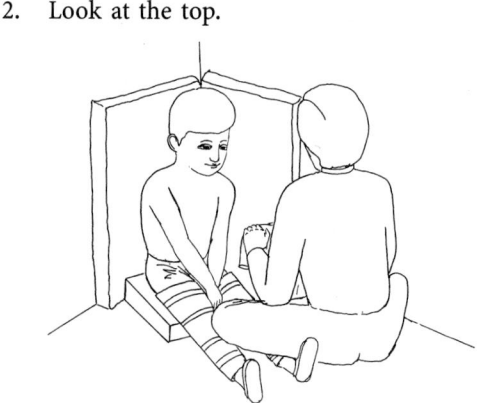	I look at top look look look	2. If the child's back is too rounded a low stool/thick book (equivalent of a telephone book)/sitting downhill on a wedge will help him gradually learn to straighten his back. 3. The care-giver shows the top to the child and names it saying pyjama top/vest/sweater. 4. She puts the top on the child and pulls it down to the middle of the trunk, then she guides his hands to grasp it and helps him pull it down. 5. Make sure the child looks at the top. 6. The care-giver says every step out loud and if possible encourages the child to speak.
3. Raise the hand and put it into the sleeve. Repeat with other hand.	Hand into sleeve 1 2 3 4 5	

4. The child bends his head and the care-giver puts the top over the child's head.

I bend head   down   down   down

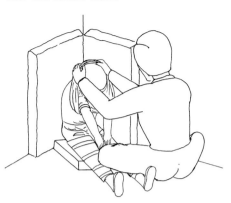

5. Pull down the top.

I pull top   pull pull pull

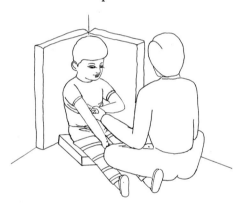

6. Repeat with the other hand.

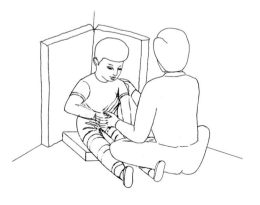

Analysis of Motor Task	*Speech/Songs/Rhymes*	*Guidelines*
1. Look at the top.	I look at the top look look look	1. The care-giver adjusts the top for the child and puts it on to below the elbows.
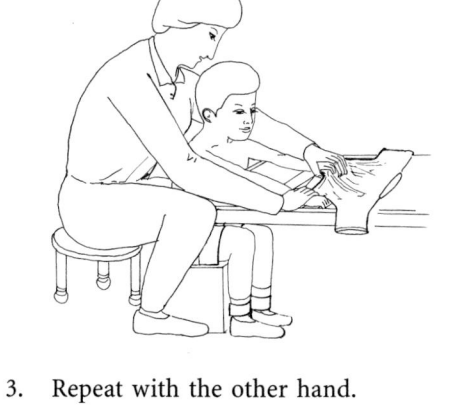		2. Make sure the child grasps the plinth with one hand while using the other to pull on the sleeve.
		3. She helps pull the top over the child's head. She encourages the child to grasp the top and pull it down.
		4. Give the child sufficient time to attempt the steps.
		5. The care-giver says each step out loud and if possible encourages the child to speak.
		6. She asks the child to look at the top as she points to it and encourages him to learn to say "top".
2. Grasp the top and pull on the sleeve.	I grasp the top and pull pull pull pull	7. Begin to teach the child the concept of "sleeve".
3. Repeat with the other hand.	I grasp the top and pull pull pull pull	

4. Bend the head.

I bend my head   down   down   down

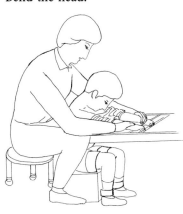

5. Fixate the child's elbows on the plinth and pull the top over the head.

I pull top over my head   pull   pull   pull

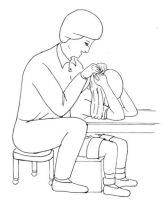

6. Grasp the top and pull it down.

I grasp and pull   1 2 3 4 5

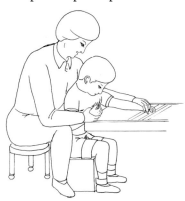

Analysis of Motor Task	*Speech/Songs/Rhymes*	*Guidelines*

1. Sitting task (see Chapter 10, Task 18, Level 3).

Sit up Straight

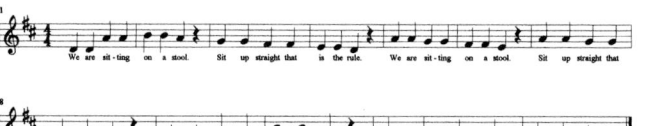

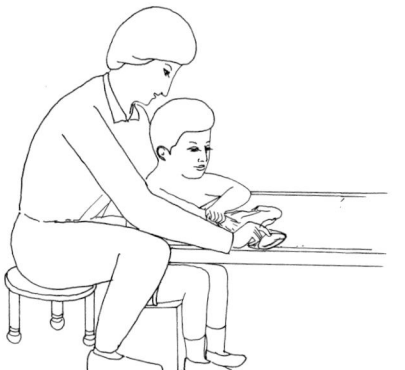

1. The care-giver adjusts the top on the bed/plinth in front of the child with the end of the top facing the child.

2. She encourages with speech but provides minimal manual facilitation. However, the child may still need help to pull the top over his head.

3. Give the child sufficient time to do each step.

4. If the top is one primary colour, ask the child if he can name the colour.

5. The child should begin to learn the concepts of different parts of the garment — "front", "back", "top", "end", "sleeve".

2. Grasp the end of the top and pull on the sleeve.

I put my hand through the sleeve   1   2   3   4   5

3. Pull up the sleeve. Repeat with the other hand.

1 pull on the sleeve   pull   pull   pull

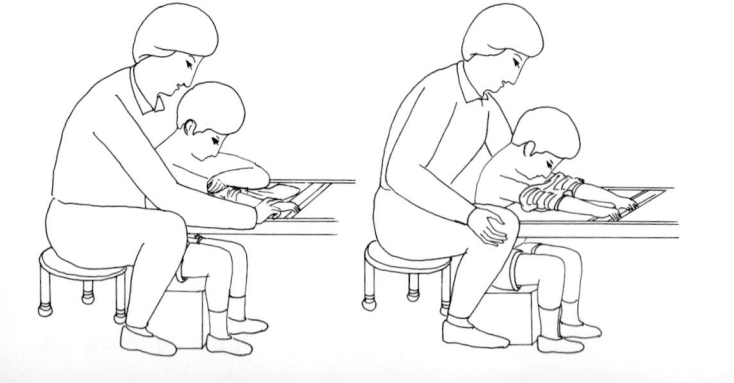

4. Grasp the top and bend the head.

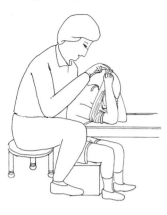

I bend my head   1   2

5. Pull the top over the head.

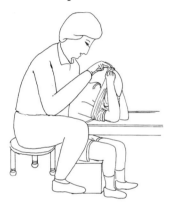

I pull the top over my head   1   2   3   4   5

6. Grasp the top and pull it down.

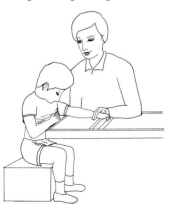

I grasp and pull   pull   pull   pull

Analysis of Motor Task	*Speech/Songs/Rhymes*	*Guidelines*

1. Long sitting/sitting on the stool task (see Chapter 16, Task 15, Levels 2–4, Chapter 10, Task 18, Level 4).

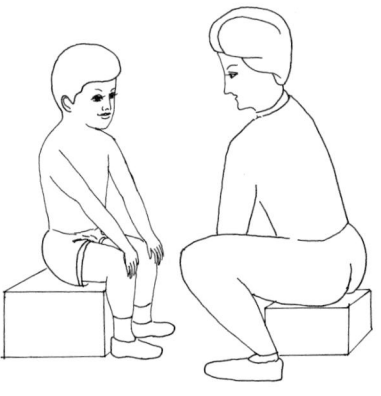

2. Grasp the top and pull on the sleeves.

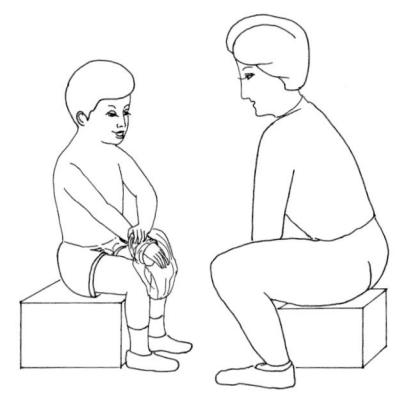

1. The child uses inner speech or may sing a song about putting on clothes.

2. The care-giver supervises the child, preferably with no manual assistance.

3. The child should begin to learn the concepts of "inside" and "outside" of the top. If the top is multi-coloured, he should begin to learn some of the colours. The child should learn clothing suitable for different weather conditions.

4. The child may also use this method to put on an anorak.

3. Pull the top over the head.

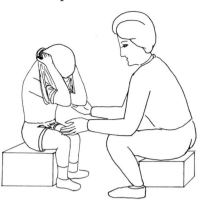

4. Pull the top down properly.

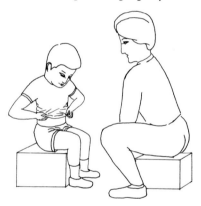

Analysis of Motor Task	*Speech/Songs/Rhymes*	*Guidelines*
1. Supine lying task (see Chapter 15, Lying Task Series, Task 3, Level 1). 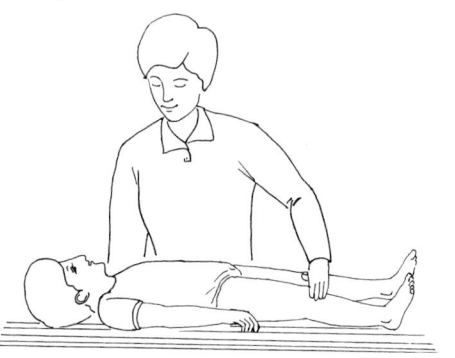	I lie straight	1. It may be easier for the child at level one to learn to put on the pants in the supine or side lying positions.
2. Lift up one leg. Repeat with the other. 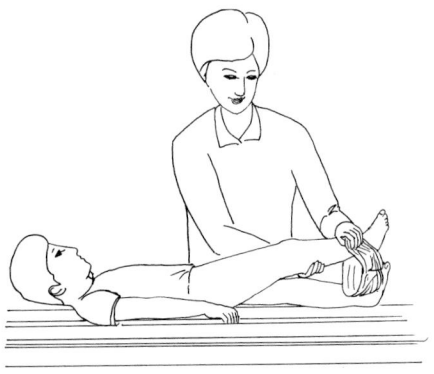	I lift my leg up up up up	2. The care-giver shows the garment to the child and names it — pyjama legs/underpants/trousers.
3. Bridging task (see Chapter 15, Lying Task Series, Task 5, Level 1). 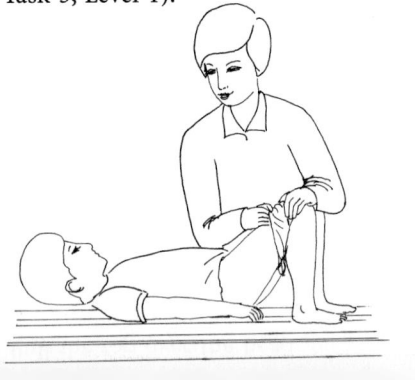	*London Bridge is Falling Down*  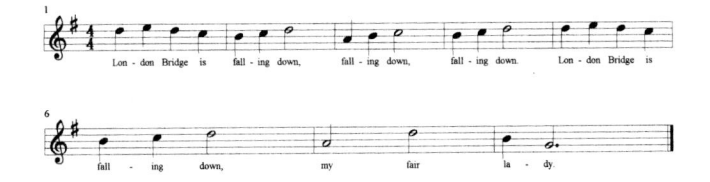	3. She puts it on to below the waist, then she guides the child's hands to grasp it and helps him pull it up.

3. She puts it on to below the waist, then she guides the child's hands to grasp it and helps him pull it up.

4. The care-giver says every step out loud and if possible encourages the child to speak.

4. Look at the pants.

I look at pants   look   look   look

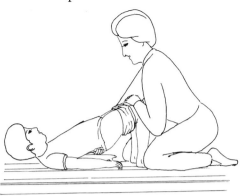

5. Grasp the pants.

I grasp pants   grasp   grasp   grasp

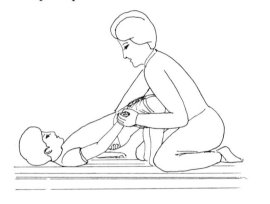

6. Pull up the pants.

I pull up   pull   pull   pull

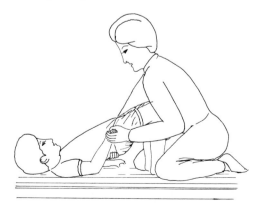

Analysis of Motor Task	*Speech/Songs/Rhymes*	*Guidelines*

1. Supine lying task (see Chapter 16, Task 8, Levels 2–4).

I lie straight   1   2   3   4   5

1. The care-giver puts on the pants to just above the knees.

2. She helps the child with the bridging task.

3. The child should be able to grasp and pull, but will need help to maintain the bridging position and pull the pants up over the bottom.

4. Give the child sufficient time to attempt the steps.

5. The care-giver says every step out loud and encourages the child to speak.

6. The child should begin to learn to name the garment.

7. Emphasise the concept of "bottom".

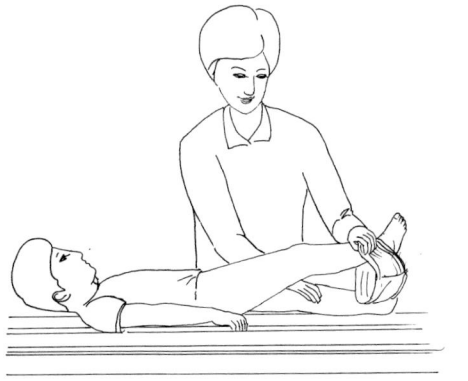

2. Lift one leg. Repeat with the other.

I lift one leg   1   2   3   4   5

3. Bridging task (see Chapter 16, Task 13, Levels 2–4).

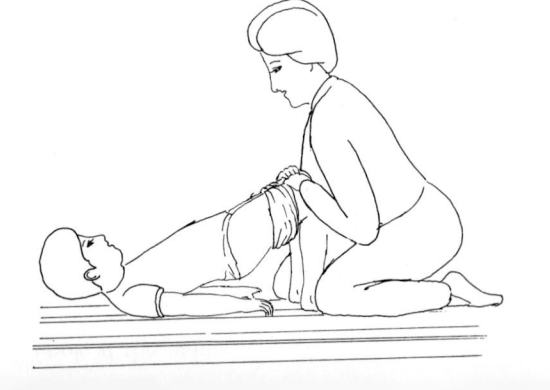

London Bridge is Falling Down

Lon - don Bridge is   fall - ing down,   fall - ing down,   fall - ing down.   Lon - don Bridge is

fall - ing   down,   my   fair   la - dy.

4. Grasp the pants.

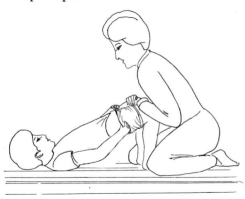

I grasp the pants   grasp grasp grasp

5. Pull up the pants.

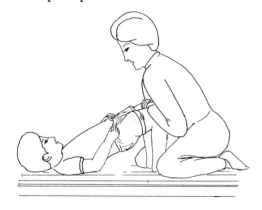

I pull up   pull pull pull

Analysis of Motor Task	*Speech/Songs/Rhymes*	*Guidelines*

1. Sitting on a stool task (see Chapter 10, Task 18, Level 1–3).

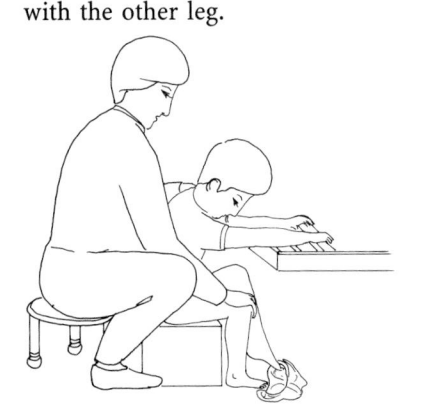

Sit up Straight

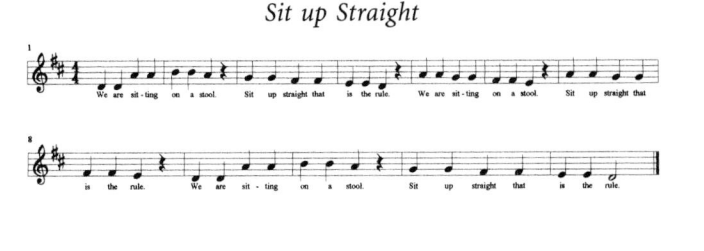

We are sit-ting on a stool. Sit up straight that is the rule. We are sit-ting on a stool. Sit up straight that is the rule. We are sit-ting on a stool. Sit up straight that is the rule.

1. The care-giver helps the child put the pants on over his feet and ankles.

2. She guides with speech.

3. Give the child sufficient time to do each step.

4. Always encourage the child to use alternate hands; this is very important for the child with hemiplegia.

5. If the pants is a primary colour, the child should begin to name the colour. The child should also begin to learn the concepts of "legs" and "waist".

2. Put the leg into the pants which is on the floor. Repeat with the other leg.

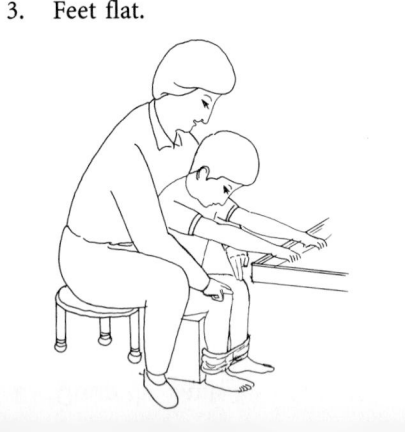

I lift one leg   1   2   3   4   5

3. Feet flat.

My feet are flat   1   2

4. Grasp the pants and pull it up.   I grasp the pants and pull   pull   pull   pull

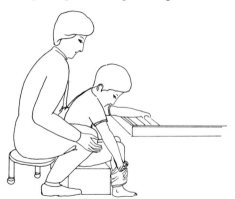

5. Stand up.   I stand up   1   2   3   4   5

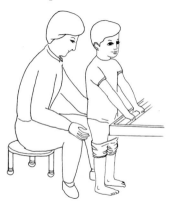

6. Grasp the pants and pull it up.   I grasp the pants and pull   pull   pull   pull

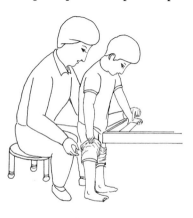

Analysis of Motor Task	*Speech/Songs/Rhymes*	*Guidelines*

1. Sitting on a stool task (see Chapter 10, Task 18, Level 4).

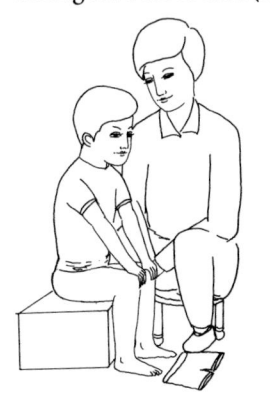

2. Bend down and grasp the pants.

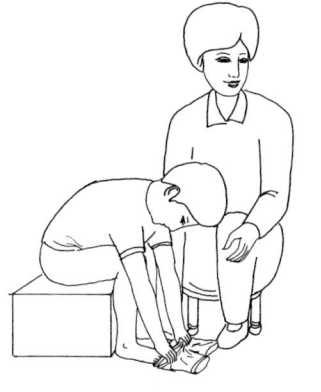

3. Put the leg into the pants. Repeat with the other leg.

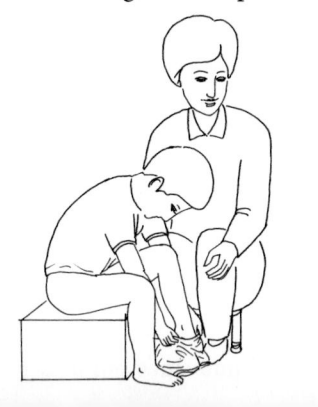

1. It is understood the child at this level has a fairly steady standing balance. However, he may still need to grasp the plinth/bed rail/wall rail/ladderback chair or some other type of furniture while standing and pulling up garment.

2. The child uses inner speech.

3. The care-giver supervises the child, preferably with no manual assistance.

4. Give the child sufficient time to do the task as independently as possible.

5. The child should begin to learn the concepts of "inside" and "outside" of pants and name different garments. If the pants is multi-coloured, he should begin to learn some of the colours.

6. He should learn clothing suitable for different weather conditions.

4. Pull up the pants.

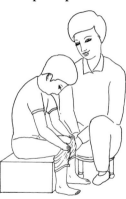

5. Grasp the wall rail/plinth/bed rail/ladderback chair and stand up.

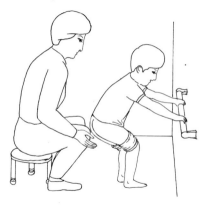

6. Pull up the pants.

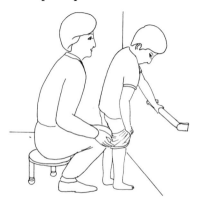

Analysis of Motor Task	*Speech/Songs/Rhymes*	*Guidelines*

1. Sitting on the care-giver's lap. Put left ankle on right knee.

   I sit well

2. Look at the sock.

   I look at sock   look   look   look

3. The care-giver puts the sock on over the toes.

   Sock on toes   look   look   look

1. Use brightly coloured socks to encourage the child to look at them and at his feet.

2. Make sure the child's hips are well flexed, his bottom pushed well back and his back straight.

3. The child may need a gaiter on the free hand to stretch the elbow and for stability.

4. Use the right hand to put the sock on the left leg and the left hand to put the sock on the right leg.

5. The care-giver encourages the child to look at the sock before helping him put it on.

6. The care-giver helps the child from the side and pulls on the sock to above the heel. She then helps him grasp the sock with his thumb inserted inside the sock and pull it up.

7. She says every step out loud and if possible encourages the child to speak. She also encourages him to try and learn to pull up the sock.

8. Encourage the child to learn to use alternate hands.

9. Emphasise the concept of "on".

4. Pull the sock over the heel.

Sock over heel   pull   pull   pull

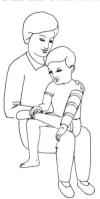

5. Pull up the sock.

I pull sock   pull   pull   pull

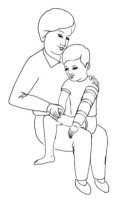

6. Repeat with the other leg.

Analysis of Motor Task	*Speech/Songs/Rhymes*	*Guidelines*

1. Sitting on the care-giver's lap. Put left ankle on right knee.

I sit well

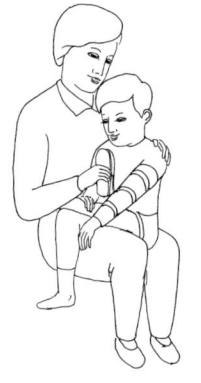

2. Look at the shoe.

I look at shoe   look   look   look

3. Put the shoe on the foot.

I put on shoe   1   2   3   4   5

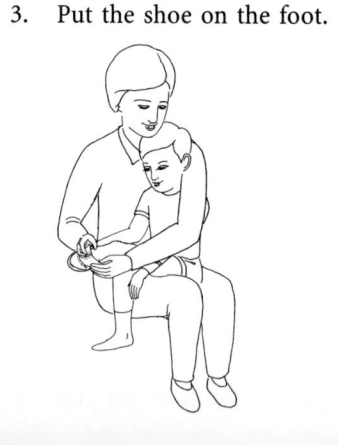

Guidelines

1. Make sure the child's hips are well flexed, his bottom pushed well back and his back straight.

2. The child may need a gaiter on the free hand to stretch the elbow and for stability.

3. Use the right hand to put on the left shoe and the left hand to put on the right shoe.

4. The care-giver supports the child from the side and guides the child's hand to grasp the shoe and put it on.

5. She says every step out loud and if possible encourages the child to speak.

6. Encourage the child to use alternate hands.

7. Emphasise the concept of "on".

4. Grasp the straps.

I grasp straps   grasp grasp grasp

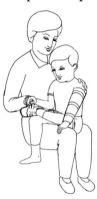

5. Affix the straps.

I affix straps   1 2 3 4 5

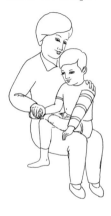

6. Repeat with the other leg.

Analysis of Motor Task	*Speech/Songs/Rhymes*	*Guidelines*

1. Long sitting/tailor sitting task (see Chapter 16, Task 18, Levels 2–4).

   I sit well

2. Bend the leg and place the heel on the opposite knee.

   I bend leg   1 2 3 4 5

3. Look at the sock.

   I look at the sock   look look look

1. Make sure the child's hips are well flexed, his bottom pushed well back and his legs apart to help him learn to sit well. At this level, some children may not be able to place the heel on the opposite knee. Do not force this movement; begin by placing the heel on the opposite ankle.

2. If the child is sitting on a mat on the floor, it may be easier at this level to sit him with his back to the wall or in a corner of the room.

3. If his back is too rounded, a low stool/thick book (equivalent of a telephone book)/sitting downhill on a wedge will help him learn to straighten his back (see Appendix).

4. If possible, the care-giver assists the child from the front to help him maintain his sitting balance.

5. The child may need a gaiter on the free hand to stretch the elbow and for stability.

6. The care-giver puts the sock over the toes and the child should be able to pull the sock onto the foot. He will need help to pull the sock over the heel. Make sure the child uses alternate hands. This is important for the child with hemiplegia.

7. The care-giver says every step out loud and encourages the child to speak.

8. Allow the child sufficient time to attempt the steps and do not help him too much.

9. Encourage the child to say "sock on".

4. Grasp the sock and pull the sock over the toes.

I grasp the sock   grasp grasp grasp

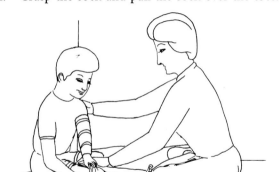

5. Pull the sock over the heel.

I pull on the sock   pull pull pull

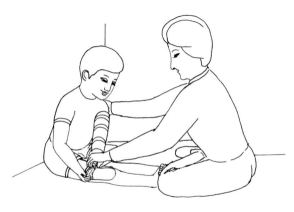

6. Pull up the sock.

I pull up the sock   pull pull pull

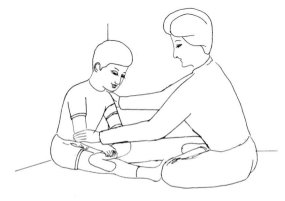

7. Repeat with the other leg.

Analysis of Motor Task	Speech/Songs/Rhymes	Guidelines
1. Long sitting/tailor sitting task (see Chapter 16, Task 18, Levels 2–4).	I sit well	1. Make sure the child's hips are well flexed, his bottom pushed well back and his legs apart to help him learn to sit well.
		2. If the child is sitting on a mat on the floor, it may be easier at this level to sit him with his back against the wall or in a corner of the room.
		3. If his back is too rounded, a low stool/thick book (the equivalent of a telephone book)/sitting downhill on a wedge will help him learn to straighten his back (see Appendix).
		4. The child may need a gaiter on the free hand to stretch the elbow and for stability.
2. Bend one knee.	I bend the knee bend bend bend	5. If possible, the care-giver assists the child from the front to help him maintain his sitting balance.
		6. The child should be able to grasp and pull. However he will need help pull on the shoe and to push it over the heel.
		7. Encourage the child to use alternate hands. This is very important for the child with hemiplegia.
		8. The care-giver says every step out loud and encourages the child to speak.
		9. Encourage the child to say "shoe on".
3. Look at the shoe.	I look at the shoe look look look	

4. Grasp the shoe and put it on.

I grasp the shoe   grasp   grasp   grasp

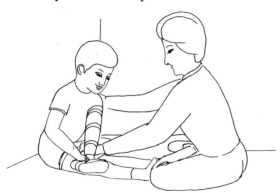

5. Pull the shoe over the heel.

I pull the shoe over the heel   1   2   3   4   5

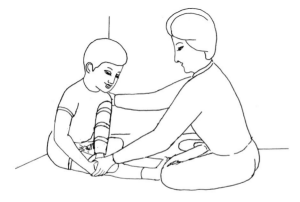

6. Grasp the straps and affix.

I grasp the straps   grasp   grasp   grasp

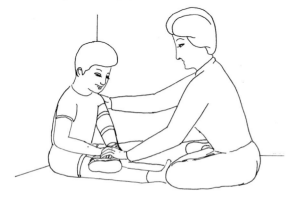

7. Repeat with the other leg.

Analysis of Motor Task	*Speech/Songs/Rhymes*	*Guidelines*
1. Long sitting task (see Chapter 16, Task 18, Levels 2–4). 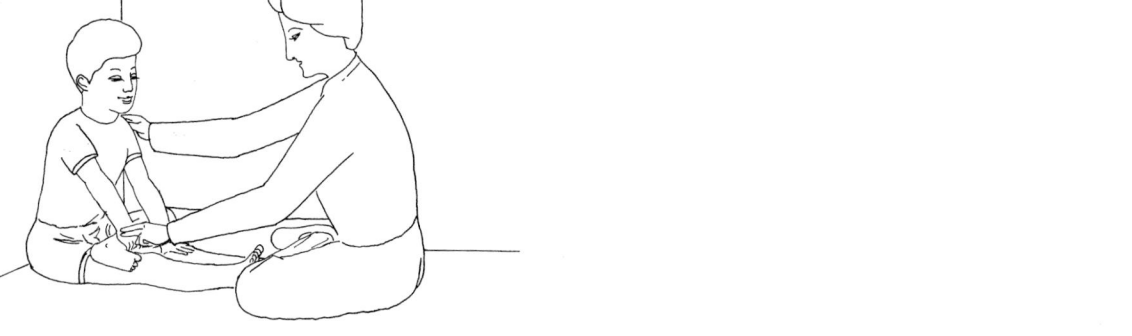	I sit well	1. Make sure the child's hips are well flexed, his bottom pushed well back and his legs apart to help him learn to sit well.
		2. If the child feels insecure sitting on the floor, he may sit against the wall or in a corner of the room for greater security.
		3. If his back is too rounded a low stool/thick book (equivalent of a telephone book)/sitting downhill on a wedge will help him learn to straighten his back (see Appendix).
2. Bend the leg and place the heel on the opposite knee. 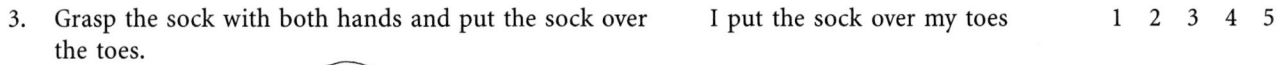	I bend my leg 1 2 3 4 5	4. Encourage the child to use alternate hands; this is very important for the child with hemiplegia as they prefer to use the unaffected hand.
		5. Use speech to facilitate the child with minimal manual assistance. However, the child may need help to pull the socks over his heels.
		6. Give him sufficient time to do task.
		7. The child should begin to learn the word "heel".
3. Grasp the sock with both hands and put the sock over the toes. 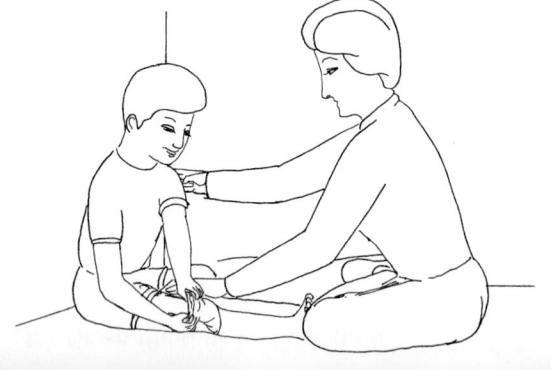	I put the sock over my toes 1 2 3 4 5	8. If the shoes/socks are in primary colours, he should begin to learn to name the colours.
		9. Teach the child the concept of pairing shoes/socks.

4. Grasp the sock and pull on.

I grasp the sock and pull   pull   pull   pull

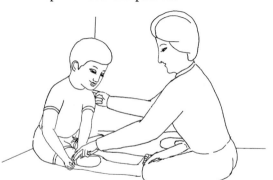

5. Grasp the shoe with both hands and put on.

I grasp the shoe and put on   1   2   3   4   5

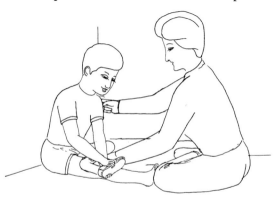

6. Grasp the straps and affix.

I affix the straps   1   2   3   4   5

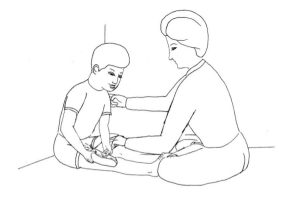

7. Repeat with the other foot.

Analysis of Motor Task	*Speech/Songs/Rhymes*	*Guidelines*

1. Sitting on the stool/long sitting task (see Chapter 10, Task 18 Level 4, Chapter 16 Task 18 Level 2–4).

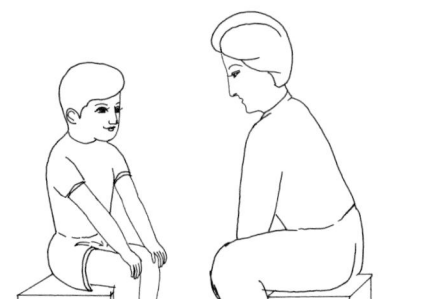

2. Place the left heel on the right knee.

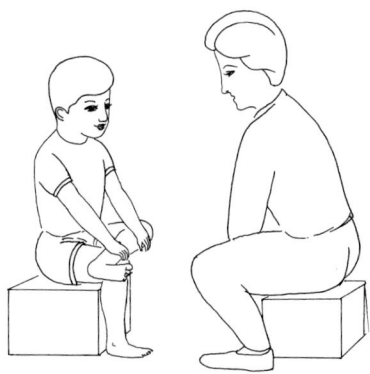

3. Grasp the sock and put on.

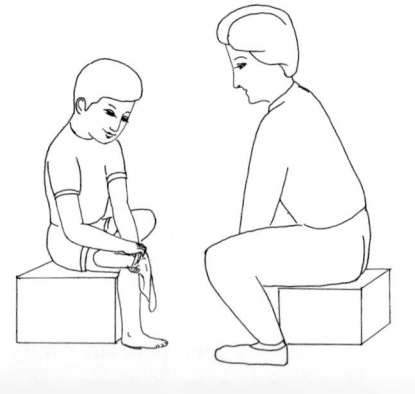

1. Depending on the ability of the child, he may sit on a stool or on a mat on the floor.

2. The child uses inner speech.

3. The care-giver supervises the child, preferably with no manual assistance.

4. Allow the child sufficient time to complete the task.

5. The child should begin to learn to differentiate right/ left foot and shoe.

6. If socks are multi-coloured he should begin to learn to name some of the colours. He should learn clothing suitable for different weather conditions.

4. Grasp the shoe and put on the shoe.

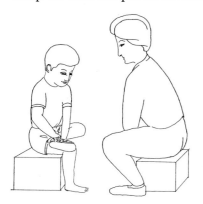

5. Affix the straps.

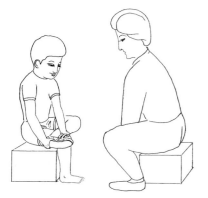

6. Repeat with the other leg.

Analysis of Motor Task	*Speech/Songs/Rhymes*	*Guidelines*
1. Sitting on the care-giver's lap. Put left ankle on right knee. 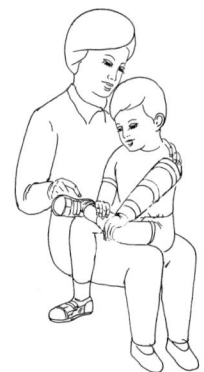	I sit well	1. Make sure the child's hips are well flexed, his bottom pushed well back and he sits firmly on the care-giver's lap with his back straight.
2. Look at the shoe.	I look at shoe look look look	2. Teach the child to use the right hand to remove the left shoe and the left hand to remove the right shoe.
3. Grasp the strap.	I grasp strap grasp grasp grasp	3. The child may need a gaiter on the free hand to stretch his elbow and for stability.

2. Teach the child to use the right hand to remove the left shoe and the left hand to remove the right shoe.

3. The child may need a gaiter on the free hand to stretch his elbow and for stability.

4. The carer-giver supports the child from the side and guides his hand step by step.

5. Encourage him to use alternate hands when learning to do this task. This is important for the child with hemiplegia as they prefer to use the unaffected hand.

6. The care-giver says every step out loud and if possible encourages the child to look and to speak.

7. Encourage the child to try to push and pull if possible.

8. Show the shoe to the child and say "shoe".

9. Emphasize the concept of "off".

10. Teach the child to play with a doll with shoes/socks as a preparation for this task.

4. Pull the strap.

I pull strap   pull pull pull

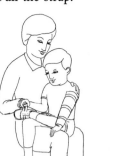

5. Grasp the back of the shoe.

I grasp shoe   grasp grasp grasp

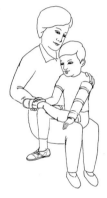

6. Push off the shoe.

I push off   push push push

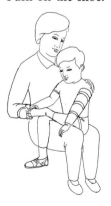

7. Repeat with the other leg.

Analysis of Motor Task	*Speech/Songs/Rhymes*	*Guidelines*
1. Sit on the care-giver's lap. Put left ankle on right knee. 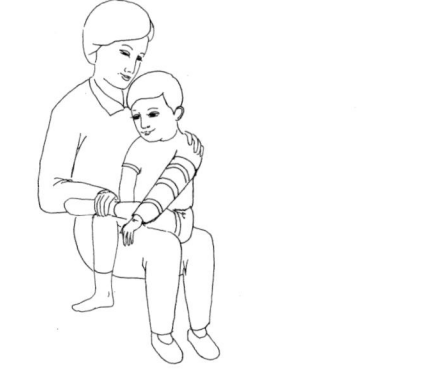	I sit well	1. The socks should be brightly coloured to encourage the child to look at his feet.
2. Look at the sock. 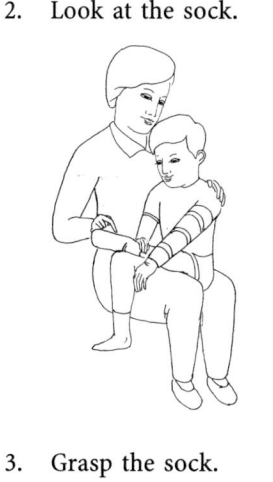	I look at sock look look look	2. Make sure the child's hips are well flexed, his bottom pushed well back and he sits firmly on the care-giver's lap with his back straight.
3. Grasp the sock. 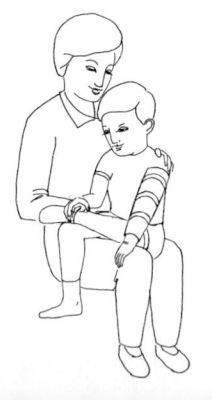	I grasp sock grasp grasp grasp	3. Teach the child to use the right hand to remove the left sock and the left hand to remove the right sock.

3. Teach the child to use the right hand to remove the left sock and the left hand to remove the right sock.

4. The child may need a gaiter on the free hand to stretch his elbow and for stability.

5. The care-giver supports the child from the side and guides his hand step by step.

6. The care-giver says every step out loud and if possible encourages the child to look and to speak.

7. Encourage him to try to push/pull if possible.

8. Show the sock to the child and say "sock".

9. Teach him to look at, touch and play with his toes.

4. Push the sock down over the heel to the toes.

I push sock   push   push   push

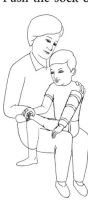

5. Grasp the sock and pull it off.

I pull sock   pull   pull   pull

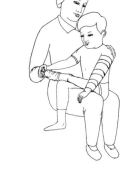

6. Put the sock in the shoe. Repeat with the other leg.

I release sock   1 2 3 4 5

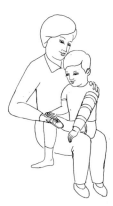

Analysis of Motor Task	*Speech/Songs/Rhymes*		*Guidelines*
1. Long sitting/tailor sitting task (see Chapter 16, Task 18, Levels 2–4).	I sit well	1 2 3 4 5	1. Make sure the child's hips are well flexed his bottom is pushed well back and his legs are apart to help him learn to sit well.
			2. At this level some children may not be able to place the heel on the opposite knee. Do not force this movement, begin by placing the heel on the opposite ankle.
			3. If the child is sitting on a mat on the floor it may be easier at this level to sit him with his back to the wall or in a corner of the room.
			4. If his back is too rounded a low stool/thick book (equivalent of telephone book)/sitting downhill on a wedge will help him learn to straighten his back (see Appendix).
2. Bend one leg and place the heel on the opposite knee.	I bend one leg	1 2 3 4 5	5. The care-giver sits opposite the child and helps him maintain the position.
			6. The child may need a gaiter on the free hand to stretch his elbow and for stability.
			7. Teach the child to use the right hand to remove the left shoe and the left hand to remove the right shoe.
			8. The child should be able to grasp the strap and pull.
			9. The child will need help to loosen the straps.
3. Look at the shoe.	I look at the shoe	look look look	10. Always make sure he uses alternate hands when learning this task. This is important for the child with hemiplegia as they prefer to use the unaffected hand.

4. Grasp the strap and pull.

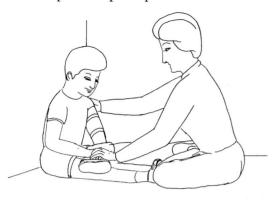

I grasp the strap and pull   pull pull pull

11. Allow the child sufficient time to attempt the steps and try not to help him too much.

12. The care-giver says every step out loud and encourages the child to look and to speak.

13. The child should try and say "shoe".

5. Grasp the back of the shoe.

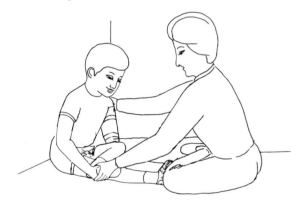

I grasp the shoe   1 2 3 4 5

6. Push off the shoe. Repeat with the other leg.

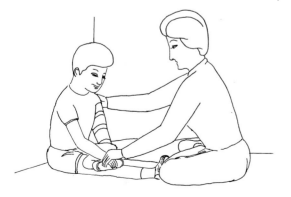

I push off the shoe   push push push

Analysis of Motor Task	*Speech/Songs/Rhymes*	*Guidelines*
1. Long sitting/tailor sitting task (see Chapter 16, Task 18, Levels 2–4).	I sit well 1 2 3 4 5	1. Make sure the child's hips are well flexed, his bottom pushed well back and his legs well parted to help him learn to sit well.

1. Make sure the child's hips are well flexed, his bottom pushed well back and his legs well parted to help him learn to sit well.

2. At this level, the child may not be able to place the heel on the opposite knee. Do not force this movement; begin by placing the heel on the opposite ankle.

3. If the child is sitting on a mat on the floor, it may be easier at this level to sit him with his back against the wall or in a corner of the room.

4. If the his back is too rounded, a low stool/thick book (equivalent of a telephone book)/sitting downhill on a wedge will help him learn to straighten his back (see Appendix).

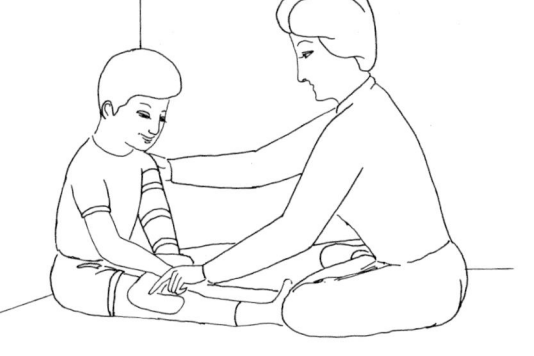

2. Bend one leg and place the heel on the opposite knee.

I bend my leg   1 2 3 4 5

5. The care-giver sits opposite the child and helps him maintain the sitting position.

6. The child may need a gaiter on the free hand to stretch his elbow and for stability.

7. Teach the child to use the right hand to remove the left sock and the left hand to remove the right sock.

8. The care-giver helps the child learn to put the thumb inside the sock and encourages him to push it down.

9. The child may need help to push the sock over the heel.

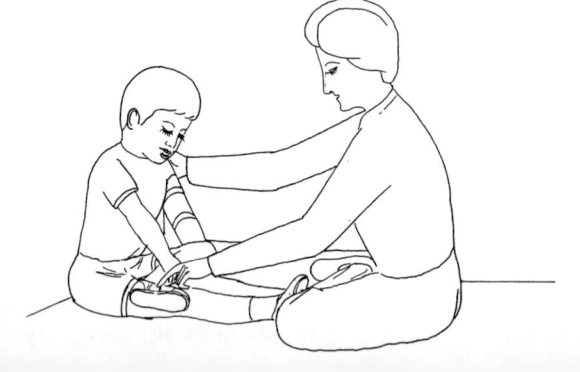

3. Look at the sock.

I look at the sock   look look look

4. Grasp the sock and push it down over the heel to the toes.

I grasp and push down   push push push

10. Allow him sufficient time to attempt each step and try not to help him too much.

11. Always ensure the child uses alternate hands.

12. If time permits, teach the child to play with his toes.

13. If possible, encourage the child to say "toes".

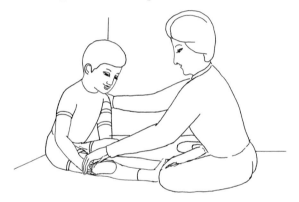

5. Grasp the sock and pull it off.

I grasp and pull   pull pull pull

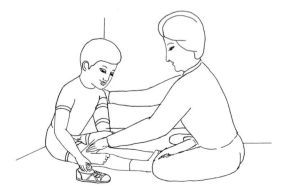

6. Put the sock in the shoe. Repeat with the other leg.

I release the sock   1 2 3 4 5

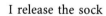

Analysis of Motor Task	Speech/Songs/Rhymes	Guidelines
1. Long sitting/tailor sitting task (see Chapter 16, Task 18, Levels 2–4).	I sit well	1. If the child feels insecure, he may sit against the wall or in a corner of the room for greater security.
2. Put left heel on right knee. Grasp the strap and pull.	I grasp the strap and pull pull pull pull	2. Make sure his hips are well flexed, his bottom pushed well back and his legs apart to help him learn to sit well.
		3. If his back is too rounded, a low stool/thick book (equivalent of a telephone book)/sitting downhill on a wedge will help him learn to straighten his back (see Appendix).
		4. Use speech to assist the child with minimal manual facilitation.
		5. Make sure the child uses alternate hands when doing this task; this is important for the child with hemiplegia as they prefer to use the unaffected hand.
3. Loosen the shoe.	I loosen the shoe 1 2 3 4 5	6. The child may still need a little help to push the sock over the heel.
		7. Allow the child sufficient time to do the task.
		8. Encourage him to play with his toes, shoes and socks.
		9. He should begin to learn to name the colour of the shoes and socks.
		10. The child should begin to learn the word "heel".
		11. He should also begin to learn the concept of pairing shoes and socks.
4. Grasp the back of the shoe and push it off.	I grasp the shoe and push push push push	

5. Grasp the sock and push it down to the toes.

I grasp the sock and push push push push

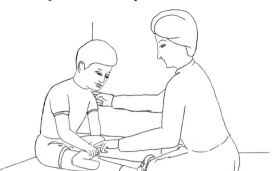

6. Grasp the sock and pull it off.

I grasp the sock and pull pull pull pull

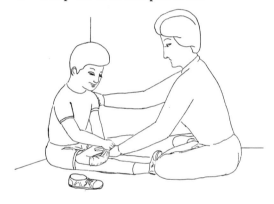

7. Put the sock in the shoe.

I release the sock 1 2 3 4 5

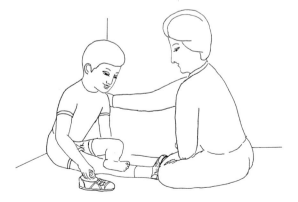

8. Repeat with the other leg.

Analysis of Motor Task	*Speech/Songs/Rhymes*	*Guidelines*

Analysis of Motor Task

1. Long sitting or sitting on a stool task (see Chapter 16, Task 18, Levels 2–4).

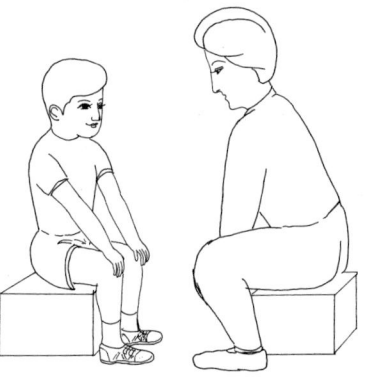

2. Undo the straps and loosen the shoe.

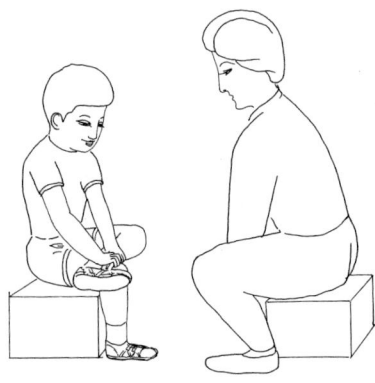

3. Push off the shoe.

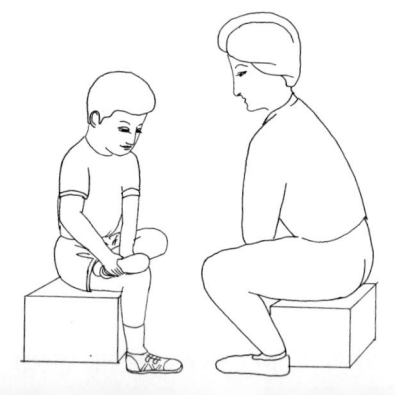

Guidelines

1. Depending on the ability of the child, he may sit on a mat on the floor or on a stool for this task.

2. The child uses inner speech.

3. The care-giver supervises the child, preferably with no manual assistance.

4. Give the child sufficient time to try and do the task as independently as possible.

5. He should begin to learn to differentiate the right and left shoe and also footwear according to weather conditions.

6. If socks are multi-coloured, encourage the child to learn to name the colours.

7. The child should begin to put away socks/shoes tidily.

4. Push down the sock.

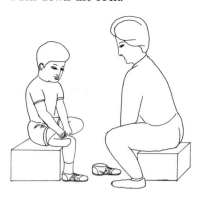

5. Pull off the sock.

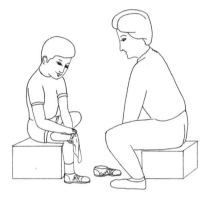

6. Put the sock in the shoe. Repeat with the other leg.

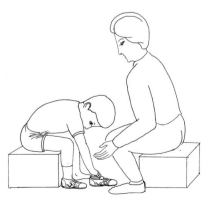

Analysis of Motor Task	*Speech/Songs/Rhymes*	*Guidelines*

1. Sitting on the care-giver's lap.

I sit well

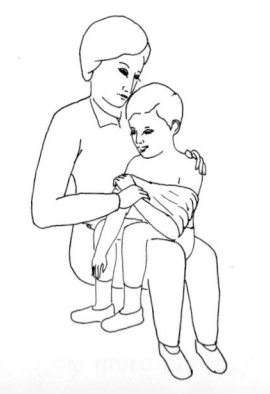

1. Make sure the child's hips are well flexed, his bottom pushed well back and his back straight.

2. The care-giver takes off the top over the child's head to below the elbows. She helps stretch his elbows and guides his hands to grasp the top and pull it off.

3. Encourage the child to look at the top.

4. The carer-giver says every step out loud and if possible encourages the child to speak.

5. She shows the top to the child and names it.

2. Bend the head. Care-giver pulls the top over the child's head.

I bend head   down   down   down

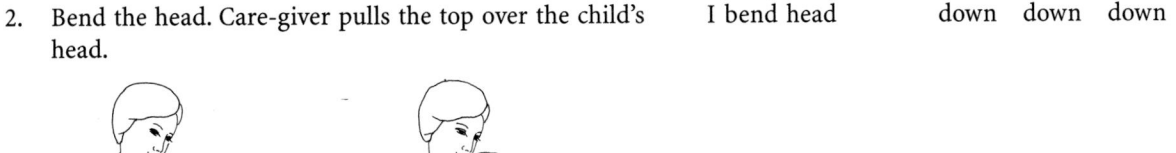

3. Grasp the top and pull off.

I pull top   pull   pull   pull

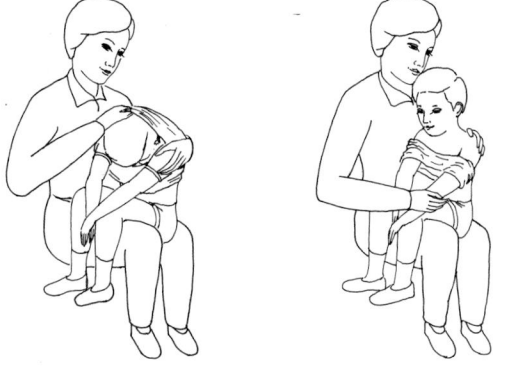

4. Repeat with the other hand.

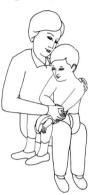

Analysis of Motor Task	*Speech/Songs/Rhymes*	*Guidelines*
1. Sitting task (see Chapter 10, Task 18, Level 2).	*I Stretch my Hands and Hold on Tight*	1. The care-giver pulls the top over the child's head leaving the face covered and asks the child to grasp it and pull it off.

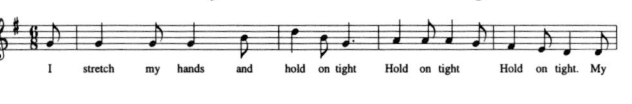

I stretch my hands and hold on tight Hold on tight Hold on tight. My

feet are flat, my bot-tom's pushed back look in the mid-dle I'm sit-ting up-right.

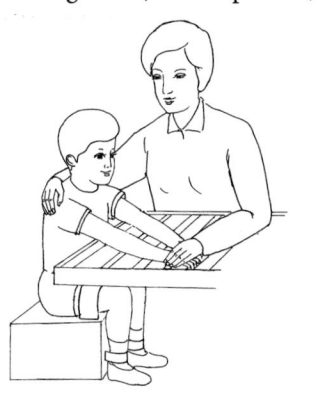

2. Make sure the child grasps the plinth while using the other hand to pull off the top.

3. Give the child sufficient time to attempt the steps.

4. The care-giver encourages the child to try and say each step with her.

5. She asks the child to look at the top and try to say "top".

6. Begin to the teach the child the concepts of "sleeve" and "off".

2. Bend the head.

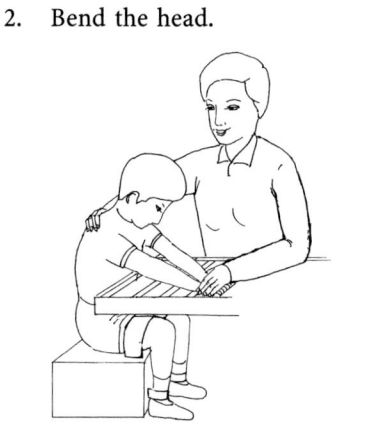

I bend my head   down   down   down

3. Grasp the top of the garment with both hands.

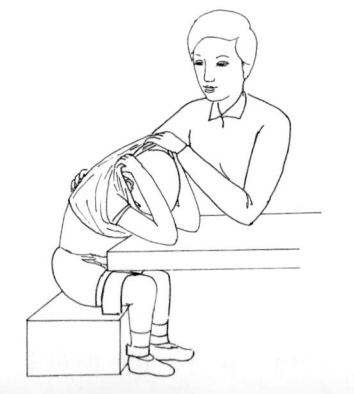

I grasp the top   grasp   grasp   grasp

4. Pull the top over the head.

I pull the top   pull pull pull

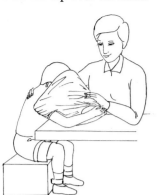

5. Grasp the sleeve and pull out the hand.

I grasp the sleeve and pull   pull pull pull

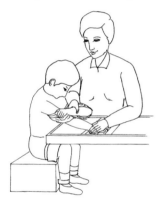

6. Repeat with the other hand.

Analysis of Motor Task	*Speech/Songs/Rhymes*	*Guidelines*
1. Sitting task (see Chapter 10, Task 18, Level 3). 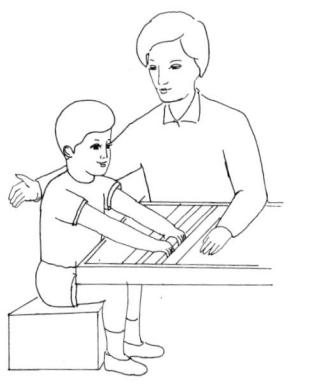	*Sit up Straight* 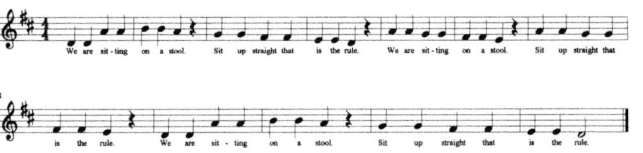 We are sit-ting on a stool. Sit up straight that is the rule. We are sit-ting on a stool. Sit up straight that is the rule. We are sit-ting on a stool. Sit up straight that is the rule.	1. The care-giver facilitates with speech and minimal manual facilitation. 2. If the top is a primary colour, ask the child if he can name the colour. 3. The child should begin to learn the following concepts: "front", "back", "top", "bottom", "sleeve". 4. Encourage the child to learn to put the top in the basket. 5. It is important at all times to encourage the child with hemiplegia to learn to use the affected hand.
2. Bend the head. 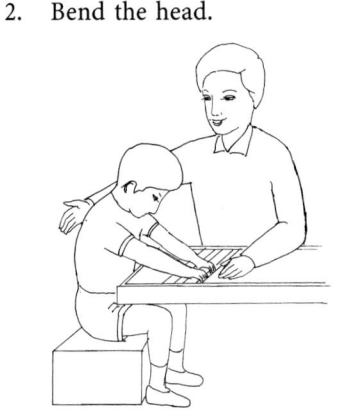	I bend my head down down down	
3. Grasp the top and pull over the head. 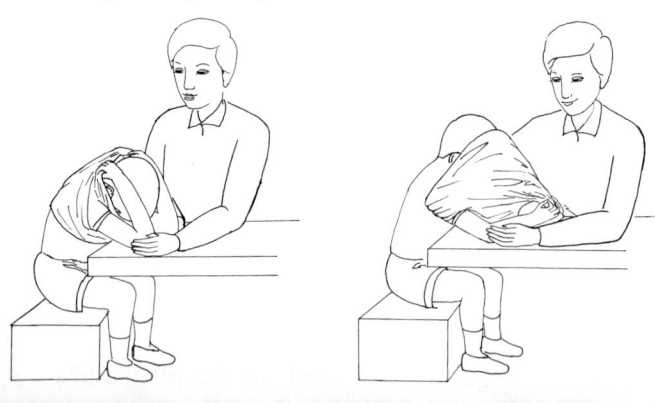	I grasp the top and pull 1 2 3 4 5	

4. Grasp the sleeve and pull off.
   Repeat with the other hand.

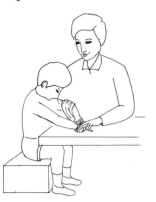

I grasp the sleeve and pull off   pull   pull   pull

| *Analysis of Motor Task* | *Speech/Songs/Rhymes* | *Guidelines* |

1. Long sitting/Sitting on stool (see Chapter 10, Task 18, Level 4, Chapter 16, Task 18, Levels 2–4).

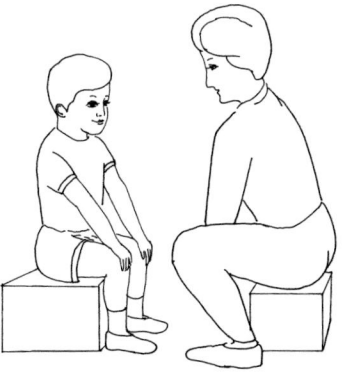

2. Pull the top over the head.

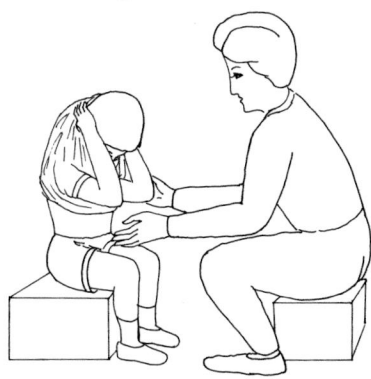

3. Grasp the sleeves and pull.

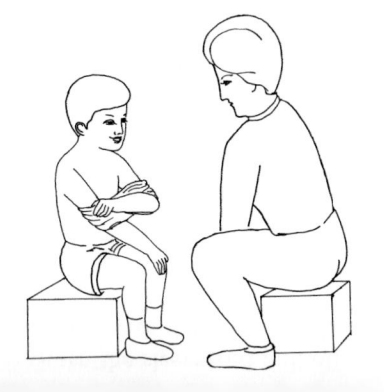

1. The child uses inner speech.

2. The care-giver supervises the child, preferaly with no manual assistance.

3. Give the child sufficient time to do the task as independently as possible.

4. The child should begin to learn the concepts of "inside", "outside", "front", "back", names of the different tops. If the top is multi-coloured, the child should learn to name some of the colours.

5. He should also learn suitable clothing for different weather conditions.

Task 12 Taking off Pyjama Legs: *Taking off Pyjama Legs/Underpants/Trousers on the Bed in Supine/Side Lying Position*

Level 1

Analysis of Motor Task	*Speech/Songs/Rhymes*	*Guidelines*

1. Lying supine task (see Chapter 15, Task 3, Level 1).

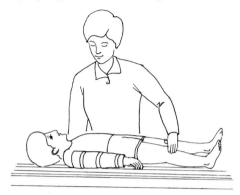

I lie straight

1. It may be easier for a child at Level 1 to learn to take off pyjama legs/underpants/trousers in the supine or side lying positions.

2. The child may need gaiters to stretch his elbows.

3. The care-giver helps the child maintain the bridging position when pushing down the pants.

4. The care-giver says every step out loud and if possible encourages the child to speak.

5. The care-giver pushes the pants down to the ankles and helps and encourages the child to kick it off.

6. Show the pants to the child and name it.

7. Emphasise the concept of "off".

2. Bridging task (see Chapter 15, Task 5, Level 1).

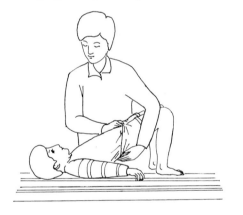

London Bridge is Falling Down

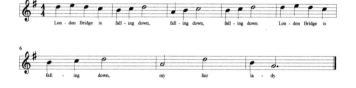

Lon - don Bridge is fall - ing down, fall - ing down, fall - ing down. Lon - don Bridge is

fall - ing down, my fair la - dy.

3. Kick off the pants.

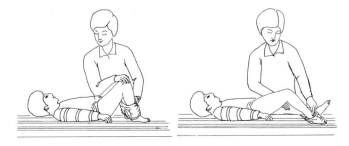

I kick off   kick kick kick

Analysis of Motor Task	*Speech/Songs/Rhymes*	*Guidelines*

1. Standing task (see Chapter 11, Task 19, Level 2).

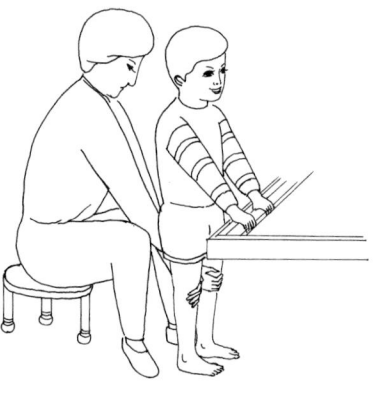

Stand up Tall

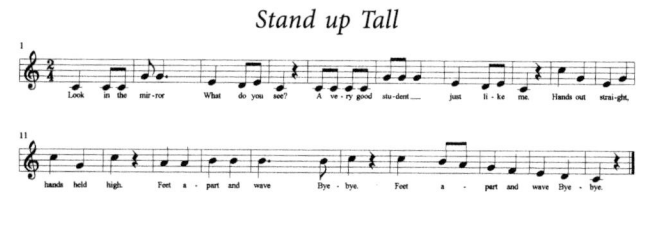

Look in the mir-ror What do you see? A ve-ry good stu-dent..... just li-ke me. Hands out strai-ght, hands held high. Feet a-part and wave Bye-bye. Feet a-part and wave Bye-bye.

2. Pull the child's pants down to below the knees.

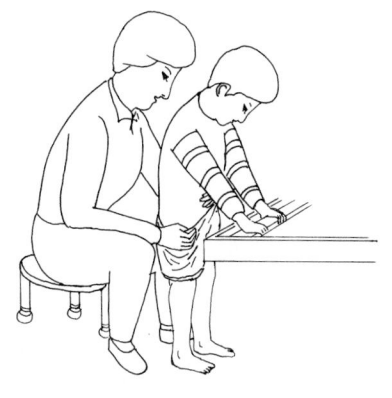

3. Sit down.

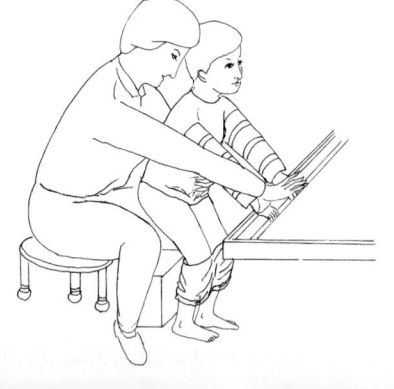

I sit down   1 2 3 4 5

1. The child at this level should be able to stand for a short period holding the plinth with both hands. If a plinth is not available, he may sit at a bed/table. However, he will need help to grasp a hand bar (see Appendix) to maintain his balance.

2. He may need gaiters to stretch the elbows and for stability.

3. The care-giver helps the child push his pants down to below his knees while he is standing.

4. She then helps him grasp the top with his thumbs out and push the pants down from below the knees.

5. Give the child sufficient time to attempt some of the steps.

6. Encourage the child to say each step and look at what he is doing.

7. Emphasise the concept of "knee".

8. If the pants is a primary colour, help the child learn to name it.

4. Grasp the top of the pants and push it down.   I grasp and push   push   push   push

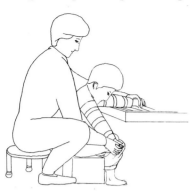

5. Kick off the pants.   I kick off   kick   kick   kick

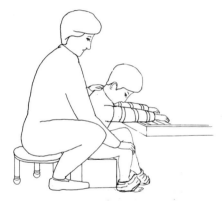

Analysis of Motor Task	*Speech/Songs/Rhymes*	*Guidelines*

1. Standing task (see Chapter 11, Task 19, Level 3).

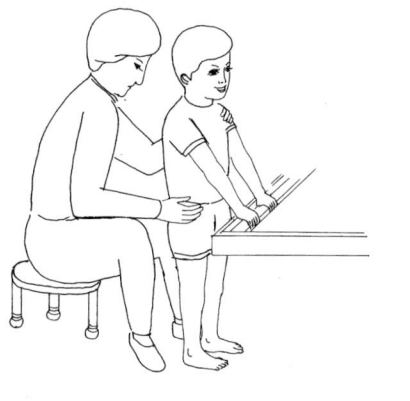

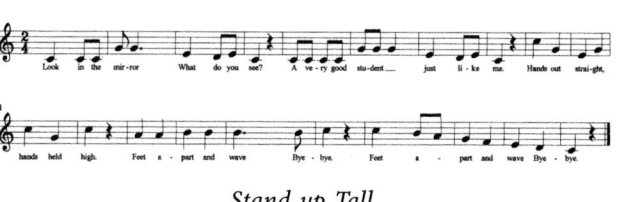

Stand up Tall

1. The care-giver guides with speech and minimal manual assistance.

2. Give the child sufficient time to do each step.

3. Encourage the child with hemiplegia to use the affected hand.

4. The child should begin to learn the concepts of "waist", "leg".

2. Grasp the pants and push it down. Repeat with the other hand.

I push down my pants   push   push   push

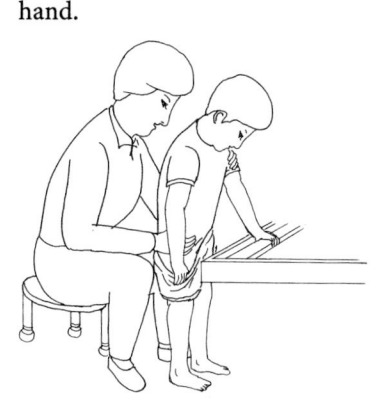

3. Sit down.

I sit down   1   2   3   4   5

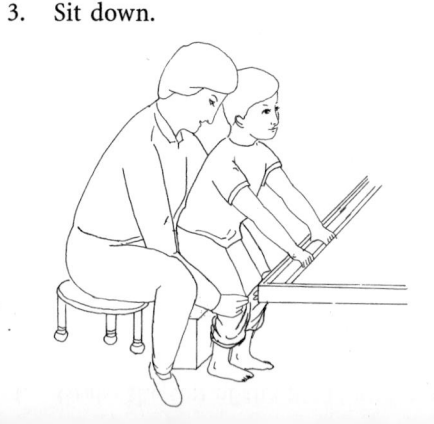

4. Push the pants down.

I push down my pants   push push push

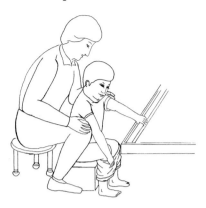

5. Kick off the pants.

I kick off my pants   kick kick kick

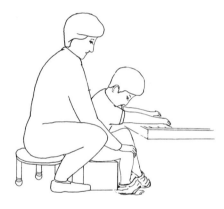

Analysis of Motor Task	*Speech/Songs/Rhymes*	*Guidelines*

1. Standing task (see Chapter 11, Task 19, Level 4).

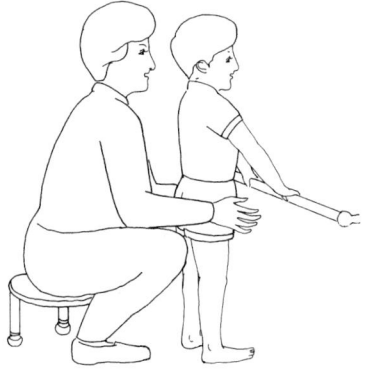

2. Grasp the pants and push it down. Repeat with the other hand.

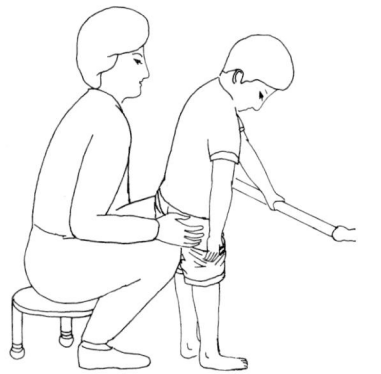

3. Step out of the pants.

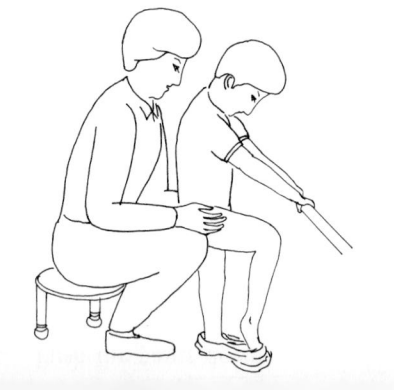

1. The child uses inner speech.

2. The care-giver supervises the child, preferably with no manual assistance.

3. Give the child sufficient time to do the task as independently as possible.

4. The child should pick up his pants and place it in a basket.

5. He should begin to learn the concepts of "inside", "outside", "front", "back", names of different garments. If the pants is multi-coloured, he should learn to name some of the colours.

6. He should also learn which clothing is suitable for different weather conditions.

4. Pick up the pants.

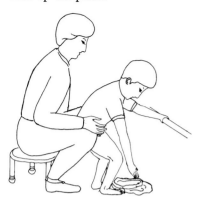

5. Put the pants in the basket.

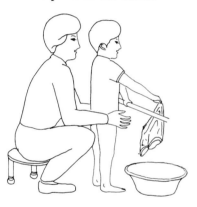

GROOMING

Analysis of Motor Task	*Speech/Songs/Rhymes*	*Guidelines*

1. Pull up the sleeve to the elbow. Repeat with the other hand.

I grasp sleeve and pull   pull   pull   pull

1. Make sure the child is sitting well for this task (see Chapter 10, Task 18, Level 1).

2. This task encourages and helps the child to learn to bring his hands into the midline.

3. Children love playing with water. If time permits give the child time to play. A toy in the water will encourage him to look at his hands in the water.

4. The care-giver helps the child with every step.

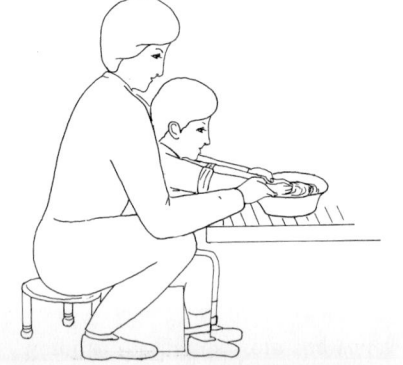

2. Stretch the elbows and put the hands in the bowl of water.

I stretch elbows   stretch   stretch   stretch

3. Rub the hands together.

Grooming Song

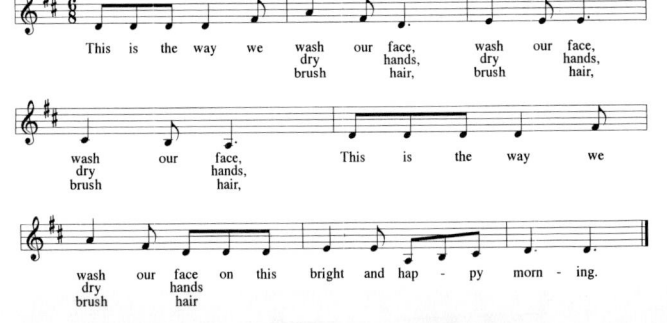

This is the way we wash our face, / dry hands, / brush hair, wash our face, / dry hands, / brush hair,

wash our face, / dry hands, / brush hair, This is the way we

wash our face / dry hands / brush hair on this bright and hap-py morn-ing.

4. Remove the hands from the water.

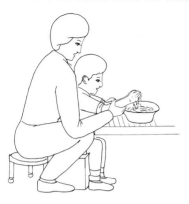

5. Dry the hands.

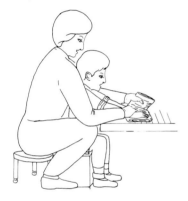

Grooming Song

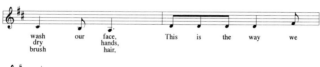

This is the way we wash our face, wash our face,
dry hands, dry hands,
brush hair, brush hair,

wash our face, This is the way we
dry hands,
brush hair,

wash our face on this bright and hap - py morn - ing.
dry hands
brush hair

Analysis of Motor Task	*Speech/Songs/Rhymes*	*Guidelines*

1. Grasp the sleeve and pull it up. Repeat with the other hand.

I grasp my sleeve and pull up   pull   pull   pull

1. Make sure the child is sitting well for this task (see Chapter 10, Task 18, Level 2).

2. This task helps the child learn to bring his hands together and cross the midline.

3. The child should be able to grasp the sleeve but will need help to push it up to the elbow.

4. The care-giver says every step out loud and encourages the child to speak and sing along with her.

5. Give the child sufficient time to attempt the step and do not over assist him.

6. The song should help the child begin to learn some body parts.

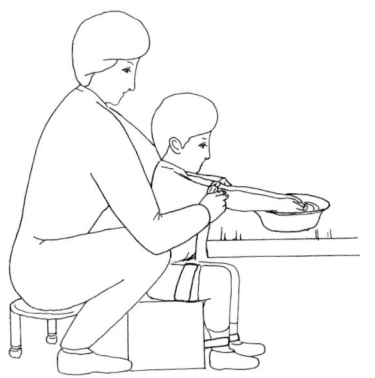

2. Stretch the elbows and put the hands in the water.

I stretch my elbows   stretch   stretch   stretch

3. Rub the hands together.

Grooming Song

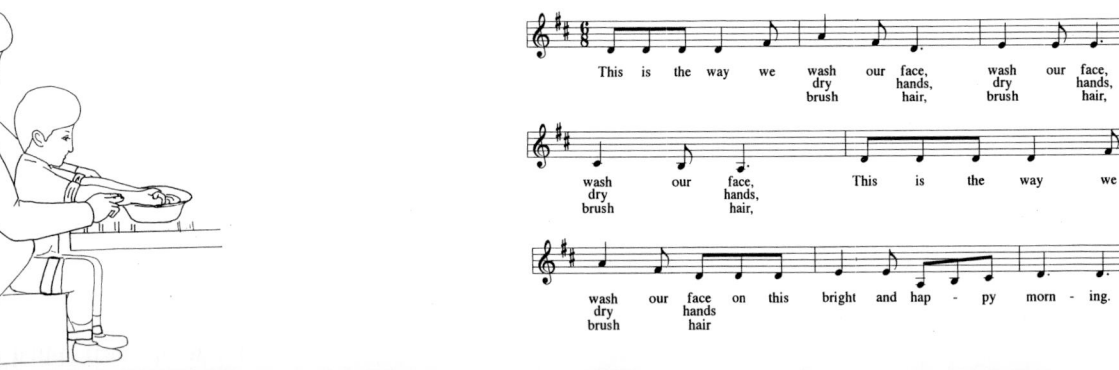

This is the way we wash our face, wash our face,
                         dry   hands,   dry   hands,
                         brush hair,   brush hair,

wash   our   face,   This   is   the   way   we
dry   hands,
brush   hair,

wash   our   face   on   this   bright   and   hap - py   morn - ing.
dry   hands
brush   hair

4. Remove the hands from the water.

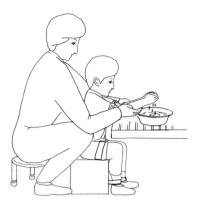

5. Grasp the flannel and place it flat on the plinth.   I grasp the flannel   grasp   grasp   grasp

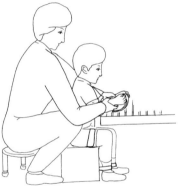

6. Dry the hands.

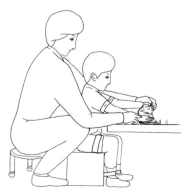

Grooming Song

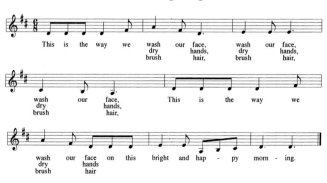

This is the way we wash our face,   wash our face,
                         dry   hands,   dry   hands,
                         brush   hair,   brush   hair,

wash   our   face,   This is the way we
dry   hands,
brush   hair,

wash   our   face   on   this   bright   and   hap - py   morn - ing.
dry   hands
brush   hair

Analysis of Motor Task	*Speech/Songs/Rhymes*	*Guidelines*
1. Pull up the sleeves to the elbows. 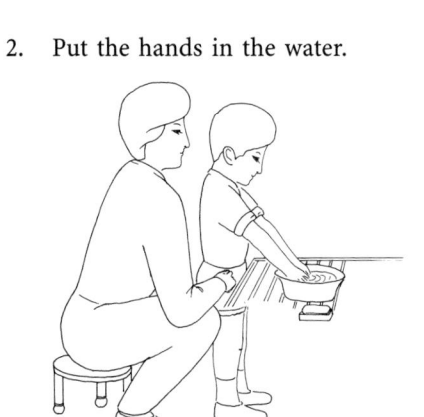	I grasp my sleeve and pull up 1 2 3 4 5	1. The child at this level may sit or stand to carry out the task. However, it is preferable if the child has the opportunity to stand as this improves his standing balance and prepares him for walking training (see Chapter 11, Task 19, Level 3).
2. Put the hands in the water.	My hands in the water 1 2 3 4 5	2. This task is excellent to help the child learn to bring his hands together and cross the midline. It also encourages the child with hemiplegia to learn to use his affected hand.
3. Grasp the soap and lather.	I grasp the soap and rub in 1 2 3 4 5	3. Children love playing with water and this task will motivate them to do each step.
		4. Encourage him to look at his hands while washing them.
		5. Give the child sufficient time to do each step and encourage him to use speech/song to guide his movements.

4. Release the soap.

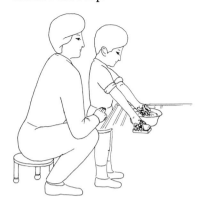

I release the soap   1 2 3 4 5

5. Rub the hands together.

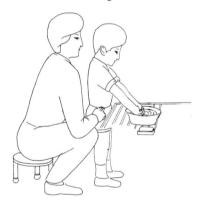

Grooming Song

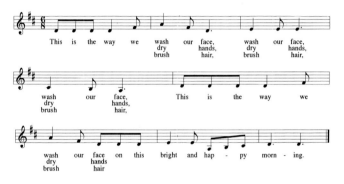

This is the way we wash our face, wash our face,
                 dry   hands,   dry   hands,
                 brush   hair,   brush   hair,

wash our face, This is the way we
dry hands,
brush hair,

wash our face on this bright and hap - py morn - ing.
dry hands
brush hair

6. Grasp the flannel and dry the hands.

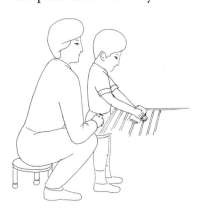

Grooming Song

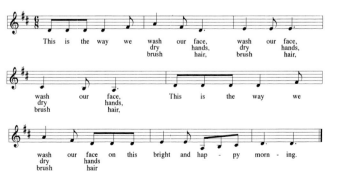

This is the way we wash our face, wash our face,
                 dry   hands,   dry   hands,
                 brush   hair,   brush   hair,

wash our face, This is the way we
dry hands,
brush hair,

wash our face on this bright and hap - py morn - ing.
dry hands
brush hair

Analysis of Motor Task	*Speech/Songs/Rhymes*	*Guidelines*

1. Pull up both sleeves.

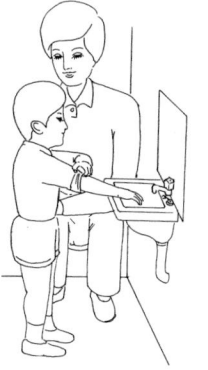

2. Put the stopper in the sink.

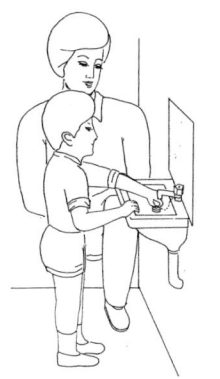

3. Turn on/off the tap.

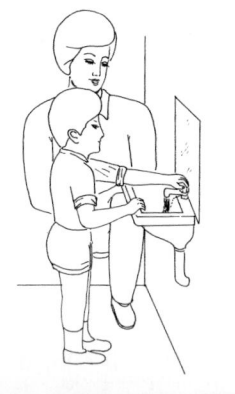

1. The child at this level should learn to walk to the sink. If there is no sink, the child can use a bowl standing at the plinth/table.

2. He uses inner speech.

3. The care-giver uses speech to supervise the child preferably with no manual assistance.

4. Give the child sufficient time to do each step and encourage him to look at his hands.

5. He should become aware of "clean hands".

4.   Put the hands in the water.

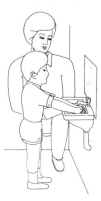

5.   Grasp the soap and wash the hands.

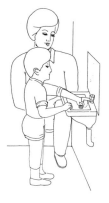

6.   Dry the hands.

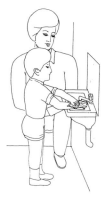

7.   Remove the stopper.

Analysis of Motor Task	*Speech/Songs/Rhymes*	*Guidelines*
1. Pull up the sleeve to the elbow. Repeat with the other hand.	I grasp and pull pull pull pull	1. Make sure the child is sitting well at the plinth or on the care-giver's lap (see Chapter 10, Task 18, Level 1).
		2. The care-giver helps the child with every step.
		3. She helps him open his hand and place the flannel on his flat hand. She then helps him bring his hand to his face and wash his face, ears and neck.
		4. Encourage the child to look in the mirror and bring his head into the midline while she washes his face.
2. Look at the flannel in the water.	I look at flannel look look look	
3. Care-giver squeezes the flannel.	I squeeze flannel squeeze squeeze squeeze	

4. Grasp the flannel.

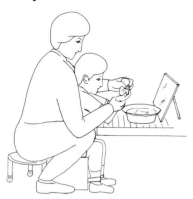

I grasp   grasp grasp grasp

5. Bring the flannel to the face and wash the face.

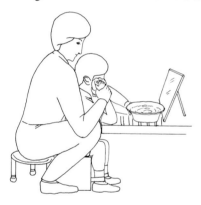

Flannel to face   up up up

Grooming Song

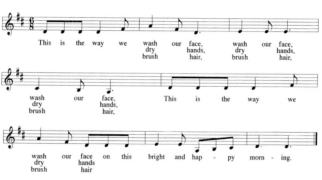

This is the way we wash our face, wash our face,
dry hands, dry hands,
brush hair, brush hair,

wash our face, This is the way we
dry hands,
brush hair,

wash our face on this bright and hap - py morn - ing.
dry hands
brush hair

6. Return the flannel to the water.

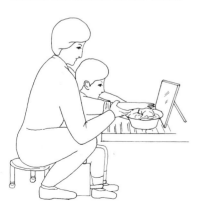

I release flannel   1 2 3 4 5

Analysis of Motor Task	*Speech/Songs/Rhymes*	*Guidelines*

1. Use the right hand to grasp the left sleeve and pull it up. Repeat with the other hand.

I pull up my sleeve   pull pull pull

1. Make sure the child is sitting well at the plinth before beginning this task (see Chapter 10, Task 18, Level 2).

2. Encourage the child to grasp the edge of the sleeve. However, the care-giver will need to help the child push up his sleeve to the elbow.

3. She will also need to help him squeeze the flannel.

4. Always encourage the child to do the step if possible and do not over assist him. However, the child may need help to hold the palm of the hand facing upwards to position the flannel.

5. Encourage the child to look in the mirror and if possible sing along with the care-giver.

2. Look at the flannel in the water.

I look at the flannel   look look look

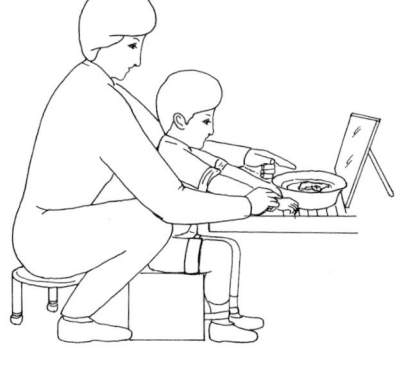

3. Squeeze the flannel.

I squeeze the flannel   1 2 3 4 5

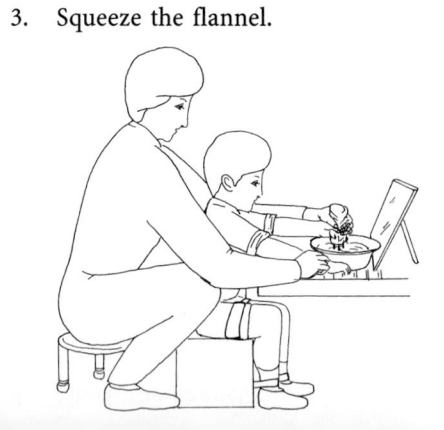

4. Spread the flannel on the palm of the hand.

I spread the flannel   1   2   3   4   5

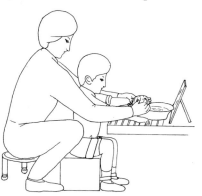

5. Bring the flannel to the face and wash the face.

Flannel to my face   1   2   3   4   5

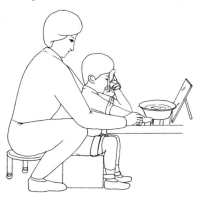

Grooming Song

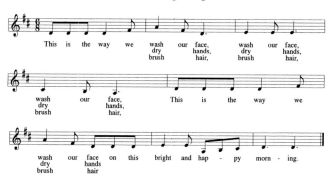

This is the way we wash our face,
dry hands, brush hair,
wash our face,
dry hands,
brush hair,

wash our face,
dry hands,
brush hair,
This is the way we

wash our face on this bright and hap - py morn - ing.
dry hands
brush hair

6. Return the flannel to the water.

I release the flannel   1   2   3   4   5

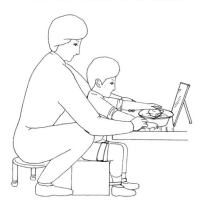

Analysis of Motor Task	Speech/Songs/Rhymes	Guidelines
1. Pull up the sleeve to the elbows.	I pull up my sleeve 1 2 3 4 5	1. The child at this level may sit or stand to carry out this task. However, it is preferable if the child has the opportunity to stand as this improves his standing balance and prepares him for walking training (see Chapter 11, Task 19, Level 3).

1. Pull up the sleeve to the elbows.

I pull up my sleeve   1   2   3   4   5

1. The child at this level may sit or stand to carry out this task. However, it is preferable if the child has the opportunity to stand as this improves his standing balance and prepares him for walking training (see Chapter 11, Task 19, Level 3).

2. Encourage the child to try and do as much of the task as possible and do not over assist him.

3. Give him sufficient time to try and do each step and encourage him to use speech/song to guide his movements.

2. Squeeze the flannel.

I squeeze the flannel   1   2   3   4   5

4. Children love playing with water and this task will motivate them to do as much as possible without assistance. This task is also a play experience for the child.

5. Encourage the child to look in the mirror.

6. Make sure the child with hemiplegia uses both hands as they usually prefer to use the unaffected hand.

3. Shake out the flannel.

I shake the flannel   1   2   3   4   5

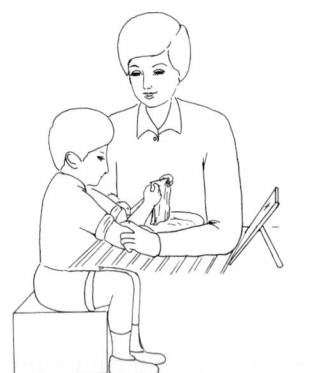

4. Spread the flannel on the palm of the hand.

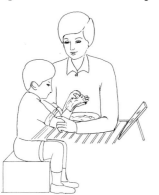

I place the flannel on my hand   1 2 3 4 5

5. Bring the flannel to the face and wash the face.

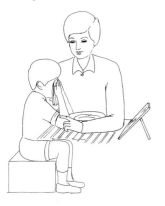

Flannel to my face   1 2 3 4 5

Grooming Song

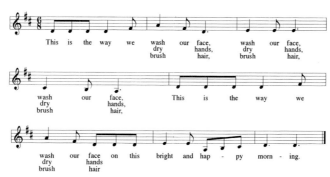

This is the way we wash our face, wash our face,
              dry hands, dry hands,
             brush hair, brush hair,

wash our face, This is the way we
dry hands,
brush hair,

wash our face on this bright and hap - py morn - ing.
dry hands
brush hair

6. Return the flannel to the water.

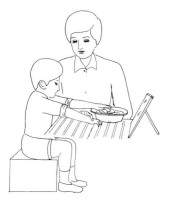

I release the flannel   1 2 3 4 5

Analysis of Motor Task	*Speech/Songs/Rhymes*	*Guidelines*

1. Pull up the sleeve.

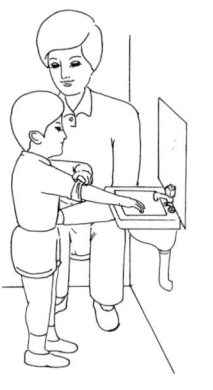

2. Put the stopper in the sink.

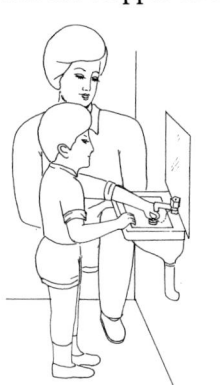

3. Turn on/off the water.

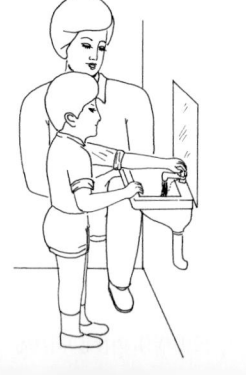

1. The child at this level should learn to walk to the sink. If there is no sink, the child can use a bowl of water standing at the plinth/table.

2. He uses inner speech.

3. Use speech to supervise him, preferably with no manual assistance.

4. Give him sufficient time to do each step and encourage him to look in the mirror and learn to become aware of "clean face".

4.   Squeeze the flannel.

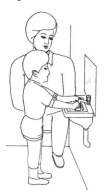

5.   Wash the face.

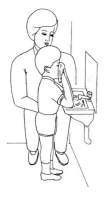

6.   Wash out the flannel.

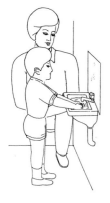

7.   Remove the stopper.

Analysis of Motor Task	Speech/Songs/Rhymes	Guidelines

1. Look at the tooth brush.

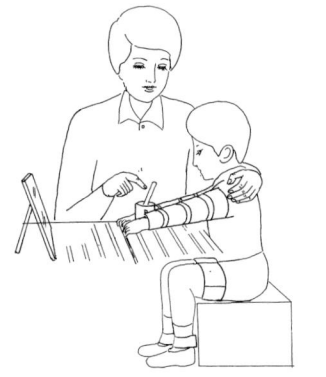

2. The care-giver grasps the tooth brush.

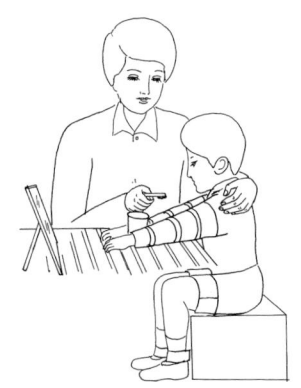

3. Open the mouth.

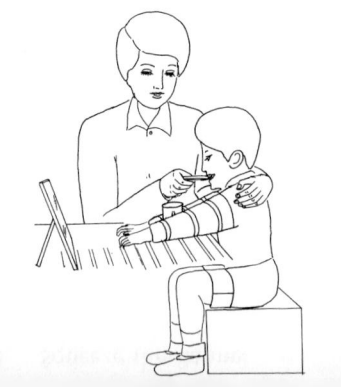

I look at tooth brush   look   look   look

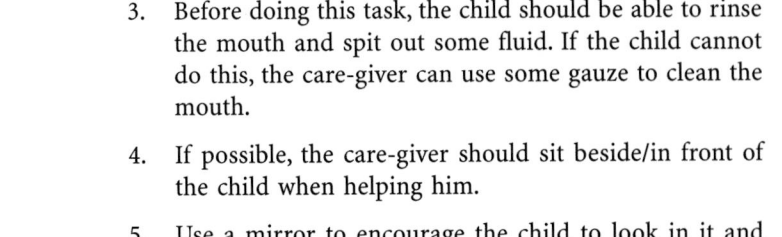

1. Make sure the child is sitting well at the plinth or on the care-giver's lap (see Chapter 10, Task 18, Level 1).

2. The care-giver helps the child with every step.

3. Before doing this task, the child should be able to rinse the mouth and spit out some fluid. If the child cannot do this, the care-giver can use some gauze to clean the mouth.

4. If possible, the care-giver should sit beside/in front of the child when helping him.

5. Use a mirror to encourage the child to look in it and bring his head into the midline while the care-giver helps him brush his teeth.

4. Brush the teeth.

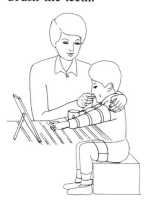

5. Rinse the mouth and spit out.

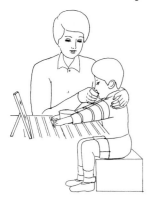

Analysis of Motor Task	*Speech/Songs/Rhymes*	*Guidelines*
1. Look at the tooth brush. 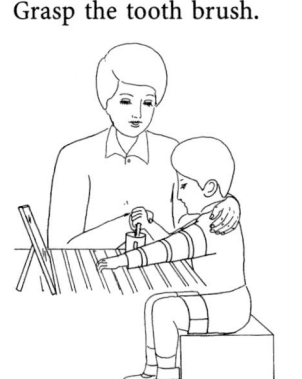	I look at the tooth brush look look look	1. Make sure the child is sitting well at the plinth (see Chapter 10, Task 18, Level 2). 2. He may still need a gaiter on the free hand to stretch his elbow and grasp the plinth. 3. The child should be able to grasp the toothbrush but may need help to bring it to his mouth and brush his teeth. 4. He may also need help to grasp the handle of the mug and bring it to his mouth. The care-giver says every step out loud. 5. Encourage the child to look in the mirror while doing the task.
2. Grasp the tooth brush.	I grasp the tooth brush grasp grasp grasp	
3. Bring the tooth brush to the mouth. 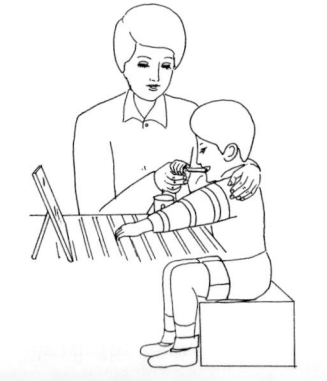	Tooth brush to my mouth 1 2 3 4 5	

4. Brush the teeth.

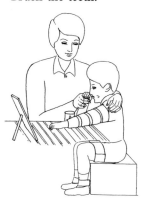

5. Rinse the mouth and spit out.

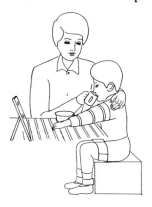

Analysis of Motor Task	Speech/Songs/Rhymes	Guidelines

1. Grasp the tooth brush.

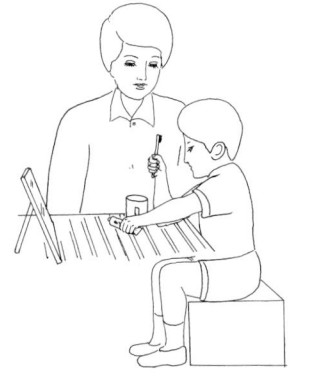

2. Grasp the tooth paste.

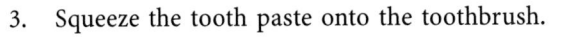

3. Squeeze the tooth paste onto the toothbrush.

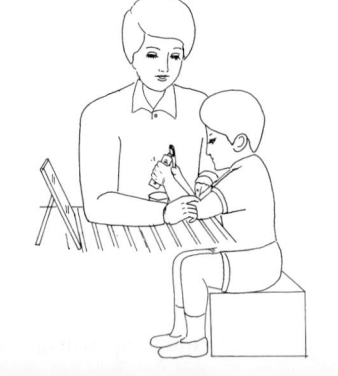

I grasp the tooth brush   1 2 3 4 5

I grasp the tooth paste   1 2 3 4 5

I squeeze the tooth paste   1 2 3 4 5

1. The child at this level may sit or stand to carry out this task. However, it is preferable if the child has the opportunity to stand as this improves his standing balance and prepares him for walking training (see Chapter 11, Task 19, Level 3).

2. If the child is standing at the sink, he may need to grasp a hand rail.

3. He may need help to squeeze the toothpaste onto the toothbrush. However, do not over assist the him.

4. Give him sufficient time to do each step and encourage him to use speech to guide his movements.

5. Encourage him to look in the mirror while doing this task.

6. Always encourage the child with hemiplegia to use his affected hand.

4. Bring the toothbrush to the mouth.   Toothbrush to my mouth   1 2 3 4 5

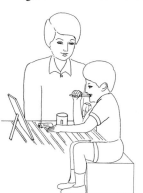

5. Brush the teeth.

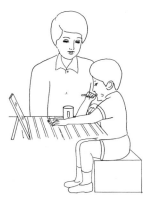

6. Rinse the mouth and spit out.

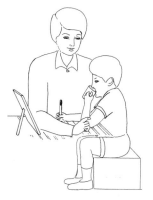

Analysis of Motor Task	*Speech/Songs/Rhymes*	*Guidelines*

1. Unscrew the cap of the tooth paste.

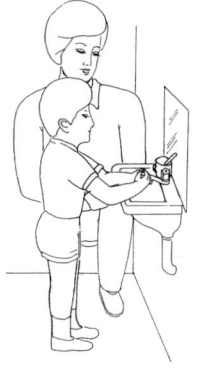

2. Grasp the tooth brush.

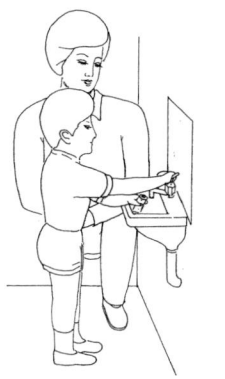

3. Squeeze the tooth paste onto the tooth brush.

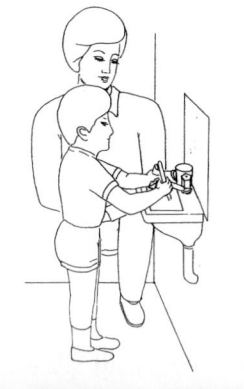

1. The child at this level should learn to walk to the sink. If there is no sink, the child can use a bowl standing at the plinth/table.

2. He uses inner speech.

3. Use speech to supervise the child, preferably with no manual assistance. However, he may need a little assistance screwing and unscrewing the cap of the toothpaste.

4. Give the him sufficient time to do each step.

5. At this level, the child with hemiplegia should spontaneously use his affected hand.

6. Encourage the child to look in the mirror while brushing his teeth.

4. Brush the teeth.

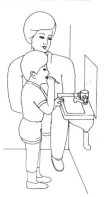

5. Rinse the mouth.

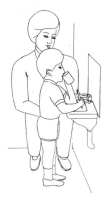

6. Replace the cap of the tube of tooth paste.

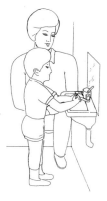

| *Analysis of Motor Task* | *Speech/Songs/Rhymes* | *Guidelines* |

1. Sitting task (Chapter 10, Task 18, Level 1).

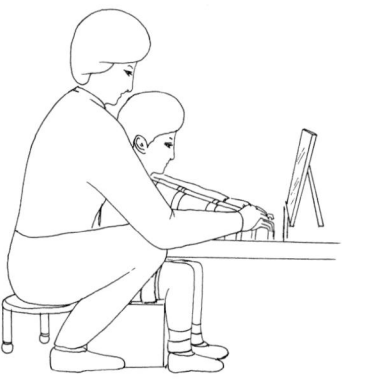

I Stretch my Hands and Hold on Tight

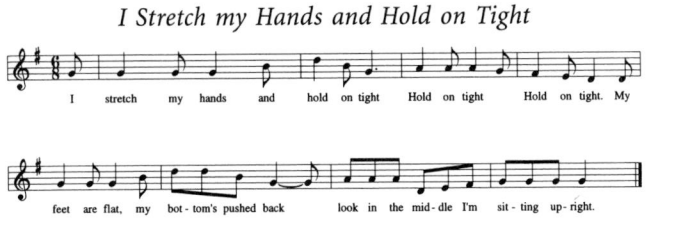

I stretch my hands and hold on tight Hold on tight Hold on tight. My feet are flat, my bot-tom's pushed back look in the mid-dle I'm sit-ting up-right.

1. Make sure the child is sitting well at the plinth or on the care-giver's lap (see Chapter 10, Task 18, Level 1).

2. The care-giver helps the child with every step.

3. Encourage the child to look in the mirror while his hair is being brushed.

2. Look at the mirror.

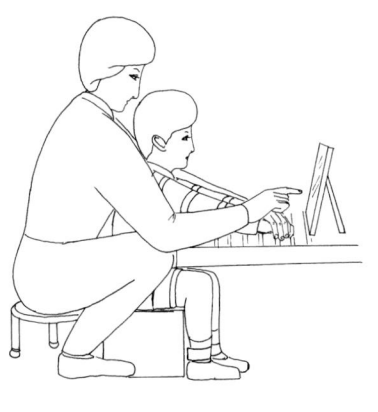

I look at mirror   look   look   look

3. Brush/Comb the hair.

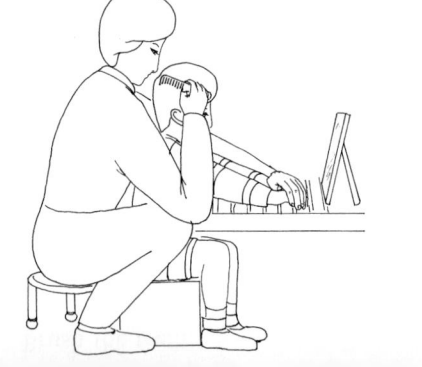

Grooming Song

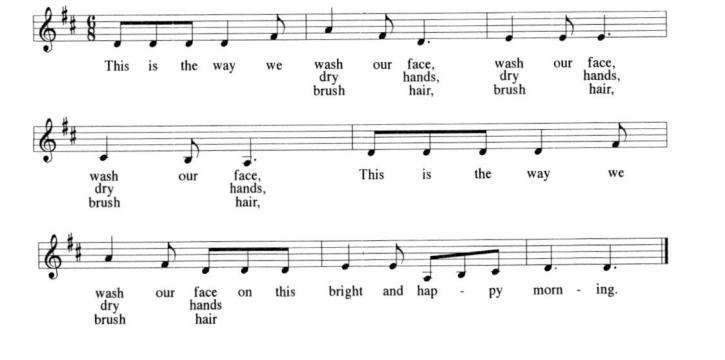

This is the way we wash our face, / dry hands, / brush hair, wash our face, / dry hands, / brush hair, wash our face, / dry hands, / brush hair, This is the way we wash our face on this bright and hap-py morn-ing. / dry hands / brush hair

Analysis of Motor Task	*Speech/Songs/Rhymes*	*Guidelines*

1. Look at the hairbrush/comb.

I look at the hairbrush   look   look   look

2. Grasp the hairbrush/comb.

I grasp the hairbrush   grasp   grasp   grasp

3. Rest the elbow on the plinth and bring the hairbrush/comb to the head.

Hairbrush to my head   1   2   3   4   5

1. Make sure the child is sitting well at the plinth (see Chapter 10, Task 18, Level 2).

2. The child should be able to look at and grasp the hair brush. However, the care-giver will have to help him bring the hair brush to his head and brush his hair.

3. Encourage the child to look in the mirror while doing this task.

4. She says every step out loud and encourages the child to speak and sing along with her.

4. Brush/Comb the hair.

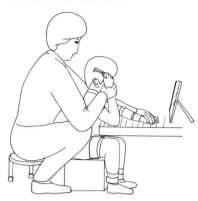

Grooming Song

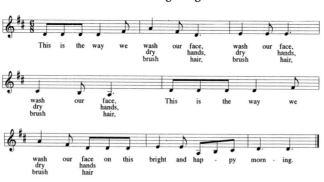

This is the way we wash our face, wash our face,
                    dry   hands, dry   hands,
                    brush   hair,   brush hair,

wash   our   face,   This is   the   way   we
dry   hands,
brush   hair,

wash   our   face   on   this   bright   and   hap - py   morn - ing.
dry   hands
brush   hair

5. Release the brush/comb.

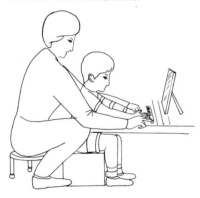

I release the hairbrush   1   2   3   4   5

Analysis of Motor Task	*Speech/Songs/Rhymes*	*Guidelines*
1. Look at the hairbrush/comb. 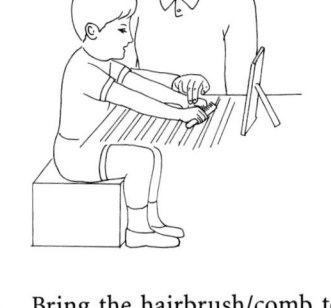	I look at the hairbrush 1 2 3 4 5	1. The child at this level may sit or stand to carry out this task. However, it is preferable if the child has the opportunity to stand as this improves his standing balance and prepares him for walking training (see Chapter 11, Task 19, Level 3). 2. The child may need some assistance to brush his hair and arrange it. However, do not over assist him. 3. Encourage the child to look in the mirror while brushing his hair. 4. Give him sufficient time to do the task and encourage him to use speech/song to guide his movements. The song should help the child begin to learn some body parts. 5. The child should begin to learn to take pride in looking neat.
2. Grasp the hairbrush/comb. 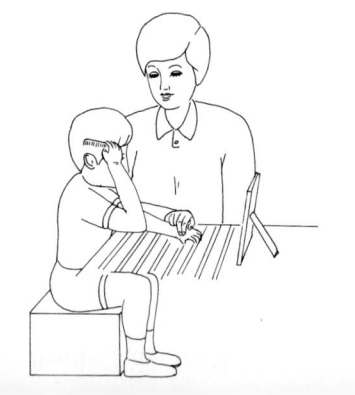	I grasp the hairbrush 1 2 3 4 5	
3. Bring the hairbrush/comb to the head.	Hairbrush to my head 1 2 3 4 5	

4. Brush/Comb the hair.

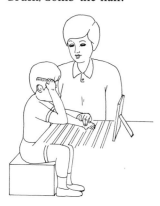

I brush my hair

Grooming Song

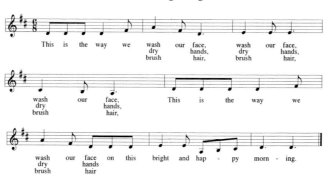

This is the way we wash our face,
dry hands,
brush hair,

wash our face,
dry hands,
brush hair,

wash our face,
dry hands,
brush hair,

This is the way we

wash our face on this bright and hap - py morn - ing.
dry hands
brush hair

5. Release the brush/comb.

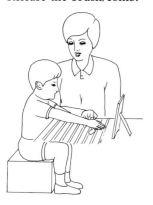

I release the brush   1 2 3 4 5

Analysis of Motor Task	Speech/Songs/Rhymes	Guidelines

1. Grasp the hairbrush/comb.

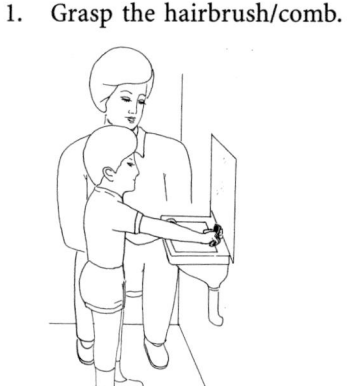

2. Brush/Comb the hair.

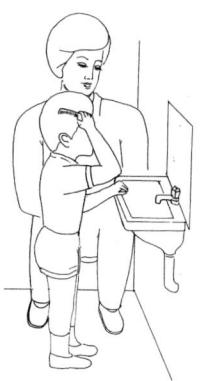

3. Return the hairbrush/comb to the ledge of the sink.

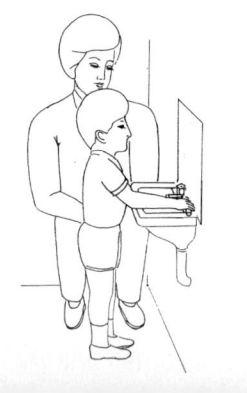

1. Make sure the child is standing well at the table/sink.

2. He uses inner speech.

3. The care-giver supervises the child, preferably with no manual assistance.

4. Encourage the child to look in the mirror and to take pride in looking neat.

Showering/Bathing

Task 17: Showering/Bathing
(Levels 1—5)

Showering/Bathing

DIFFERENT POSITIONS WHEN BATHING A CHILD WITH CEREBRAL PALSY (LEVELS 1 AND 2)

a. Use the same method as when bathing a new born baby. Hold the child around the shoulders.

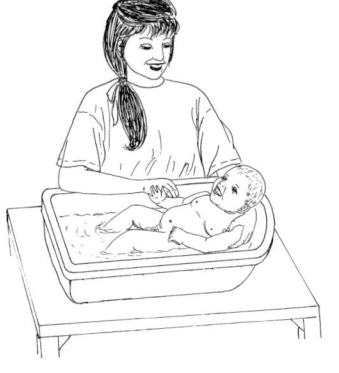

b. Lifting the child in/out of bathtub/basin.

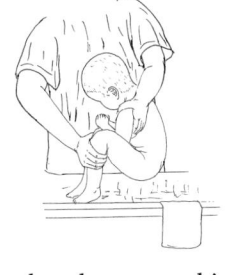

c. It is preferable if the care-giver kneels on a cushion at the bathtub when bathing the child to prevent strain on the back.

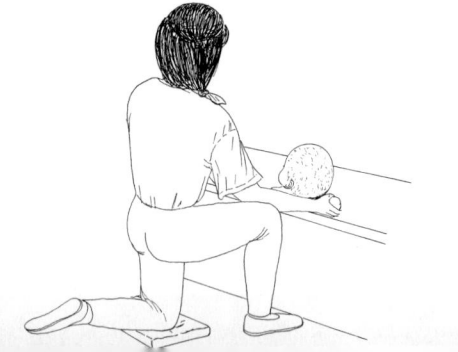

d. Other positions for bathing a child with cerebral palsy.

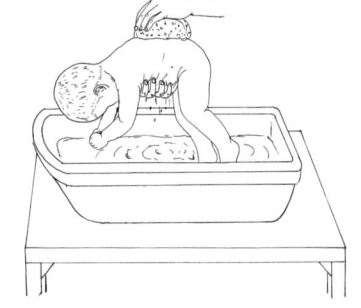

e. Keep the child's hips well bent when bathing.

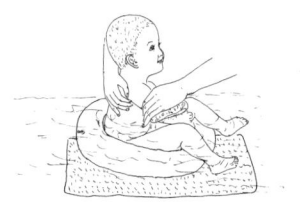

GUIDELINES

1. The care-giver prepares everything necessary beforehand. Never leave the child unattended during the task.

2. Children at Levels 1 and 2 are dependent on the care-giver to bathe them. If using a bath tub, use a nonslip bath mat to prevent the child slipping in the tub. Also prevent him from hitting his head against sharp edges of the water taps.

3. Check the water is at a suitable temperature before bathing. If the water is either too hot or too cold it can cause a child with spasticity to increase the muscle tone. This makes it more difficult to bathe him.

4. Depending on the child, there are various ways to position him. One common way is to place the child supine with the care-giver's forearm holding his shoulders to keep them forward and his head above the water. If possible, the child may grasp a fixed bar with both hands. If appropriate, use flexion mitts to help him maintain his grasp (see Appendix).

5. Use slow even movements while bathing the child to help him relax. Talk to the him and if appropriate, give him some time to play with the water.

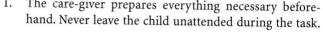

Analysis of Motor Task	*Speech/Songs/Rhymes*	*Guidelines*

1. Sitting task (see Chapter 10, Task 18, Level 3).

I sit well   1 2 3 4 5

1. The care-giver prepares everything necessary beforehand. Never leave the child unattended during the task.

2. The child sits on a low plastic stool/chair and grasps the hand rail for security. Make sure his feet are flat on a non-slip mat on the floor.

3. Check that the water is at a suitable temperature.

4. Avoid directing the water towards the child's face as this may upset him and cause him to become tense.

5. The care-giver showers and dries the child. The child learns to shift his body on the stool/chair as required during showering and drying.

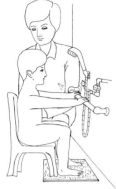

2. Grasp the hand rail with both hands.

I grasp the hand rail   1 2 3 4 5

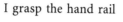

Analysis of Motor Task	*Speech/Songs/Rhymes*	*Guidelines*

1. Sitting task (see Chapter 10, Task 18, Level 4).

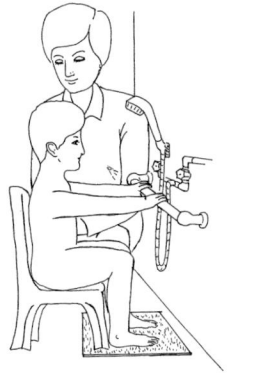

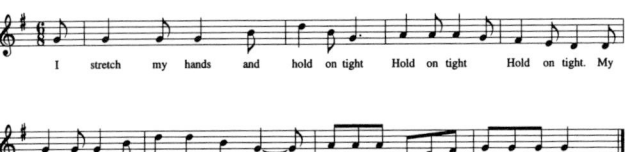

I Stretch my Hands and Hold on Tight

I stretch my hands and hold on tight Hold on tight Hold on tight. My

feet are flat, my bot-tom's pushed back look in the mid-dle I'm sit-ting up-right.

1. The care-giver prepares everything necessary beforehand. Never leave the child unattended during the task.

2. Make sure the child is sitting well with his feet flat on a non-slip mat. The child should learn to maintain grasp of the rail with one hand while using the other hand to learn to shower himself.

3. He will need help to learn to test and adjust the temperature of the water.

4. The child will also need assistance to rub in the soap, shower and dry.

5. Make sure he grasps the hand rail with both hands when he has to stand up to prevent him from slipping.

2. Grasp the shower head with one hand.

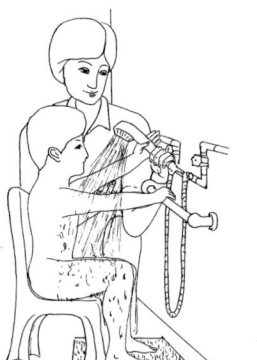

I grasp the shower head   1 2 3 4 5

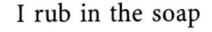

3. Grasp the soap and rub in.

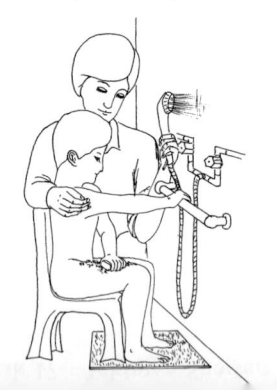

I rub in the soap

4. Grasp the shower head and shower.

I grasp the shower head

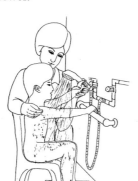

| *Analysis of Motor Task* | *Speech/Songs/Rhymes* | *Guidelines* |

1. Adjust the water temperature and test it.

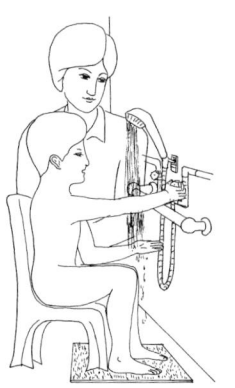

2. Shower the body.

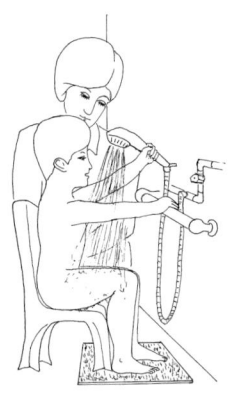

3. Grasp the soap and rub it in.

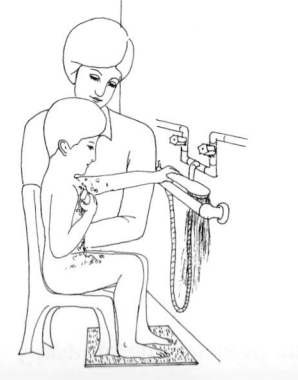

1. The care-giver prepares everything before-hand. Never leave the child unattended during the task.

2. He should be able to sit freely without grasping the hand rails. Use a non-slip mat on the floor to prevent him from slipping.

3. He may still need help to adjust the temperature of the water and test it.

4. Encourage him to name his body parts as he is showering and drying.

4. Wash the body.

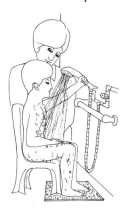

5. Turn off the tap.

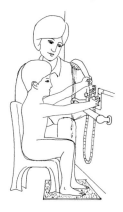

6. Grasp the towel and dry the body.

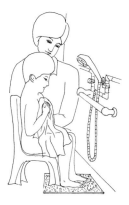

Chapter 10

Sitting

TASK 18: SITTING ON A STOOL/CHAIR
(LEVELS 1—4)

Analysis of Motor Task	*Speech/Songs/Rhymes*	*Guidelines*

1. Grasp the plinth.

I grasp plinth   grasp grasp grasp

1. It is important from the outset the child learns to sit well. He will need this position for many activities of daily living, eg., playing, eating, drinking, grooming, transferring from one position to another, attending class, etc.

2. At this level, the child may need a chair with sides and back support (see Appendix). The chair/stool should be of a suitable height whereby the child can place his feet firmly on the floor. The height of the plinth (see Appendix) should lend the child support for his trunk if needed and should also be suitable for play/meals etc.

2. Feet flat.

My feet flat   flat flat flat

3. The child may need gaiters (Appendix) to stretch his elbows and for stability. He may also need ankle straps and thigh straps (see Appendix) to help him stabilise his feet and thighs, part his knees and give him a good sitting base. The straps will also prevent him pushing himself off the chair at the beginning when he is learning to sit.

4. If he cannot grasp the slats of the plinth use a horizontal handbar (see Appendix) which may be easier for him to learn to grasp. He may also need flexion mitts (see Appendix) to maintain his grasp of the handbar/plinth.

5. The care-giver helps the child with every step. She says every step out loud and if possible encourages him to speak.

3. Feet apart.

My feet apart   apart apart apart

4. Push the bottom back.

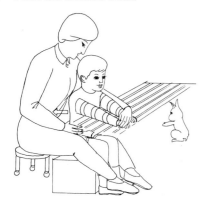

My bottom back   push push push

6. Encourage the child to look at the care-giver's face/toy to help him sit up straight. If the child is learning to sit on a stool, he may still need ankle and thigh straps for fixation.

7. The child should not be allowed to sit in the same position for more than twenty to thirty minutes. Encourage him to shift his position e.g. teaching him to stand up (see Chapter 12, Task 21, Level 1).

5. Back straight.

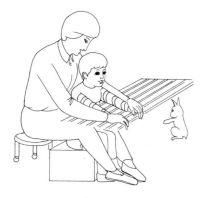

My back straight   straight straight straight

6. Sit straight.

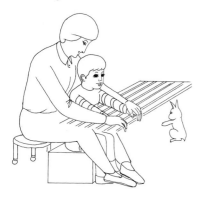

I Stretch my Hands and Hold on Tight

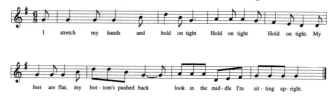

I stretch my hands and hold on tight Hold on tight Hold on tight. My

feet are flat, my bot-tom's pushed back look in the mid-dle I'm sit-ting up-right.

Analysis of Motor Task	*Speech/Songs/Rhymes*	*Guidelines*

1. Grasp the slats.

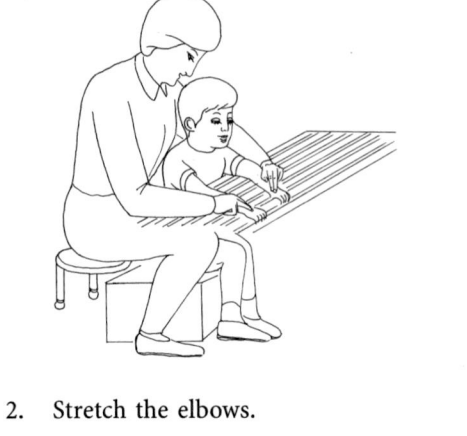

2. Stretch the elbows.

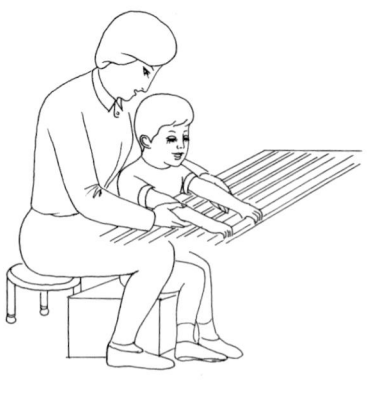

3. Feet flat.

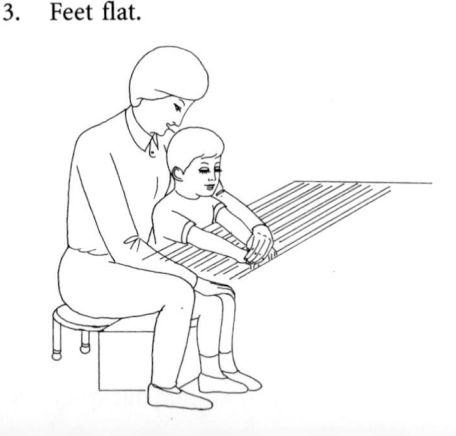

I grasp the slats   grasp grasp grasp

I stretch my elbows   stretch stretch stretch

My feet are flat   1   2

1. The stool/plinth should be of a suitable height to ensure the child has both feet flat on the floor and he can play/eat with comfort.

2. He may need gaiters on one or both arms to stretch his elbows and for stability.

3. He may still need ankle/thigh straps. However, remove the use of the straps as soon as he has learnt to stabilise himself in the sitting position.

4. Encourage the child who constantly pushes himself off the chair to push his bottom well back and try and learn to keep his feet apart and flat on the floor.

5. Always encourage the child to stretch his elbows to help him sit up straight and do not allow him to lean across the plinth.

6. The child may feel insecure when learning to sit on a stool; always remind him to maintain his grasp of the handbar/plinth.

7. The care-giver says every step out loud and encourages the child to speak.

8. Give him sufficient time to try and attempt each step.

4. Feet apart.

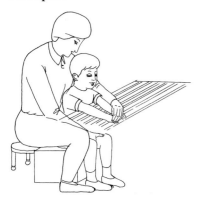

My feet are apart   1 2 3 4 5

9. Encourage him to sit well by asking him to look at the care-giver's face/toy.

10. Do not allow the child to sit in one position for more than twenty to thirty minutes. Give him the opportunity to transfer from one position to another.

5. Push the bottom back.

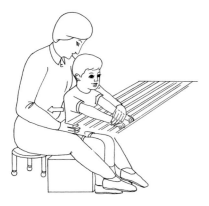

I push my bottom back   1 2 3 4 5

6. Sit straight.

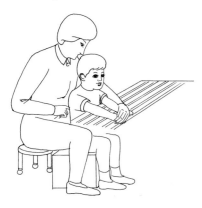

I Stretch my Hands and Hold on Tight

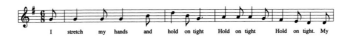

I stretch my hands and hold on tight Hold on tight Hold on tight. My

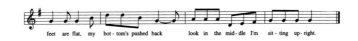

feet are flat, my bot-tom's pushed back look in the mid-dle I'm sit-ting up-right.

Analysis of Motor Task	*Speech/Songs/Rhymes*	*Guidelines*

1. Grasp the plinth.

I grasp the plinth   1   2   3   4   5

1. The child uses speech to guide his steps with minimal manual facilitation.

2. Always encourage the child to stretch his elbows to help him sit up straight, keep his feet well apart and flat on the floor and his bottom pushed well back.

3. Give the child sufficient time to do each step.

4. Do not allow the child to sit in one position for more than twenty to thirty minutes. Give him the opportunity to learn to transfer from one position to another.

2. Stretch the elbows.

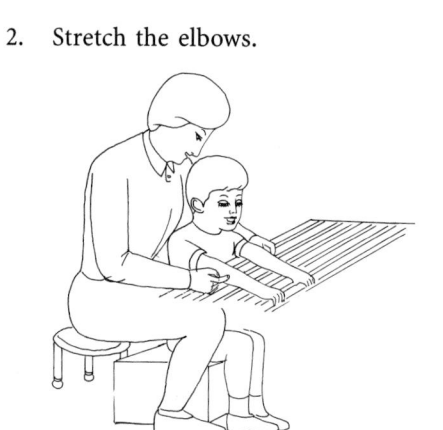

I stretch my elbows   1   2   3   4   5

3. Feet flat.

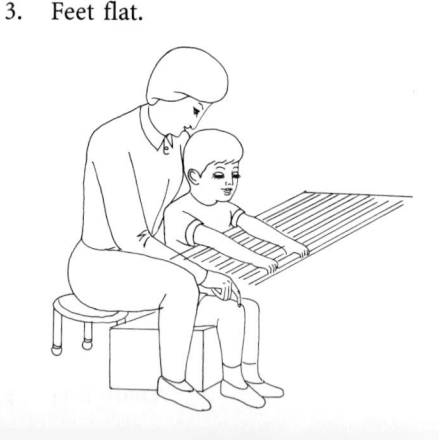

My feet are flat   1   2

4. Feet apart.

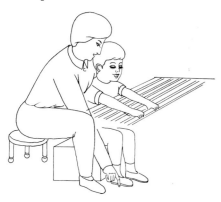

My feet are apart   1   2   3   4   5

5. Push the bottom back.

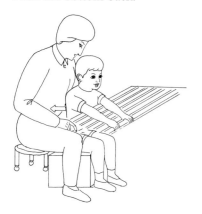

I push my bottom back   1   2   3   4   5

6. Sit straight.

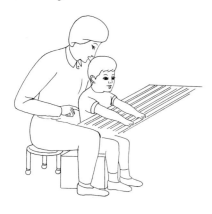

I Stretch my Hands and Hold on Tight

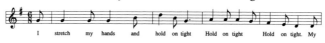

I   stretch   my   hands   and   hold   on   tight   Hold   on   tight   Hold   on   tight.   My

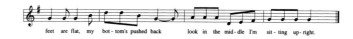

feet   are   flat,   my   bot - tom's   pushed   back   look   in   the   mid - dle   I'm   sit - ting   up - right.

Analysis of Motor Task	*Speech/Songs/Rhymes*	*Guidelines*

1. Feet flat and apart.

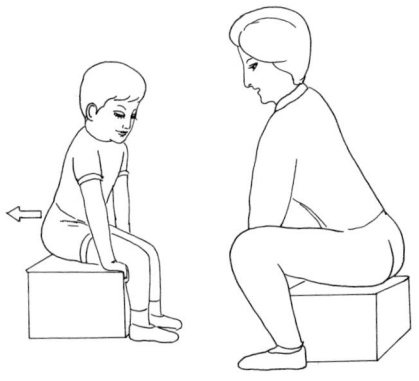

2. Push the bottom back.

3. Sit straight.

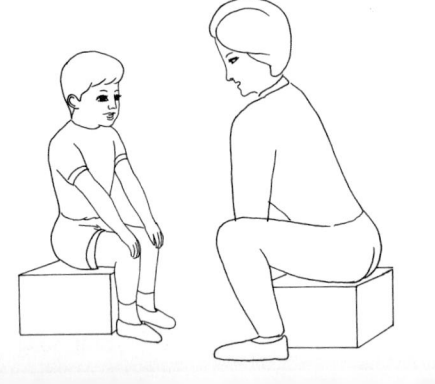

Sit up Straight

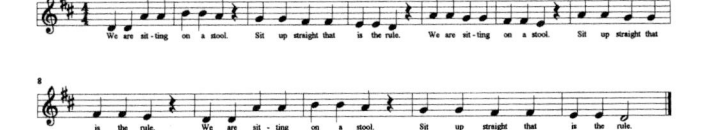

1. The child uses inner speech.

2. The care-giver supervises the child, preferably with no manual facilitation.

3. Give the child sufficient time to do each step.

4. The child can use this position for play, attending class or transferring from one position to another etc.

5. Do not allow the child to sit in one position for more than twenty to thirty minutes.

Chapter 11

Standing and Walking

TASK 19: STANDING
(LEVELS 1—4)

TASK 20: WALKING
(LEVELS 1—4)

Analysis of Motor Task	*Speech/Songs/Rhymes*	*Guidelines*
1. Grasp the ladderback chair.	I grasp chair grasp grasp grasp	1. Some children may be unable to stand without assistance. We should give them every opportunity to learn to stand, especially children over 12 months, as early standing is essential for development of the hip joints. However, children who stand on tip toes with the legs crossed, the hips, knees and elbows bent are not standing. Likewise, children who excessively pull backwards or whose knees excessively extend backwards are not standing. Such children are using an incorrect motor pattern. If these positions are encouraged and used regularly, they will eventually lead to contractures and deformity.
2. Feet flat.	Feet flat flat flat flat	2. Standing prepares the child for many activities of daily living. It gives the child important sensory feedback. It stimulates the respiratory, cardiovascular, digestive and excretory systems of the body. It improves weight bearing and is a preparation for walking training. Grasping the ladderback chair in front in the standing position helps the child with asymmetrical tonic neck reflex (ATNR) learn to bring the head into the midline. It helps prevent deformity at the trunk, hips, knees and ankles.
		3. If the child cannot weight bear through his legs, he will need long leg gaiters (see Appendix).
3. Feet apart.	Feet apart apart apart apart	4. Two care-givers assist the child. One care-giver supports the child from behind while the other helps the child grasp the rung of the ladder back chair (see Appendix) in front. Depending on the child, the care-giver may have to support him at the shoulders or upper arms. If the child cannot grasp the rung of the chair, use a flexion mitt (see Appendix) to help him sustain grasp of the rung. Make sure the child's weight falls through his body and not behind his feet. Pushing the chair a little forward will ensure this.

4. Knees straight.

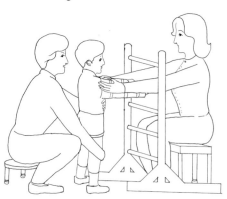

My knees straight   straight straight straight

5. If the child's head control is poor, encourage him to learn to lift his head by dangling a brightly coloured toy in front or by singing. Usually at this level, the care-giver's face is the best stimulation.

6. The child will need maximum assistance and the care-givers help the child do each step.

5. Look at the care-giver/toy.

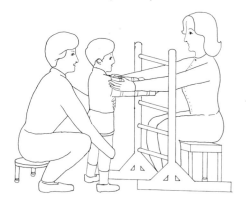

I look at toy   look look look

6. Stand straight.

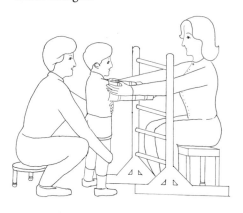

Look at me

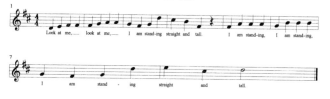

Look at me,____ look at me,____ I am stand-ing straight and tall. I am stand-ing, I am stand-ing,

I am stand - ing straight and tall.

Analysis of Motor Task	*Speech/Songs/Rhymes*	*Guidelines*
1. Grasp the rung.	I grasp the rung grasp grasp grasp	1. The child may still need gaiters to extend his elbows and for stability.

2. He should be able to weight bear and also to grasp the rung of the chair.

3. The care-giver makes sure the child's feet are flat and apart, his knees and back are straight and his head in the midline.

4. If the child pulls back, facilitate him by asking him to push the chair forward to help him bring his weight over his feet. However, do not allow him lean too far forward as this may cause him to collapse in flexion.

2. Feet flat.

My feet are flat   1 2

5. The child who cannot keep his feet flat on the floor and is constantly moving will need the care-giver to fixate his feet by pressing down on his feet gently but firmly with her foot.

6. Use toy/song to encourage the child to learn to lift his head.

7. Encourage the child to learn to release one hand and raise it up to answer to his name or to participate in a game. Repeat with the other hand.

3. Feet apart.

My feet are apart   apart apart apart

4. Knees straight.

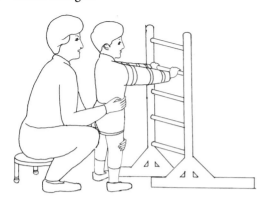

My knees are straight   straight straight straight

5. Look at the care-giver/toy and stand straight.

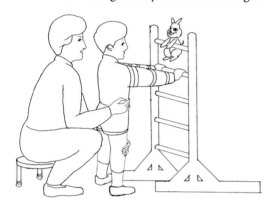

I look at the toy   look look look

Look at me

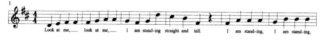

Look at me,   look at me,   I am stand-ing straight and tall.   I am stand-ing, I am stand-ing,

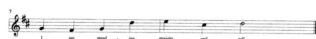

I   am   stand - ing   straight   and   tall.

Analysis of Motor Task	*Speech/Songs/Rhymes*	*Guidelines*

1. Stretch the elbows and grasp the chair.

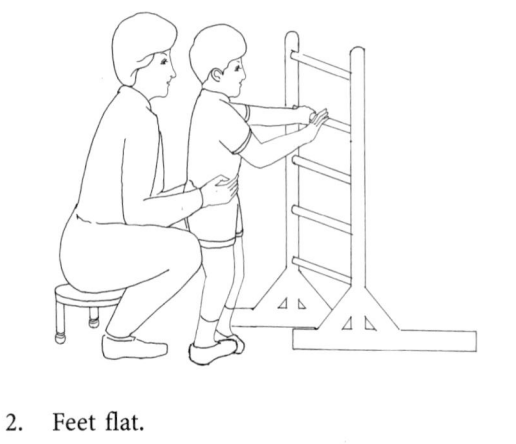

I stretch my elbows and grasp   1 2 3 4 5

1. The care-giver facilitates with speech and minimal manual facilitation.

2. Make sure the child's weight falls through his body and not behind his feet. Pushing the chair forward a little will help ensure this. However, do not allow the child to push too far forward as this may cause him to collapse in flexion.

3. Remind the child at all times to stretch his elbows to keep his back straight.

4. Encourage the child to keep his head in the midline, feet flat and apart, and knees and back straight.

5. If the child has difficulty keeping his feet flat on the floor, the care-giver encourages him with speech and minimal manual facilitation of her feet pressing down on his feet. However, remove help when the child can do it independently.

6. Give the child every opportunity to stand as to improve his standing balance and facilitate his walking training. He may stand for play, classroom activities, watching TV, singing, reciting, etc.

2. Feet flat.

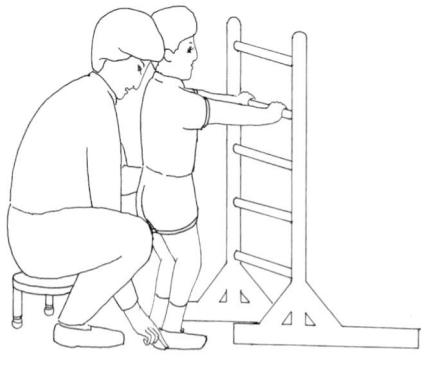
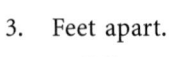

My feet are flat   1 2

3. Feet apart.

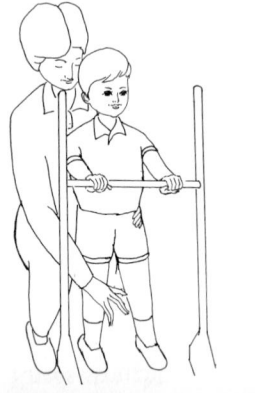

My feet are apart   1 2

Stand up Tall

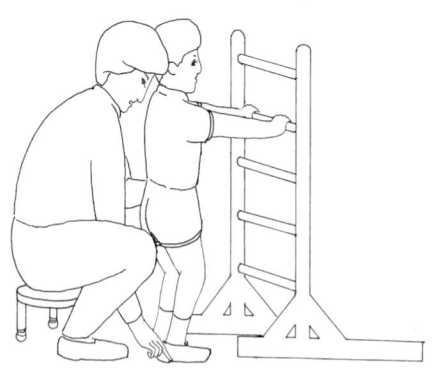

Look in the mir-ror What do you see? A ve-ry good stu-dent just li-ke me. Hands out strai-ght,

hands held high. Feet a-part and wave Bye-bye. Feet a-part and wave Bye-bye.

4.   Knees straight.

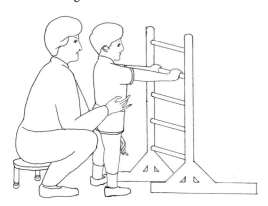

My knees straight   1 2 3 4 5

5.   Look at the toy.

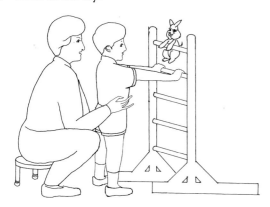

I look at the toy   look look look

Stand up Tall

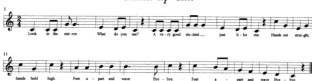

Look in the mir-ror What do you see? A ve-ry good stu-dent...... just li-ke me. Hands out strai-ght,

hands held high. Feet a-part and wave Bye-bye. Feet a-part and wave Bye-bye.

Analysis of Motor Task	*Speech/Songs/Rhymes*	*Guidelines*

1. Stretch the elbows and grasp the quoit.

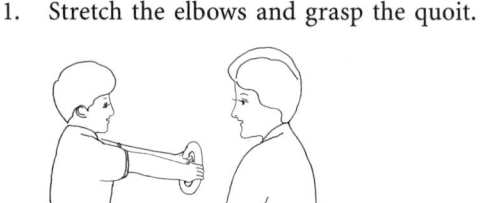

2. Feet flat and apart.

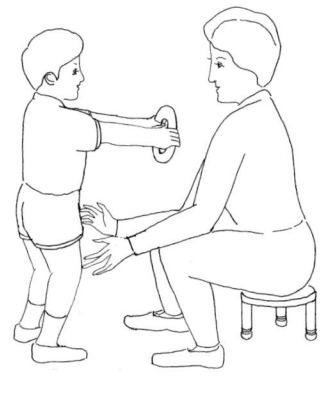

3. Knees straight.

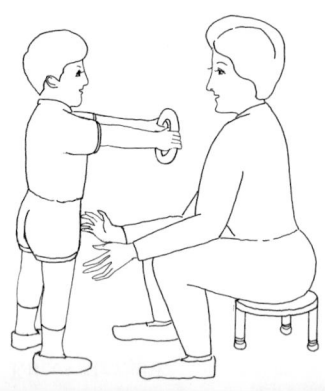

1. The child uses inner speech and preferably no manual assistance.

2. The child may grasp stick/quoit or clasp the hands for stability. Prior to using stick/quoit, the child may stand with his back against the wall/furniture for support. However, encourage him not to lean too heavily against the wall and gradually move away from using the wall/furniture as support.

3. When the child is standing grasping the stick/quoit, the care-giver should not support him but sit in front of him with her arms outstretched in a protective manner to give him security.

4. Remind the child to stand straight with head in the midline, feet flat and apart, and knees and back straight.

5. Give him every opportunity to stand to improve his standing balance and facilitate his walking training.

Stand up Tall

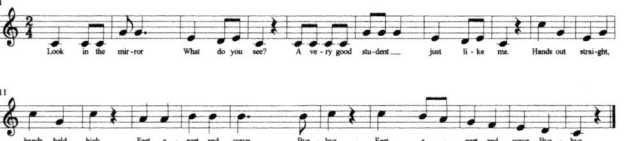

Look in the mir-ror What do you see? A ve-ry good stu-dent ____ just li-ke me. Hands out strai-ght,
hands held high. Feet a - part and wave Bye - bye. Feet a - part and wave Bye - bye.

Analysis of Motor Task	*Speech/Songs/Rhymes*	*Guidelines*

1. Standing task (see Task 19, Level 1).

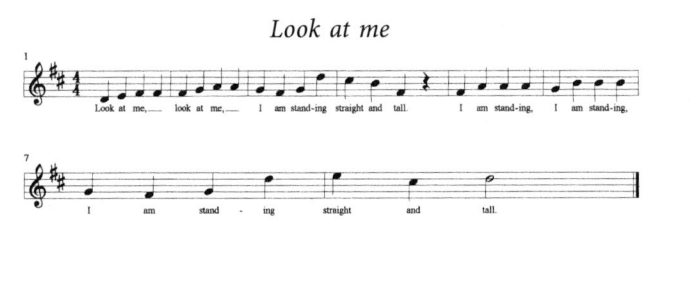

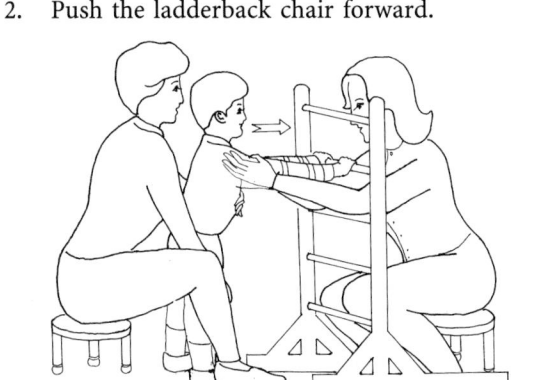

2. Push the ladderback chair forward.

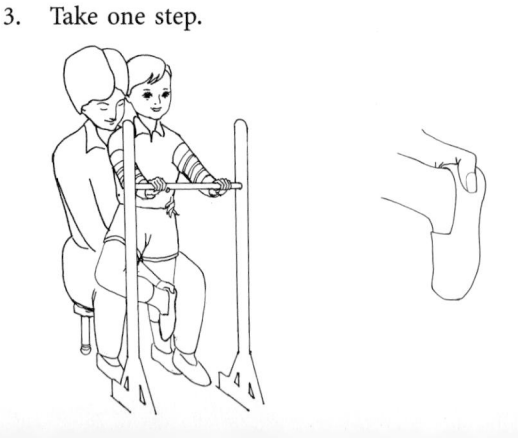

3. Take one step.

Look at me

Look at me,— look at me,— I am stand-ing straight and tall. I am stand-ing, I am stand-ing,

I am stand - ing straight and tall.

I push chair   push push push

I step one

1. Some children may be unable to walk without assistance. However, we should not deprive them of the opportunity to move from one point to another in the upright position. This gives the child important sensory feedback. It also stimulates the respiratory, cardiovascular, digestive and excretory systems of the body. At this level, it improves weight bearing. Grasping the ladderback chair in front helps the child with asymmetrical tonic neck reflex (ATNR) learn to bring the head into the midline.

2. Walking training at Level 1 involves maximum assistance from the care-givers. The child with poor or no weight bearing needs gaiters on both arms and legs for stability (see Appendix).

3. Two care-givers assist the child, one supports the child from behind sitting on a low stool, the other helps the child grasp the ladderback chair in front. Depending on the child, she may need to support him at the shoulders or upper arms. The child who constantly pushes himself backwards will need to be grasped firmly at the shoulders to help him maintain a good starting position.

4. Use flexion mitts to help the child who cannot grasp learn to sustain grasp of the rung of the chair (see Appendix).

5. The care-giver in front helps the child learn to push the chair. This ensures that the child's weight falls through his body and not behind his feet. However, before helping the child initiate a step, make sure his trunk is not pushed too far forward otherwise the balance of weight throughout the body is not distributed evenly.

6. Encourage the child to keep his head in the neutral position.

4. Foot on the floor.

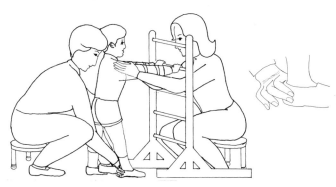

5. Take the second step. Repeat steps 3 and 4 with the other leg.

I step two

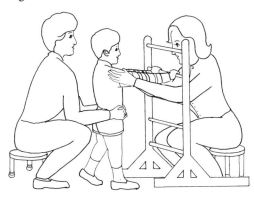

6. Stand straight.

I stand straight   straight   straight   straight

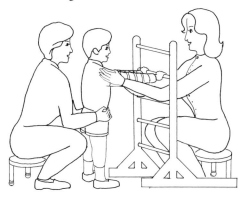

7. Repeat.

7. When helping the child learn to take a step while using long leg gaiters, the care-giver grasps the child's ankle and pushes the weight onto the other leg. She will not be able to lift the child's leg too high as the long leg gaiter will prevent this. Repeat with the other leg.

8. If the child does not need long leg gaiters, the care-giver can help the child initiate a step by grasping the child's ankle. She moves the leg slightly backwards to extend the hip, then flexes the knee while moving the heel of the foot upward towards the knee of the opposite leg. Make sure the knee of the moving leg is turning outwards. Return the foot to the floor taking care the heel is flat on the floor. Repeat with the other leg. Use this movement for the child with crossed legs (scissors gait).

9. Encourage the child to learn to initiate a step by putting a hand in front of the child's hip and pressing gently but firmly to stimulate the child to lift his leg off the floor. Help the child put his foot down with the heel flat on the floor and feet apart.

10. When a child is beginning his training in walking, twenty to thirty steps is sufficient at any one time.

11. From the outset, the child should learn to walk towards a goal, e.g., play, meals, toilet, etc.

12. When facilitating children from behind during walking training, it is preferable if the care-giver sits on a low stool, otherwise standing behind the child will encourage him to pull backwards into extension.

Analysis of Motor Task	*Speech/Songs/Rhymes*	*Guidelines*
1. Standing task (see Task 19, Level 2). 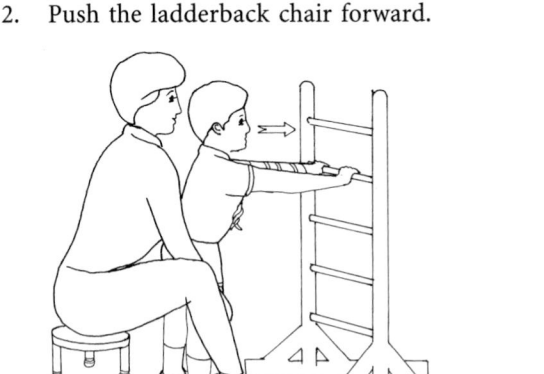	*Look at me* 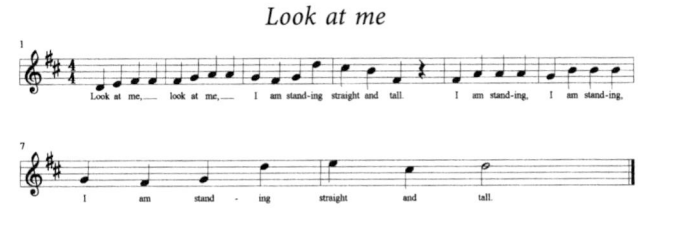 Look at me,___ look at me,___ I am stand-ing straight and tall. I am stand-ing, I am stand-ing, I am stand - ing straight and tall.	1. The child should be able to bear weight. 2. He may still need gaiters on one or both arms to stretch his elbows and for stability. 3. The care-giver sits on a low stool and helps the child from behind. She encourages the child initiate a step and at the same time helps keep straight the knee of the leg which is taking weight. See Level 1 on learning to take steps (see Task 20, Level 1). 4. If the resistance level of the ladderback chair is too low, the child will push it too far forward and as a result may collapse in flexion. Correct this by hanging a sandbag over the rung of the chair.
2. Push the ladderback chair forward.	I push the chair push push push	5. Always encourage the child to learn to stand straight, i.e., back/hips/knees straight, feet flat and apart. 6. If the child cannot keep his feet flat on the floor, the care-giver stabilises them by pressing gently but firmly down on the child's foot with her own foot. This gives the child the sensation of his feet making contact with the surface of the floor. 7. Always encourage the child to try and learn to push the ladderback chair. 8. The child should always walk towards a goal, e.g., play, meals, toilet, etc.
3. Take one step. 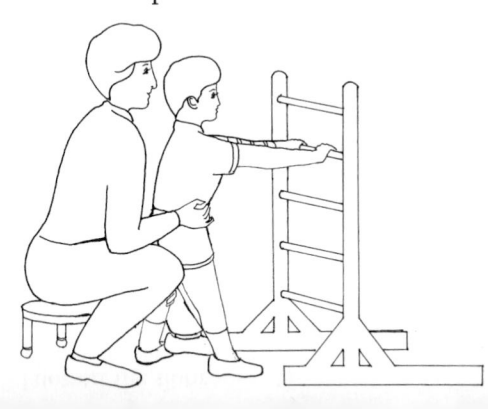	I step one step step step	

4. Take the second step.

I step two   step step step

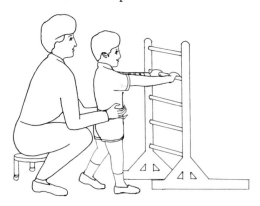

5. Stand straight.

I stand straight   straight straight straight

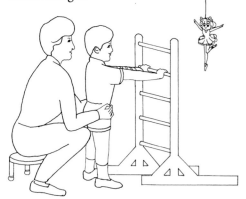

6. Repeat.

Analysis of Motor Task	*Speech/Songs/Rhymes*	*Guidelines*

1. Standing task (see Task 19, Level 3).

Stand up Tall

Look in the mir-ror What do you see? A ve-ry good stu-dent____ just li-ke me. Hands out strai-ght,

hands held high. Feet a-part and wave Bye - bye. Feet a - part and wave Bye - bye.

1. The child should be able to push the ladderback chair and take steps without assistance. However, make sure he maintains a correct posture and gait at all times.

2. The care-giver may still need to help the child keep his feet flat and apart, and his knees and back straight.

3. At each step, the child should be encouraged to release one hand and then the other and clap once in mid-air to prepare for walking without the aid of the ladderback chair. To encourage the child to release his hand, hang objects from the ceiling, e.g., a ball, and ask the child to hit it.

4. If possible, the care-giver may position herself in front with her arms outstretched in a protective manner in order to give security when the child is learning to release both hands.

5. The child should always have a goal when walking, e.g., play, meals, toilet, etc.

2. Push the chair.

I push the chair   push push push

3. Take one step.

I step one

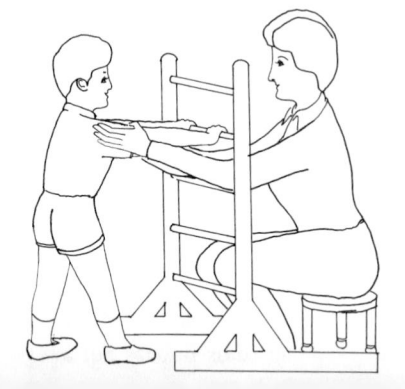

4. Take the second step.

I step two

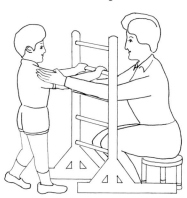

5. Stand straight and raise up one hand.

I raise one hand   1   2   3   4   5

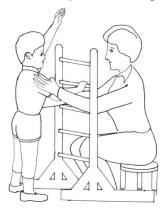

6. Repeat with the other hand.

I raise the other hand   1   2   3   4   5

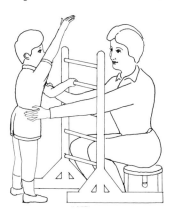

Analysis of Motor Task	*Speech/Songs/Rhymes*	*Guidelines*

1. Standing task (see Task 19, Level 4).

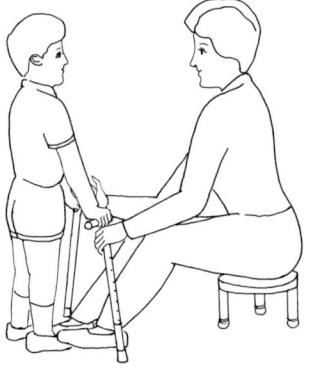

2. Put the right quadripod forward.

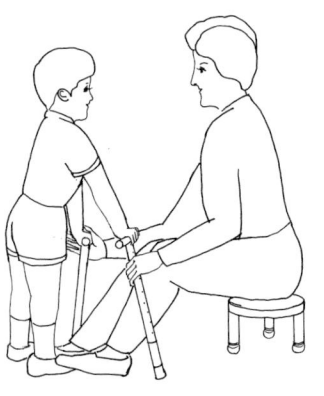

3. Put the left foot forward.

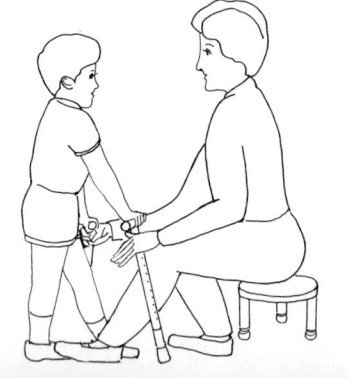

Stand up Tall

Look in the mir-ror What do you see? A ve-ry good stu-dent.... just li-ke me. Hands out strai-ght,

hands held high. Feet a-part and wave Bye-bye. Feet a-part and wave Bye-bye.

I put the right quadripod forward   1   2

I put my left foot forward   1   2

1. Some children may learn to walk independently. How-ever, many children have to use walking aids, e.g., ladderback chair, two walking sticks, quadripods, tripods, one tripod, one walking stick.

2. The care-giver sits on a low stool in front of the child and helps by guiding the child's hand which is grasping the quadripod/stick.

3. Make sure the child keeps his legs well parted and does not lean forward too heavily onto the aid. Insist on straight knees, straight back, feet flat on the floor and apart and the child takes the weight through his feet.

4. The care-giver may need to stabilise the child by fixating the weight bearing foot or the quadripods with her foot.

5. When the child's sense of security and balance improves, the child may use one quadripod/stick if possible.

6. The child's walking will deteriorate if he habitually walks too fast and is not reminded at all times to maintain a good walking gait.

4. Put the left quadripod forward.

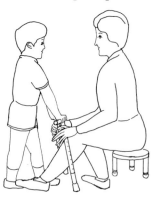

I put the left quadripod forward   1   2

5. Put the right foot forward.

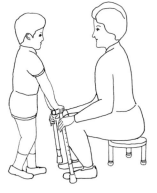

I put my right foot forward   1   2

6. Stand straight.

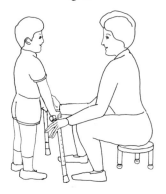

I stand straight   1   2   3   4   5

7. Repeat.

Analysis of Motor Task	*Speech/Songs/Rhymes*	*Guidelines*

1. Stretch the elbows and grasp the quoit.

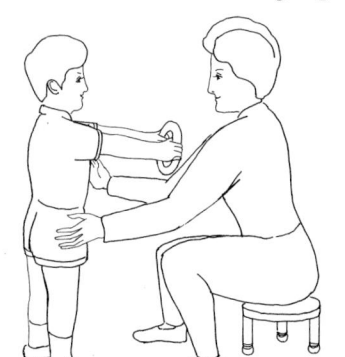

2. Take one step.

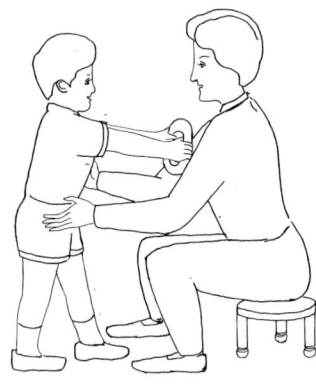

3. Take the second step.

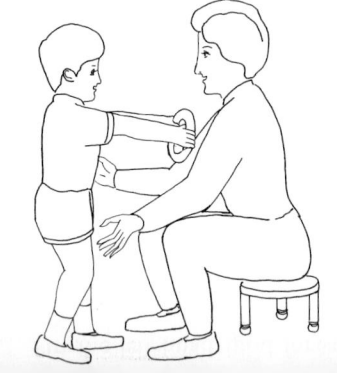

1. The child uses inner speech.

2. If the child feels insecure or unsteady, the care-giver may give him a little support at the shoulders.

3. Do not over assist the child and gradually reduce assistance as soon as he can do it independently.

4. The child may need the security of the care-giver in front with her arms outstretched in a protective manner to help him in case he stumbles and falls.

5. It is important to give the child sufficient time to do this task as independently as possible.

6. For children learning to improve their balance and as a preparation for independent walking, they should be encouraged at all times to cruise along the walls. This decreases their dependence on, e.g., hand rail/furniture for support.

4. Stand straight.

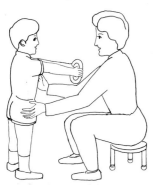

Transfers

Analysis of Motor Task	*Speech/Songs/Rhymes*	*Guidelines*

1. Put both hands at the edge of the plinth.

I grasp plinth   grasp   grasp   grasp

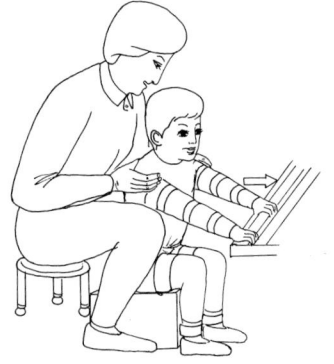

1. It is important to give the child as many opportunities as possible to learn to transfer from sitting to standing. The child should not be picked up but should learn to move from one position to another.

2. At this level the child will need gaiters to stretch his elbows and for stability.

3. If possible, two care-givers will need to help the child.

4. One care-giver helping the child from behind places the child's hands at the edge of the plinth and helps him push it forward. Before standing up the other care-giver helps the child from the front sustain his grasp of the plinth and stabilises his arms and shoulders.

2. Push the plinth forward.

I push   push   push   push

5. Encourage the child to look at his feet and make sure his body weight is well over the feet before he attempts to stand up.

6. The care-giver in front helps him sustain his grasp of the plinth as he stands up. Depending on the ability of the child, she may need to stabilise him at the shoulders or elbows.

7. The care-giver helping the child from behind will need to stabilise his lower limbs and help him maintain the upright position.

3. Look at the feet.

I look at feet   look   look   look

4. Untie the straps and lift up the bottom.

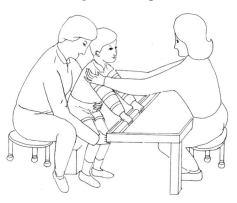

I lift bottom   up   up   up

8. When the child is in the standing position, help him stretch his knees, keep his feet flat and apart, his back straight and his head in the midline. Do not allow him pull backwards into extension.

9. If the child's feet are constantly moving and he cannot put them flat on the floor, the care-giver stabilises them by pressing down gently with her own feet. This will give the child the experience of his feet flat on the floor.

5. Stand up slowly.

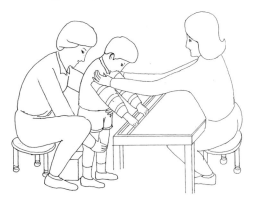

I stand up   up   up   up

6. Standing task (see Chapter 11, Task 19, Level 1).

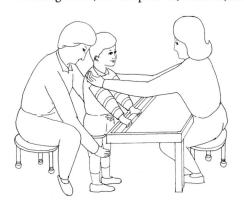

Look at me

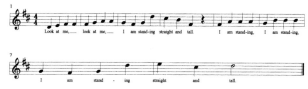

Look at me,____ look at me,____ I am stand-ing straight and tall. I am stand-ing, I am stand-ing,

I am stand - ing straight and tall.

Analysis of Motor Task	*Speech/Songs/Rhymes*	*Guidelines*

1. Put both hands at the edge of the plinth.

I grasp the plinth   grasp grasp grasp

1. It is important that the child has as many opportunities as possible to transfer from sitting to standing.

2. The child may still need gaiters to stretch his elbows and for stability.

3. The care-giver will need to help the child place both hands at the edge of the plinth and push it forward.

4. Make sure the child's body weight is well over his feet before he attempts to stand up.

5. Help him sustain his grasp of the plinth as he stands up.

6. If the child cannot initiate lifting up his bottom, the care-giver helps him by pressing down gently but firmly on his knees. However, remove assistance if the child actively initiates the movement.

2. Push the plinth forward.

I push the plinth   push push push

7. Make sure the child has both feet flat and apart, knees and back straight and head in the midline when standing. Do not allow him to pull backwards into extension.

8. The care-giver may still need to stabilise the child's feet with her own feet.

9. She says every step out loud and encourages him to speak.

3. Look at the feet.

I look at my feet   look look look

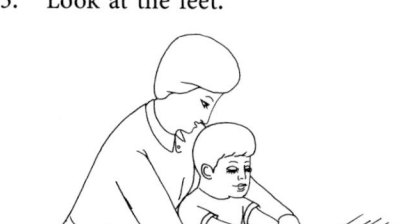

4. Lift up the bottom.

I lift up my bottom   1   2   3   4   5

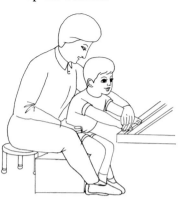

5. Stand up slowly.

I stand up slowly   1   2   3   4   5

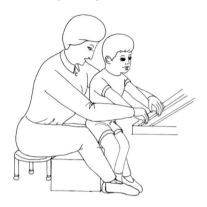

6. Standing task (see Chapter 11, Task 19, Level 2).

Look at me

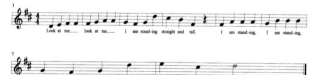

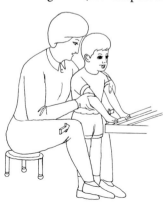

Analysis of Motor Task	*Speech/Songs/Rhymes*	*Guidelines*

1. Put both hands at the edge of the plinth.

I grasp the plinth   1 2 3 4 5

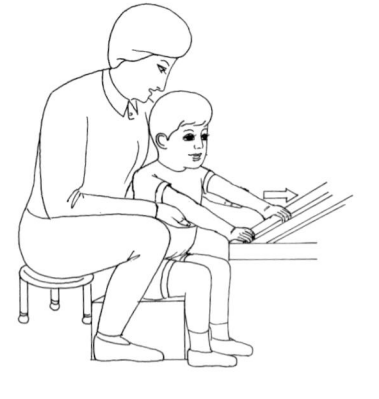

2. Push the plinth forward.

I push the plinth   push push push

3. Look at the feet.

I look at my feet   look look look

1. It is important the child has as many opportunities as possible to transfer from sitting to standing.

2. The child should be able to place both hands at the edge of the plinth and push.

3. Make sure the child's body weight is well over his feet before he attempts to stand up and sustains grasp of the plinth as he stands up.

4. Always carry out the standing task after the transfer.

5. Encourage the child to stretch his elbows in order to help him stand up straight.

6. Encourage him to try and keep his feet flat on the floor.

7. Give the child sufficient time to do each step and encourage him to use speech to guide his movements.

8. Use every opportunity to encourage the children to stand i.e. morning greeting, answering a question in the classroom, listening to a story etc.

4. Lift up the bottom.

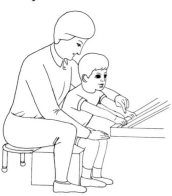

I lift up my bottom   1 2 3 4 5

5. Stand up slowly.

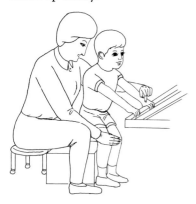

I stand up slowly   1 2 3 4 5

6. Standing task (Chapter 11, Task 19, Level 3).

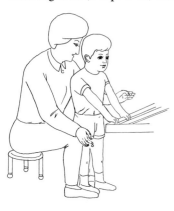

Stand up Tall

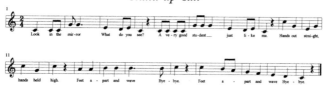

Analysis of Motor Task	*Speech/Songs/Rhymes*	*Guidelines*

1a. Stretch the elbows and grasp the stick or

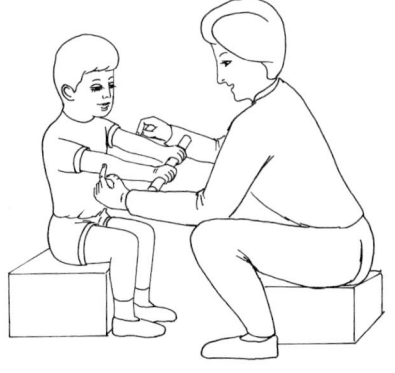

1b. stretch the elbows and clasp the hands.

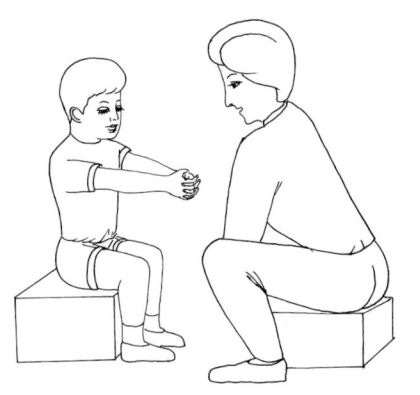

2. Look at the feet and lean forward.

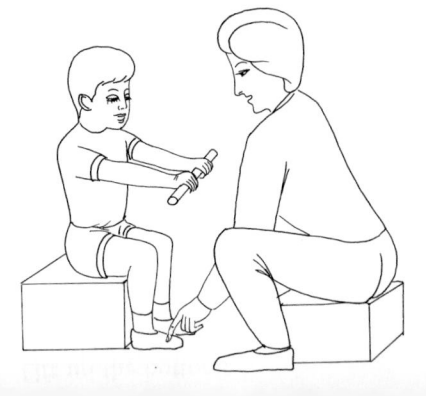

1. The child uses inner speech.

2. The care-giver supervises the child and preferably no manual assistance.

3. Always do the standing task when the child is standing.

4. Use every opportunity to encourage the child to stand.

3. Stand up slowly.

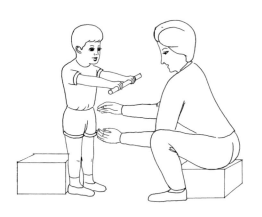

Stand up Tall

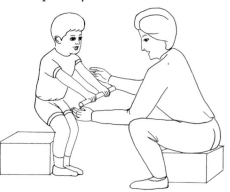

Look in the mir-ror What do you see? A ve-ry good stu-dent ___ just li-ke me. Hands out strai-ght,

hands held high. Feet a - part and wave Bye - bye. Feet a - part and wave Bye - bye.

Analysis of Motor Task	*Speech/Songs/Rhymes*	*Guidelines*
1. Grasp the plinth.	I grasp plinth grasp grasp grasp	1. It is important to give the child as many opportunities as possible to transfer from standing to sitting. The child should not be picked up and put sitting on a chair/stool but should learn to move from one position to another.
		2. If the child has gaiters on the lower limbs for weight bearing, remove them before the child prepares to sit down. However he may need gaiters on the hands to stretch the elbows and for stability.
		3. If possible two care-givers will need to help the child. One care-giver helps the child from behind learn to weight bear by keeping the knees and the back straight, the other care-giver stabilises the child from the front and helps him learn to grasp the slatted plinth.
2. Feet apart.	Feet apart apart apart apart	4. Make sure the child sustains grasp as he sits down.
		5. When sitting down many children cannot bend at the hips. The care-giver will need to help the child bend at the hips and sit down slowly. Do not allow the child to collapse when doing this movement.
		6. At this level some children may need a chair with back and side support. If the child consistently pushes out of the chair he will need ankle and thigh straps to stabilise him and give him the experience of maintaining a good sitting position on the chair (see Appendix). Make sure the child learns to push his bottom well back in the sitting position.
3. Feet flat.	Feet flat 1 2 1 2	7. Some children may be able sit on a stool but may need thigh and ankle straps for stabilisation (see Appendix). Place a toy in front of the child to encourage him to look at it and keep his head in midline.

4. Look at the feet.

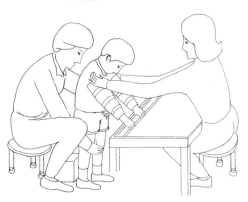

Look at feet   look   look   look

5. Bend the hips and knees.

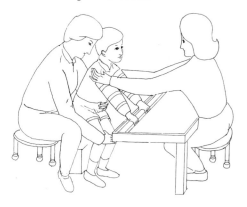

Bend knees   bend   bend   bend

6. Sit down slowly.

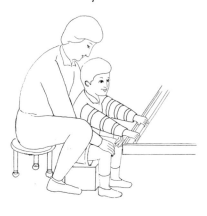

I sit down   down   down   down

I Stretch my Hands and Hold on Tight

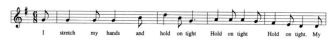

I stretch my hands and hold on tight Hold on tight Hold on tight. My

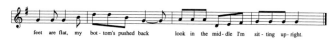

feet are flat, my bot-tom's pushed back look in the mid-dle I'm sit-ting up-right.

Analysis of Motor Task	*Speech/Songs/Rhymes*	*Guidelines*

1. Standing task (Chapter 11, Task 19, Level 2).

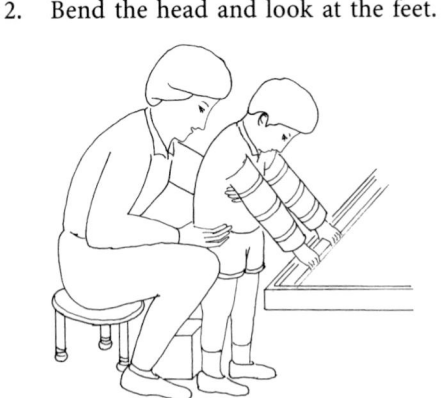

Look at me

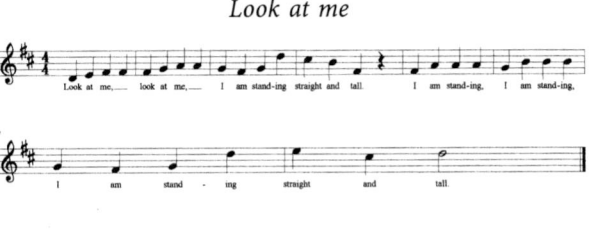

Look at me,—— look at me,—— I am stand-ing straight and tall. I am stand-ing, I am stand-ing,

I am stand - ing straight and tall.

1. The child should be able to weight bear with minimal assistance.

2. He may still need gaiters to stretch the elbows and for stability.

3. Make sure the child's feet are flat and apart and he grasps the plinth standing well forward.

4. Make sure the child sustains grasp of the plinth as he sits down.

5. He may still need help to bend his hips and avoid collapsing as he sits down.

6. He may still need ankle and thigh straps to maintain a good sitting posture.

7. Children who push themselves off the chair/stool will need to be constantly reminded to keep their bottom pushed well back, and feet flat and apart in order to learn to sit well.

8. Place a toy in front of the child to help him keep his head in midline.

2. Bend the head and look at the feet.

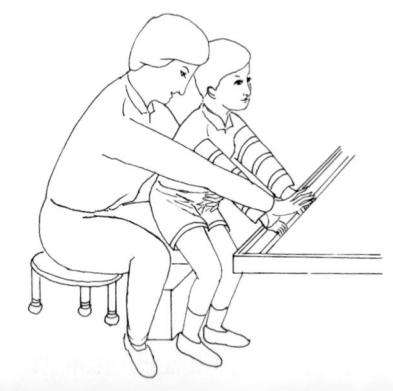

I look at my feet   look   look   look

3. Bend the hips and knees.

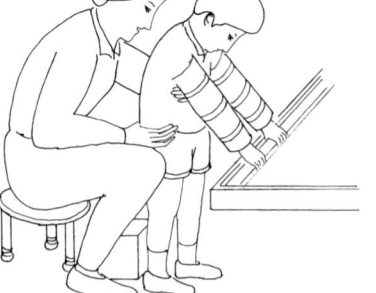

I bend my knees   1   2   3   4   5

4. Sit down slowly.

I sit down   1   2   3   4   5

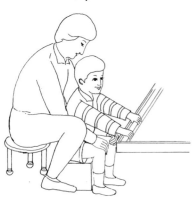

5. Sitting task (see Chapter 10, Task 18, Level 2).

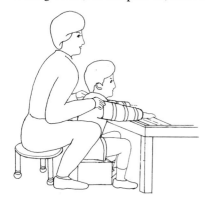

I Stretch my Hands and Hold on Tight

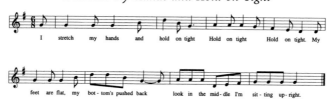

I stretch my hands and hold on tight Hold on tight Hold on tight. My

feet are flat, my bot-tom's pushed back look in the mid-dle I'm sit-ting up-right.

Analysis of Motor Task	*Speech/Songs/Rhymes*	*Guidelines*

1. Standing task (see Chapter 11, Task 19, Level 3).

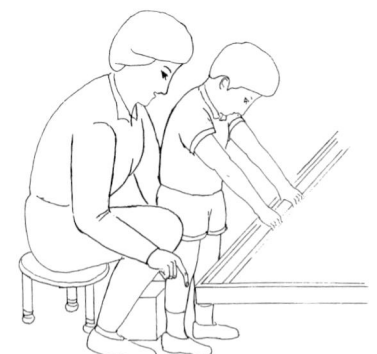

Stand up Tall

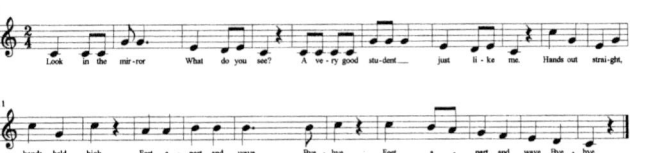

Look in the mir-ror What do you see? A ve-ry good stu-dent___ just li-ke me. Hands out strai-ght,

hands held high. Feet a - part and wave Bye - bye. Feet a - part and wave Bye - bye.

1. Use speech to facilitate the child and use minimal manual assistance.

2. Encourage the child to sit down slowly.

3. If the child's feet are constantly moving, he may still need ankle straps to stabilise them. However remove the straps as soon as the child learns to keep his feet flat on the floor (see Appendix). Make sure he pushes his bottom well back to help him maintain the sitting position.

4. Always encourage the child to stretch the elbows to help him sit up straight.

5. Give the child sufficient time to perform each step.

6. Remind the child at all times to sit well.

2. Look at the feet.

I look at my feet   look   look   look

3. Sit down. Sitting task (see Chapter 11, Task 18, Level 3).

I sit down   1   2   3   4   5

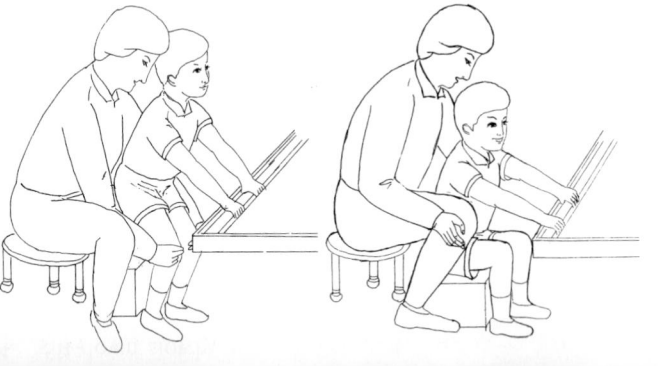

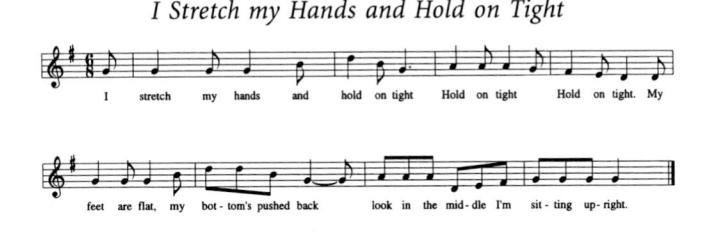

I Stretch my Hands and Hold on Tight

I   stretch   my   hands   and   hold on tight   Hold on tight   Hold on tight. My

feet   are flat,   my   bot-tom's pushed back   look in the mid-dle I'm   sit-ting up-right.

Analysis of Motor Task	*Speech/Songs/Rhymes*	*Guidelines*
1. Standing task (see Chapter 11, Task 19, Level 4).	*Stand up Tall*	1. The child uses inner speech.

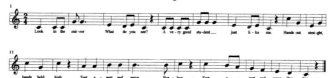

Look in the mir-ror What do you see? A ve-ry good stu-dent..... just li-ke me. Hands out strai-ght,

hands held high. Feet a-part and wave Bye-bye. Feet a-part and wave Bye-bye.

2. The care-giver supervises the child and preferably no manual assistance is given.

3. Insist on good standing and sitting at all times and make sure the child keeps his back straight.

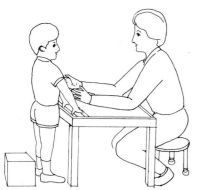

2. Sit down.

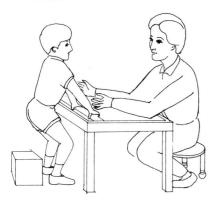

3. Sitting task (Chapter 10, Task 18, Level 4).

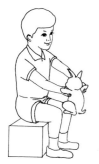

Analysis of Motor Task	*Speech/Songs/Rhymes*	*Guidelines*

1. Standing task (see Chapter 11, Task 19, Level 2).

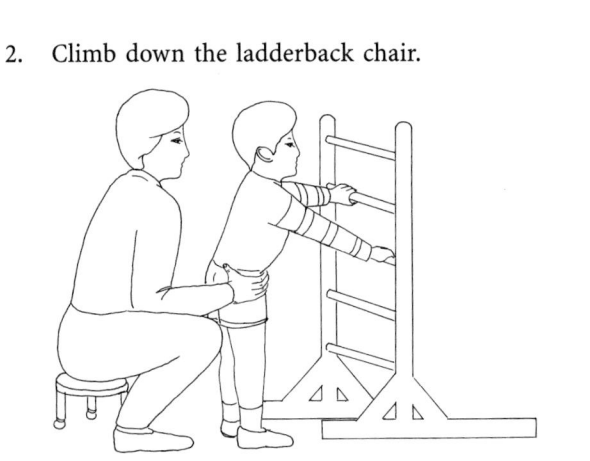

Look at me

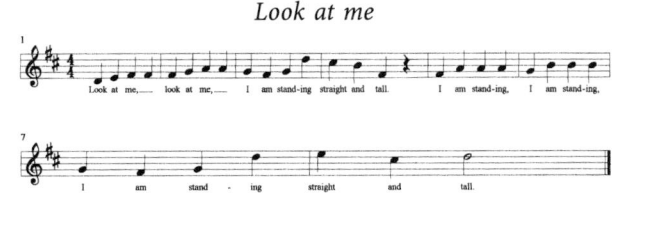

1. The child should be able to weight bear through the lower limbs.

2. He may need gaiters to stretch his elbows and for stability.

3. The care-giver may need to help the child to initiate bending the knees before kneeling down.

4. Make sure the child has his bottom tucked well in while he is learning to kneel up straight.

2. Climb down the ladderback chair.

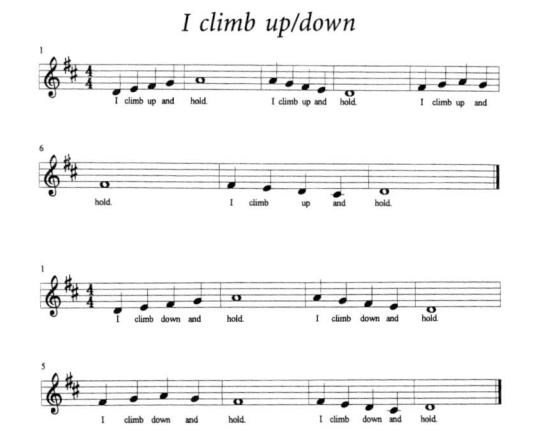

I climb up/down

3. Bend the right leg and kneel down.

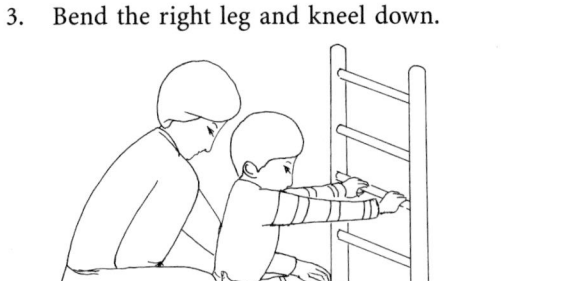

I bend the right leg   1   2   3   4   5

4. Bend the left leg and kneel down.

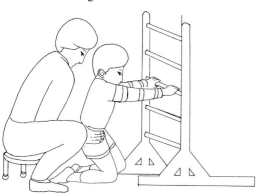

I bend the left leg   1   2   3   4   5

5. Kneel straight.

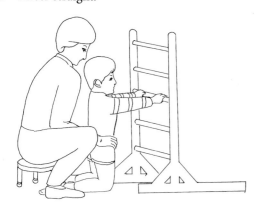

I kneel straight   straight   straight   straight

Analysis of Motor Task	*Speech/Songs/Rhymes*	*Guidelines*

1. Push the chair forward.

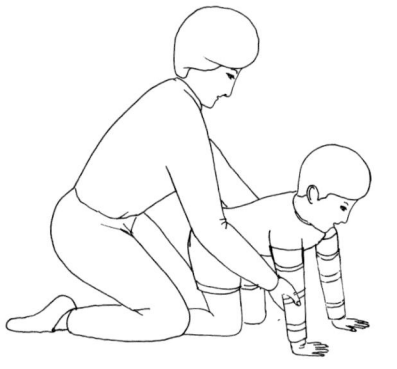

2. Put both hands flat on the floor.

3. Side sit to the left.

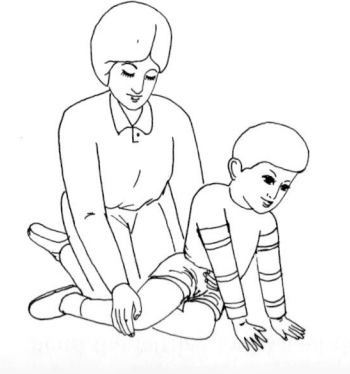

I push the chair   push   push   push

My hands are flat   1   2

I sit to the side   1   2   3   4   5

5. The care-giver will need to help the child get into the side sitting position.

6. Make sure the child learns from the beginning to push through the arms, lift up the bottom slightly and push back. Encourage the child to play with a toy placed between his legs to help him part his legs. This is essential in order to give the child a stable base from which he can maintain the long sitting position.

7. If his back is too rounded, he may sit on a low stool/ thick book (equivalent of a telephone book) or sit downhill on a wedge to help him learn to straighten his back.

8. This position is used to help the child learn to part his legs and stretch his knees, improve his trunk balance, put on/take off shoes, socks, for play, socialisation, cognitive learning e.g. rhymes and songs etc.

4. Put the right hand to the right side, put the left hand to the left side.

My hand to the side   1 2 3 4 5

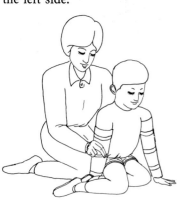

5. Both legs straight and apart.

I stretch my knees   stretch stretch stretch

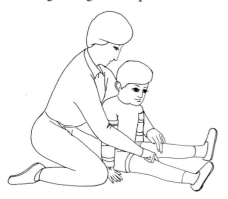

6. Push through the hands and push the bottom back.

I push back   push push push

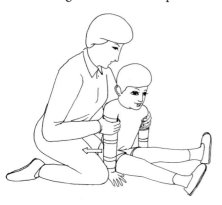

249

Analysis of Motor Task	*Speech/Songs/Rhymes*	*Guidelines*

1. Climb down the ladderback chair.

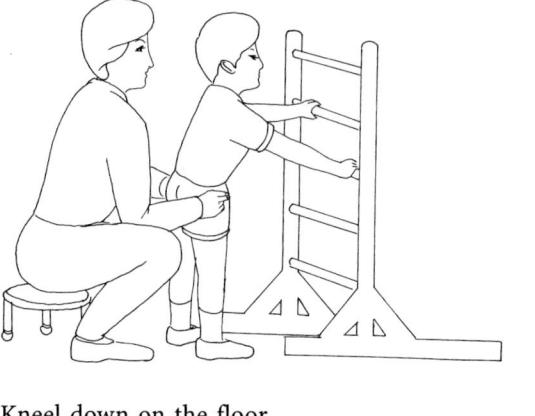

I climb up/down

1. The care-giver facilitates with speech and minimal manual assistance.

2. While kneeling, encourage the child to stretch his elbows and kneel up straight with his bottom tucked well in.

3. Make sure the child pushes through his arms, lifts up his bottom slightly and pushes back. Encourage him to part his legs by placing a toy between his legs for play.

4. If he still sits with a rounded back, a low stool/thick book (equivalent of a telephone book)/sit downhill on a wedge will help him learn to straighten his back.

5. Make sure the child stretches his elbows when sitting in this position as this will help him to sit up straight.

2. Kneel down on the floor.

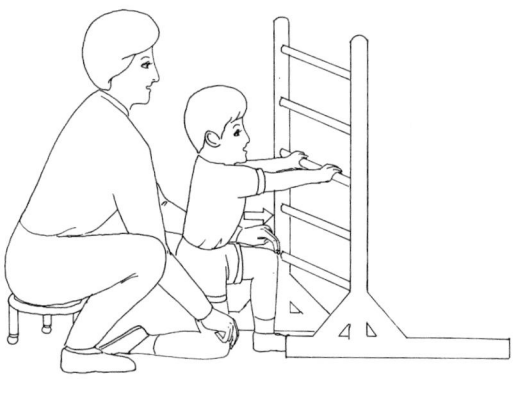

I kneel down   1   2   3   4   5

6. This position helps the child learn trunk balance and is also used to put on/take off shoes and socks, for socialisation, play, cognitive learning e.g. rhymes, songs etc.

7. In this position the child may cross the legs with the knees well apart in order to adopt the tailor-sitting position.

3. Kneel straight and push the chair forward.

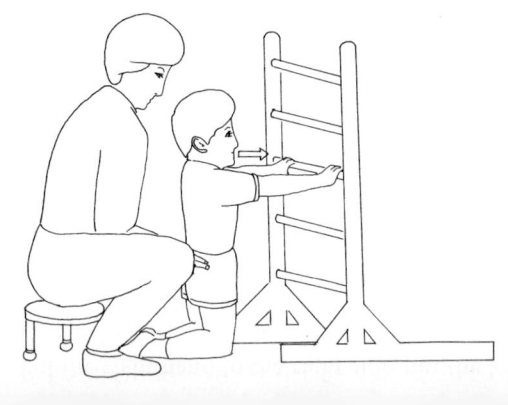

I push the chair   1   2   3   4   5

4. Put both hands flat on the floor (four-point kneeling).   My hands are flat   1   2

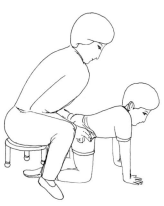

5. Side sit to the right.   I sit to the right   1   2   3   4   5

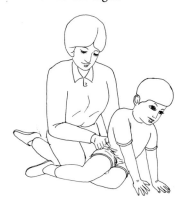

6. Put hands by each side and straighten the legs.   I stretch my knees   1   2   3   4   5

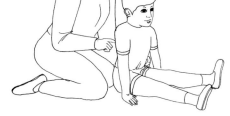

Analysis of Motor Task	*Speech/Songs/Rhymes*	*Guidelines*

1. Stand with clasped hands.

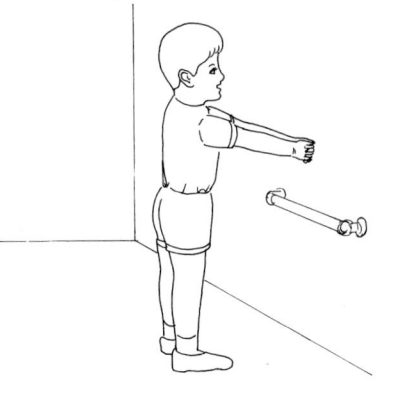

2. Grasp handrail and half kneel.

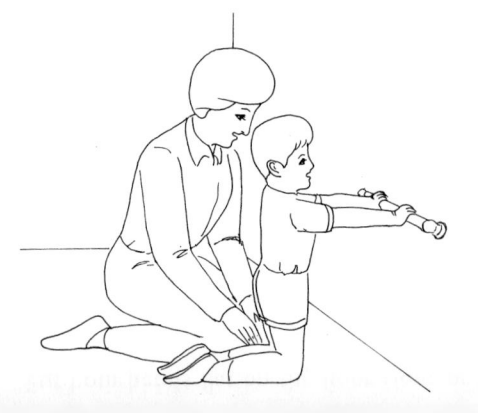

3. Kneel straight and release hands.

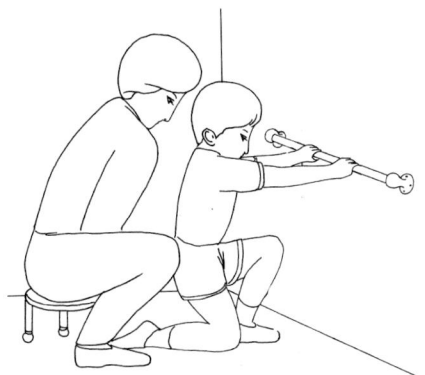

Stand up Tall

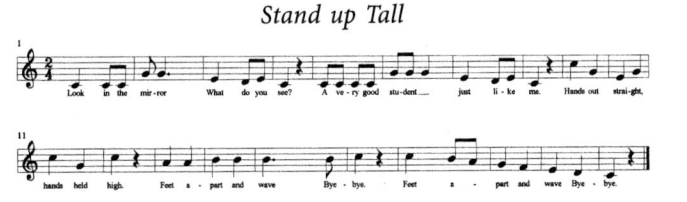

Look in the mir-ror What do you see? A ve-ry good stu-dent ...... just li-ke me. Hands out strai-ght,

hands held high. Feet a-part and wave Bye - bye. Feet a - part and wave Bye - bye.

1. The child uses inner speech.

2. The care-giver supervises the child and preferably no manual facilitation. However the child may need assistance when kneeling down.

3. Encourage the child to move and explore his immediate environment.

4. In this position the child may cross the legs with the knees well apart in order to adopt the tailor-sitting position.

4. Sit to one side.

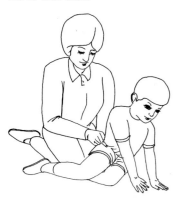

5. Bottom back and sit well.

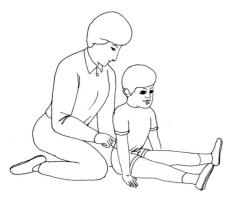

Analysis of Motor Task	*Speech/Songs/Rhymes*	*Guidelines*

1. Long sitting task (see Chapter 16, Task 18, Levels 2–4).

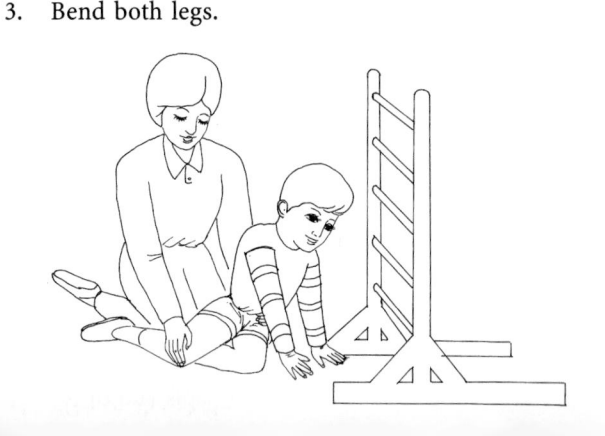

       1. The child should be able to weight bear through the lower limbs.

       2. He may still need gaiters to stretch his elbows and for stability.

       3. Place a toy at the side towards which the child is moving to encourage him to move in that direction.

       4. The care-giver may need to help the child to move into the side sitting position.

       5. The child may need help to sustain his grasp of the rung of the chair when he is transferring from the side sitting position into the kneeling position.

2. Put both hands to one side and press down on the mat.　　My hands to the side　　1　2　3　4　5

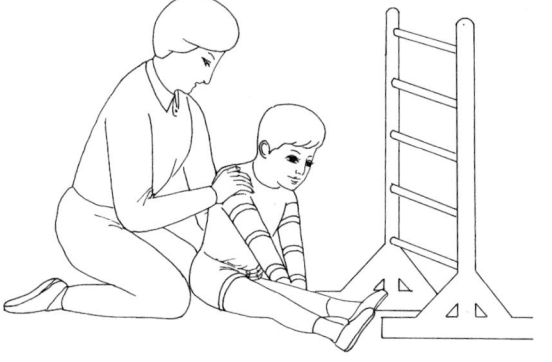

3. Bend both legs.　　I bend my legs　　1　2　3　4　5

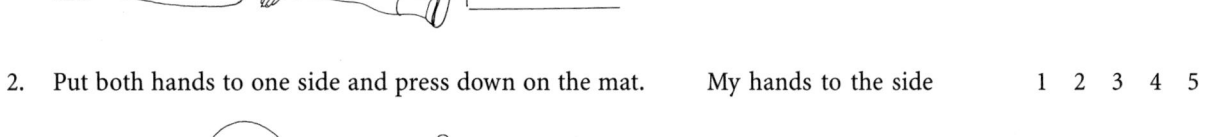

4. Grasp the chair.

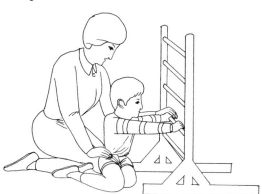

I grasp the chair   grasp   grasp   grasp

5. Kneel up.

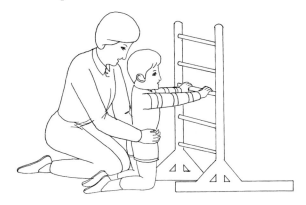

I kneel up   1   2   3   4   5

Analysis of Motor Task	*Speech/Songs/Rhymes*	*Guidelines*
1. Kneel up.	I kneel up 1 2 3 4 5	6. Make sure the child's body weight is well over his knees as he learns to stand up.

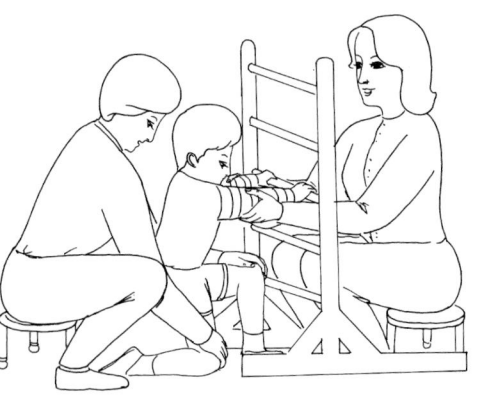

7. If he has difficulty initiating standing up, help him by pressing down gently but firmly on his knees and asking him to stand up slowly. Make sure he sustains grasp of the rung while doing this step.

8. Give him sufficient time to grasp and release as he climbs up the ladderback chair.

9. Help the child stand straight with feet flat and apart, knees and back straight and head in the midline. Do not allow him to pull backwards into extension when standing.

2. Place one foot flat in front to half kneeling position.   My foot flat   1 2

10. The care-giver says every step out loud and encourages the child to speak.

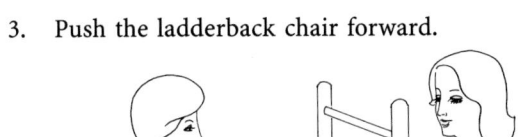

3. Push the ladderback chair forward.   I push the chair   1 2 3 4 5

4. Stand up.   I stand up   1 2 3 4 5

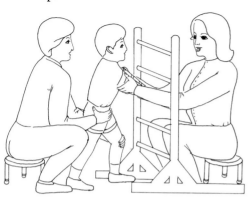

5. Use both hands to climb up the ladderback chair.

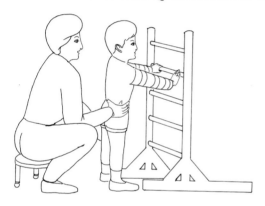

I climb up/down

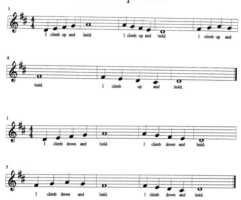

I climb up and hold. I climb up and hold. I climb up and hold. I climb up and hold.

6. Standing task (see Chapter 11, Task 19, Level 2).

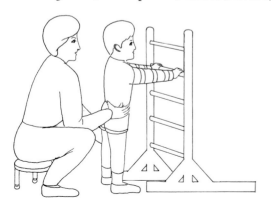

Look at me

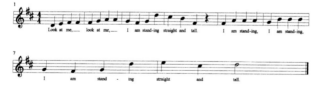

Look at me,___ look at me,___ I am stand-ing straight and tall. I am stand-ing, I am stand-ing, I am stand-ing straight and tall.

Analysis of Motor Task	Speech/Songs/Rhymes	Guidelines
1. Long sitting task (see Chapter 16, Task 18, Levels 2–4).	I sit well 1 2 3 4 5	1. The care-giver helps the child with speech and minimal manual assistance.

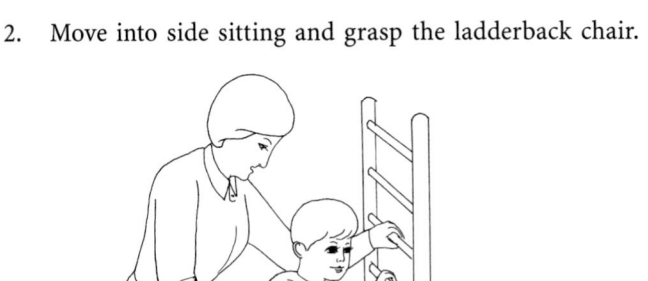

2. Make sure the child pushes the ladderback chair well forward his elbows are straight and his body weight is well over his feet before he attempts to stand up.

3. Do not allow the child to climb up the ladderback chair and then pull himself up.

4. Give him sufficient time to do the task and try not to help him too much. Encourage him to use speech to guide his movements.

5. Insist on good standing, making sure his elbows are straight, feet flat and apart, knees and back straight.

2. Move into side sitting and grasp the ladderback chair.   I grasp the rung   grasp   grasp   grasp

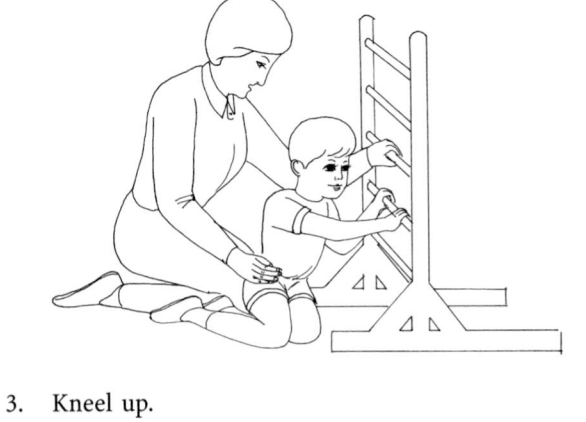

3. Kneel up.   I kneel up   1 2 3 4 5

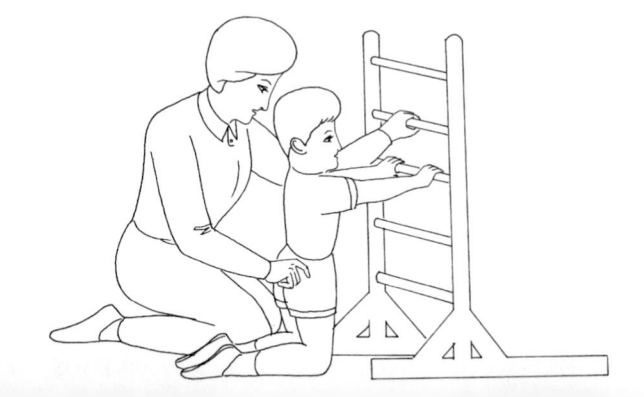

4. Put one foot flat to half kneeling position and stand up.　　　My foot is flat　　1 2 3 4 5

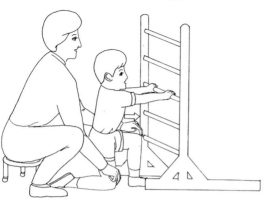

5. Use both hands to climb up the ladderback chair.

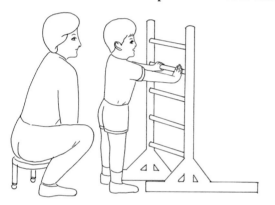

I climb up/down

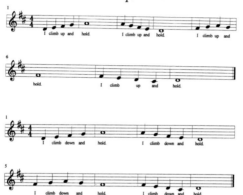

6. Standing task (see Chapter 11, Task 19, Level 3).

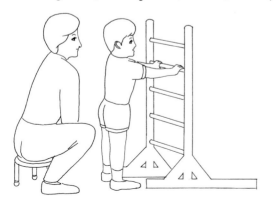

Stand up Tall

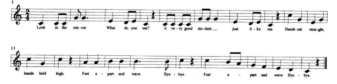

Analysis of Motor Task	*Speech/Songs/Rhymes*	*Guidelines*

1. Long sitting task (see Chapter 16, Task 18, Levels 2–4).

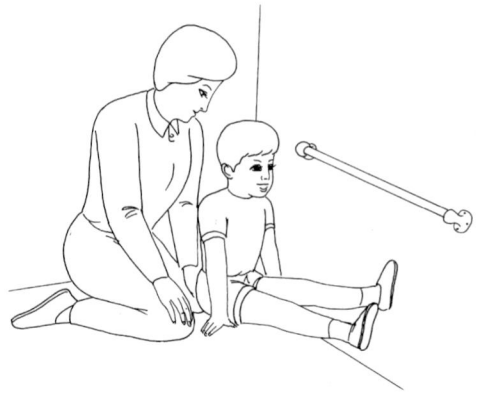

2. Move into the side sitting position.

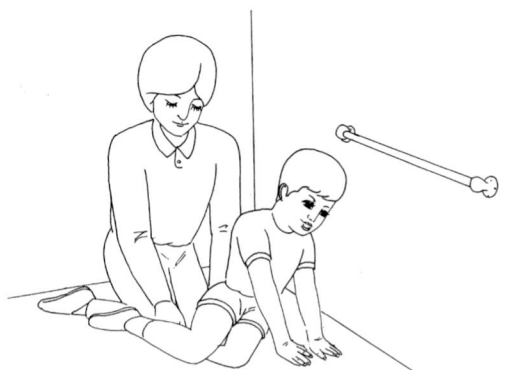

3. Kneel up.

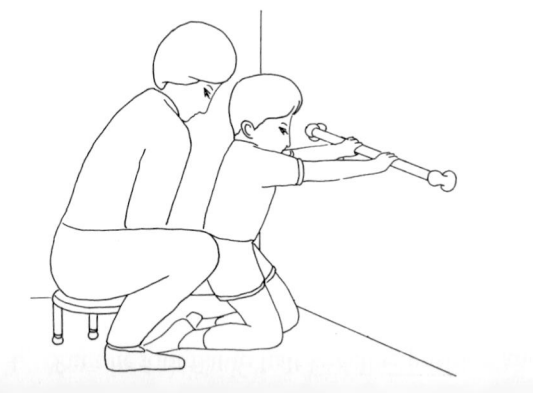

1. The child uses inner speech.

2. The care-giver supervises the child and preferably no manual facilitation.

3. Give the child sufficient time to do the task as independently as possible.

4. Move into the half kneeling position.

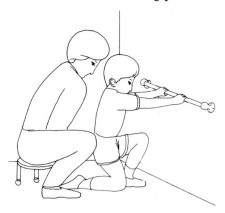

5. Stand up.

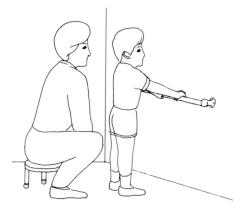

6. Release both hands and stand.

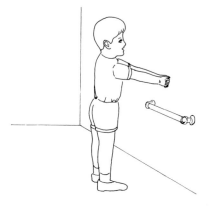

Chapter 13

Getting In and Out of Bed

TASK 25: GETTING ONTO THE BED
(LEVELS 1—4)

TASK 26: GETTING FROM THE BED TO THE FLOOR
(LEVELS 1—4)

Analysis of Motor Task	*Speech/Songs/Rhymes*	*Guidelines*

1. Stand at the bed with hands resting on the bed.

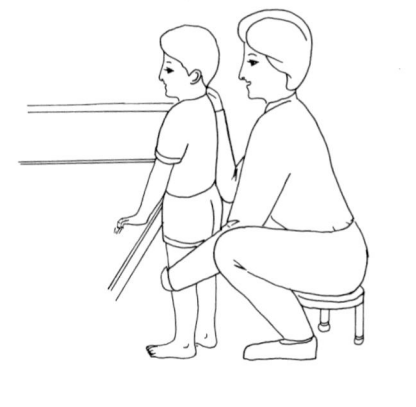

Look at me

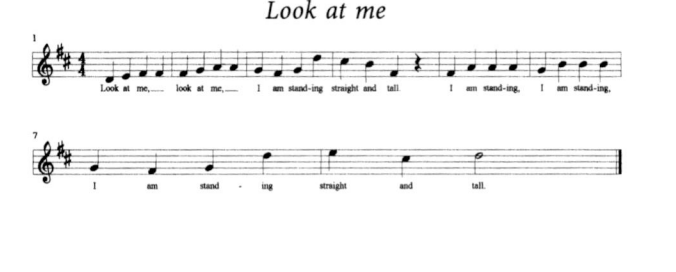

Look at me,____ look at me,____ I am stand-ing straight and tall. I am stand-ing, I am stand-ing,

I   am   stand - ing   straight   and   tall.

1. The child may still need gaiters to stretch his elbows and for stability.

2. The care-giver will have to help the child sustain grasp of the bed clothes when he is pulling onto the bed.

3. Place a toy on the bed to encourage him to lift up his head as he pulls onto and pivots on the bed.

4. Make sure the child learns to part his legs when pivoting.

5. The care-giver says every step out loud and encourages the child to speak.

2. Bend down and pull onto the bed.

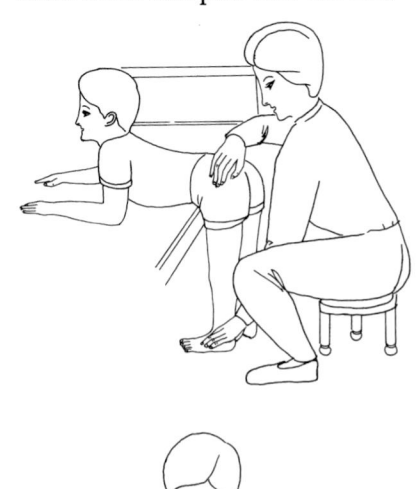

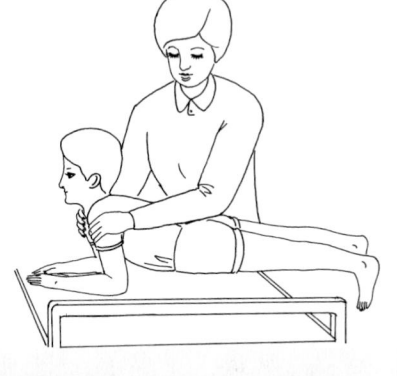

I pull onto bed   pull pull pull

3. Pivot (see Chapter 16, Task 22, Levels 2–4).

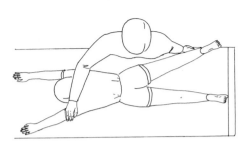

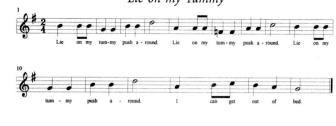

Lie on my Tummy

Lie on my tum-my push a - round. Lie on my tum-my push a - round. Lie on my tum - my push a - round. I can get out of bed.

4. Roll over.

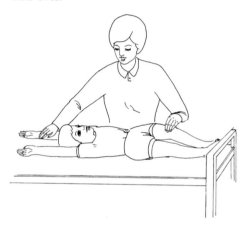

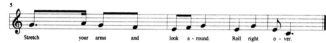

Stretch your Arms

Stretch your arms and look a - round, look a - round, look a - round. Stretch your arms and look a - round. Roll right o - ver.

5. Lie straight.

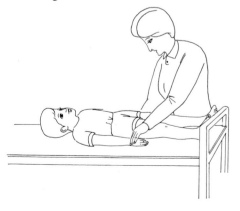

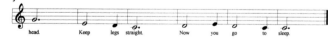

Go to Sleep

Rest your head. Both arms straight. You can go to sleep. Rest your head. Keep legs straight. Now you go to sleep.

Analysis of Motor Task	Speech/Songs/Rhymes	Guidelines
1. Stand at the bed with hands resting on the bed.	I grasp the bed 1 2 3 4 5	1. The care-giver may have to help the child pull onto the bed.

2. Encourage the child to lift up his head as he pulls on.

3. Make sure the child learns to part his legs when pivoting.

4. Give the child sufficient time to do the task and encourage him to use speech/song to guide his movements.

2. Bend down and pull onto the bed.

I pull on   1   2   3   4   5

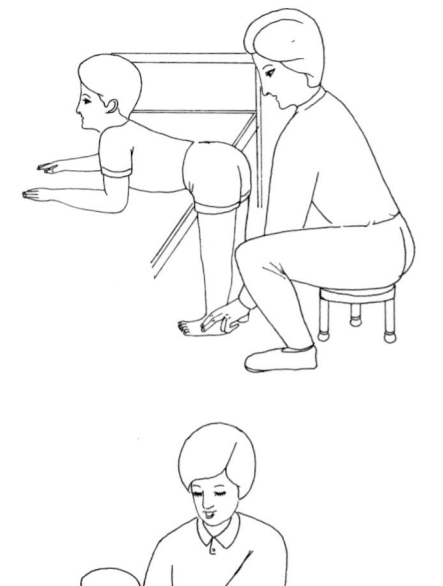

3. Pivot (see Chapter 16, Task 22, Levels 2–4).

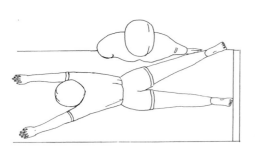

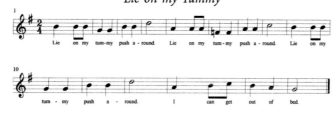

Lie on my Tummy

Lie on my tum-my push a-round. Lie on my tum-my push a-round. Lie on my tum-my push a-round. I can get out of bed.

4. Roll over.

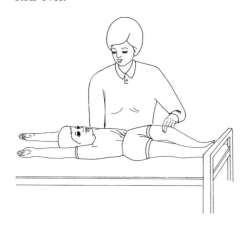

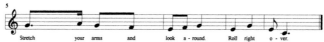

Stretch your Arms

Stretch your arms and look a-round, look a-round, look a-round. Stretch your arms and look a-round. Roll right o-ver.

5. Lie straight.

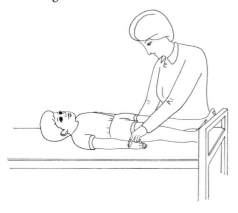

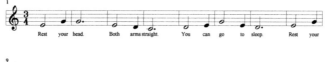

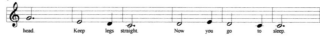

Go to Sleep

Rest your head. Both arms straight. You can go to sleep. Rest your head. Keep legs straight. Now you go to sleep.

267

Analysis of Motor Task	*Speech/Songs/Rhymes*	*Guidelines*

1. Release one quadripod and grasp the bed.

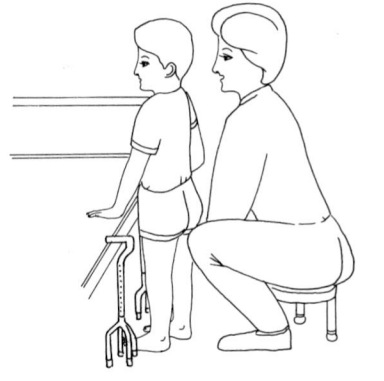

2. Release the other quadripod and grasp the bed.

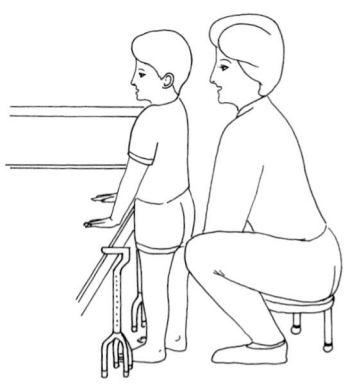

3. Pull onto the bed.

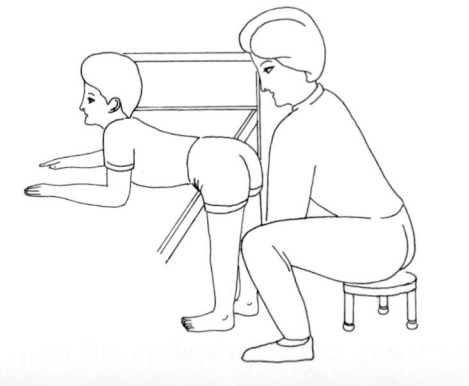

1. The child uses inner speech.

2. The care-giver supervises the child and preferably gives no manual assistance.

3. Encourage the child to keep his legs apart as he pulls onto the bed.

4. Give the child sufficient time to do the task.

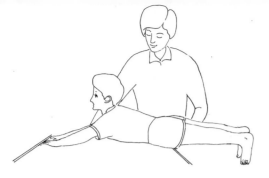

4. Pivot (see Chapter 16, Task 22, Levels 2–4).

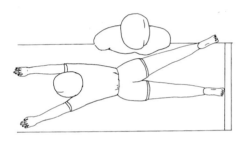

5. Roll over.

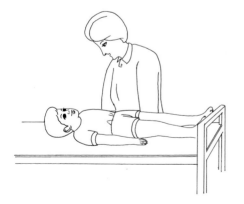

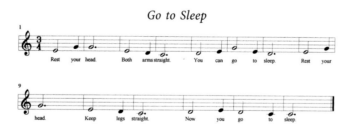

Go to Sleep

Rest your head. Both arms straight. You can go to sleep. Rest your head. Keep legs straight. Now you go to sleep.

Analysis of Motor Task	*Speech/Songs/Rhymes*	*Guidelines*

1. Both hands above the head.

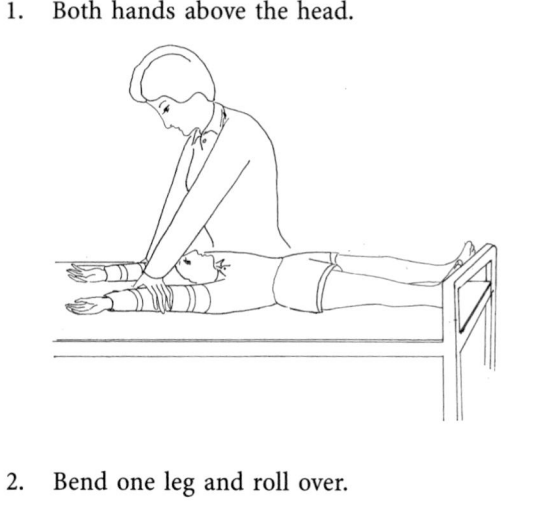

Hands above head   up   up   up

1. Always give the child the opportunity to learn to push off the bed, and as far as possible do not lift him out of the bed.

2. The child may need gaiters to extend the elbows and for stability.

3. The care-giver helps the child raise the hands above the head and bend one leg.

4. Place a toy on the side towards which the child is rolling and encourage him to look at it. She will also need to help the child to pivot and push off the bed.

2. Bend one leg and roll over.

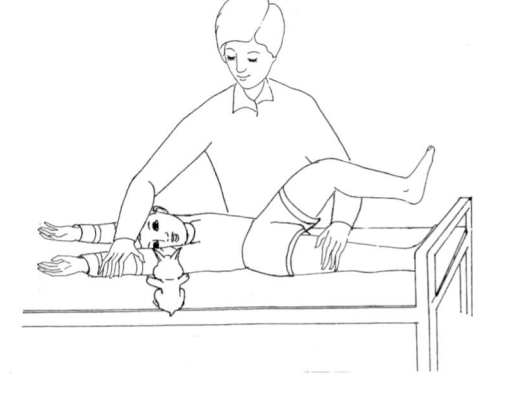

I bend leg   bend   bend   bend

5. If the child has poor weight bearing the care-giver facilitates the child at the knees and makes sure the feet are flat and apart. If the child cannot keep his feet flat she may need to stabilise him with her own feet. At this level the child may lean across the bed.

6. Encourage the child to stretch his arms across the bed and gradually stand up straight.

7. This is a preparation for walking training and is excellent to teach children take weight through the legs with the feet flat on the floor.

3. Pivot 90 (see Chapter 15, Task 8, Level 1).

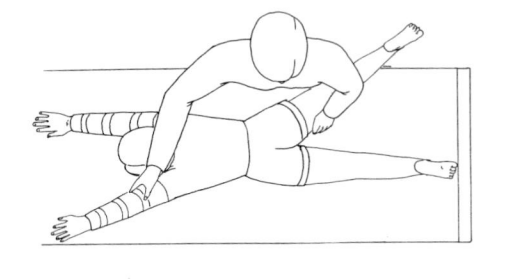

Lie on my Tummy

Lie on my tum-my push a-round. Lie on my tum-my push a-round. Lie on my

tum-my push a-round. I can get out of bed.

4. Push off the bed.   I push off   push   push   push

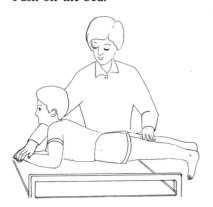

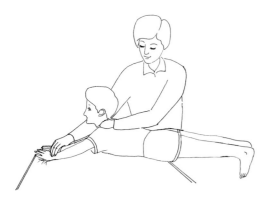

5. Feet flat and knees straight.   Feet flat   flat   flat   flat

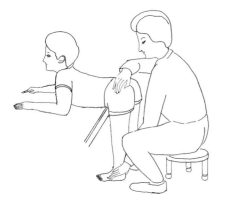

Analysis of Motor Task	Speech/Songs/Rhymes	Guidelines
1. Both hands above the head. 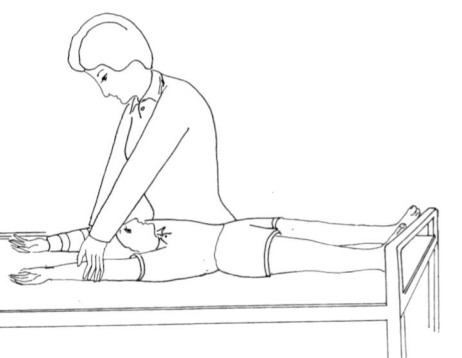	Hands above head 　1　2　3　4　5	1. The care-giver may need to help the child to raise his arms above the head. The child should be able to bend his leg.
2. Bend the leg and roll over. 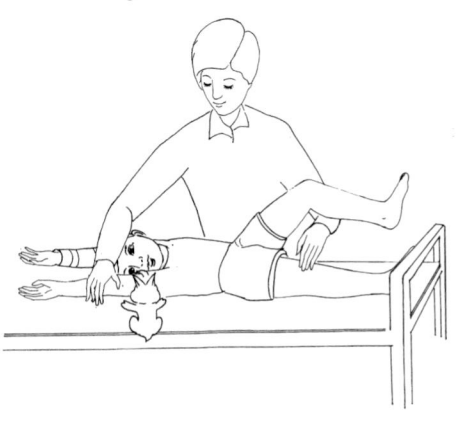	I bend leg and roll over 　1　2　3　4　5	2. The care-giver may still need to help the child to pivot and push off the bed. 3. The child may still need gaiters to extend the elbows and for stability. 4. Make sure the child's feet are flat and apart and his knees are straight. If the child's feet are constantly moving, the care-giver stabilises them by placing her own feet over the child's feet. 5. This task is excellent for helping the child part their legs and learn to keep their feet flat on the floor. 6. The care-giver says every step out loud and encourages the child to speak.
3. Pivot 90 (see Chapter 16, Task 22, Levels 2–4). 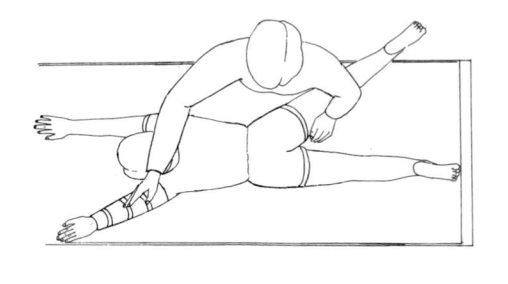	*Lie on my Tummy* 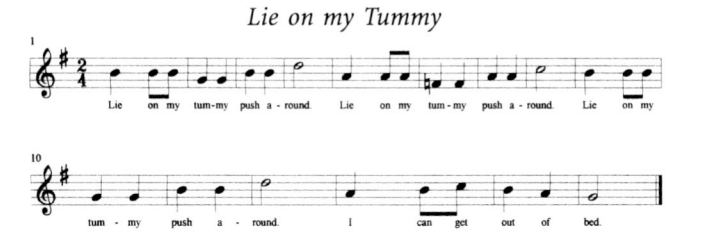 Lie on my tum-my push a-round. Lie on my tum-my push a-round. Lie on my tum-my push a-round. I can get out of bed.	

4. Push off the bed.

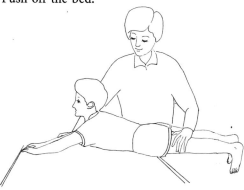

I push off   push   push   push

5. Part one hand part one leg.

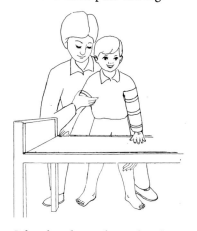

Right Hand First

Right hand first,   right leg then,   left hand fol - low   left   a - gain. La   la

la   la   la   la   la   la   la   la   la   la   la   la   la   la   la   la   la.

6. Other hand together other leg together. (Repeat).

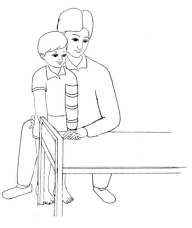

Analysis of Motor Task	*Speech/Songs/Rhymes*	*Guidelines*

1. Both hands above the head.

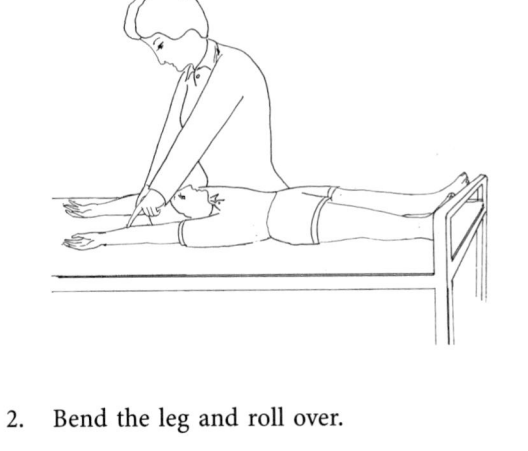

My hands above my head   1   2   3   4   5

1. Use speech to the facilitate the child and give minimal manual assistance.

2. Insist on feet flat and knees straight.

3. Encourage the child to use speech to guide his steps.

4. While the child is learning to move along the side of the bed, the care-giver sits behind the child to give him security. However try not to help him too much.

5. Make sure he parts his legs and puts his feet flat on the floor.

2. Bend the leg and roll over.

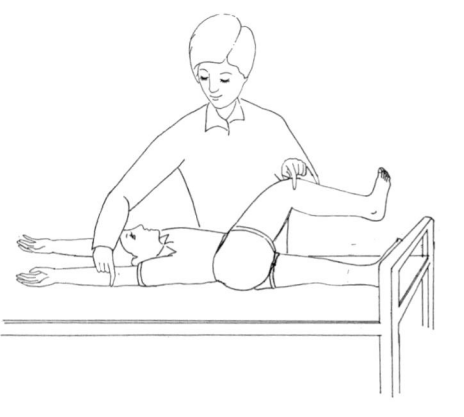

I bend my leg I roll over   1   2   3   4   5

3. Pivot (see Chapter 16, Task 22, Levels 2–4).

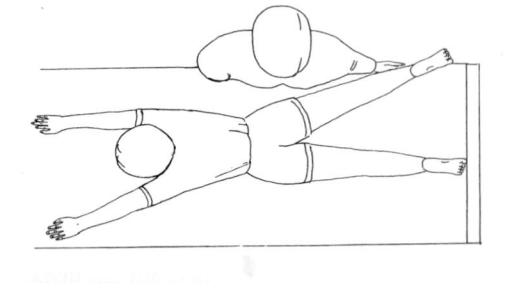

Lie on my Tummy

Lie on my tum-my push a-round. Lie on my tum-my push a-round. Lie on my

tum-my push a-round. I can get out of bed.

4. Push off the bed.

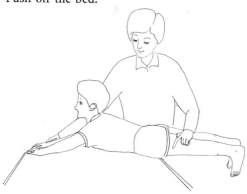

I push off   push push push

5. Part one hand part one leg.

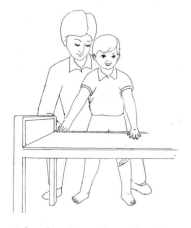

Right Hand First

Right hand first, right leg then, left hand fol-low left a-gain. La la la la la la la la la la la la la la la la la la la la.

6. Other hand together other leg together. (Repeat).

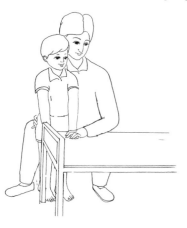

Analysis of Motor Task	*Speech/Songs/Rhymes*	*Guidelines*

1. Both hands above the head, bend the leg and roll over.

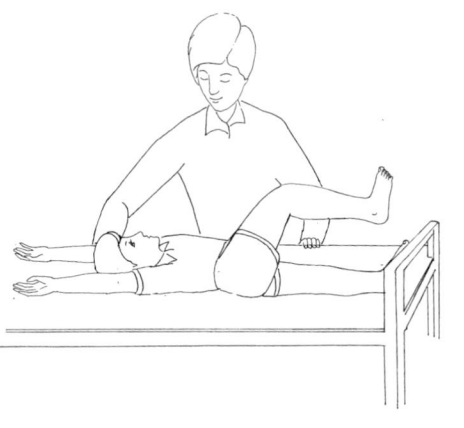

2. Pivot and push off.

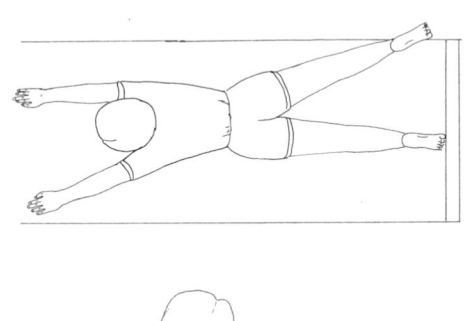

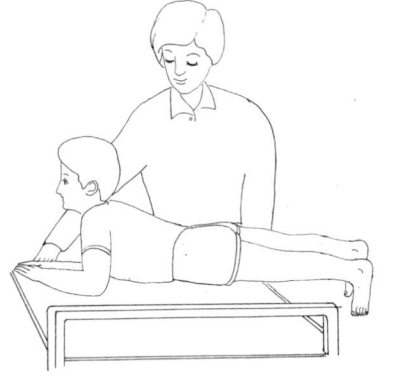

1. The child uses inner speech to direct his movements.

2. The care-giver supervises the child and preferably gives no manual facilitation.

3. Give the child sufficient time to walk to the toilet and do not rush him.

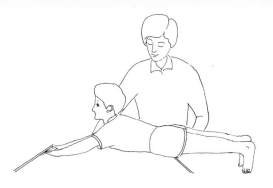

3. Walk to the toilet with clasped hands or grasp quadripod.

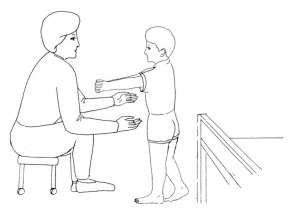

Mother and Baby Group

- LYING TASK SERIES
  (TASKS 1—9)

- SITTING TO STANDING TASK SERIES
  (TASKS 1—4)

- HAND TASK SERIES
  (TASKS 1—5)

Mother and Baby Group

The mother and baby group is geared mainly towards babies below two years of age. It aims to stimulate a natural mother-child interaction and gives the mother and by extension the family the confidence and skills to take an active role in guiding the baby's overall development. Primarily, it lays the groundwork for the mother to acquire a positive and constructive attitude towards the emotional, social, physical and cognitive development of her child.

The mother is the key mediator between the baby and his environment. From the beginning, great emphasis is placed on her facial and body gestures to stimulate her child to respond appropriately and help him develop ways of communicating. Gradually, she learns how to direct him to concentrate on the task at hand, attend to the care-giver and most importantly enjoy the programme/routine. No activity should be forced on the baby. Rather, the baby group is exposed to toys, games, songs and rhymes to encourage them to achieve the desired movement or activity.

The programme focuses on helping them experience the **Basic Motor Pattern** and prepares them for increasing involvement in the **activities of daily living**. In particular, they are introduced to habits of self-care. It is important to be aware of the baby's level of tolerance. At the beginning, the programme usually lasts from one to one-and-a-half hours and it can be extended to about two-and-a-half hours after a year. The process should be gentle and gradual. However, great emphasis is placed on guiding the mother on how to manage the baby throughout the whole day in the home situation.

The group situation, as well as being a new experience for the babies, also provides support for the mothers and offers them an indispensable opportunity for interaction amongst each another. As the group develops and progresses, the mother's role should gradually decrease allowing the child to interact with the care-givers and with other children. This prepares them eventually for work in the nursery/kindergarten groups.

The tasks in this chapter includes:

Lying Task Series (Tasks 1—9)

Sitting to Standing Task Series (Tasks 1—4)

Hand Tasks Series (Tasks 1—5)

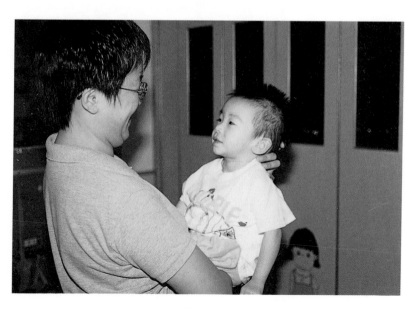

Fig. 14.1

Analysis of Motor Task	*Speech/Songs/Rhymes*	*Guidelines*

Analysis of Motor Task

1. Feet flat and apart and bottom back.

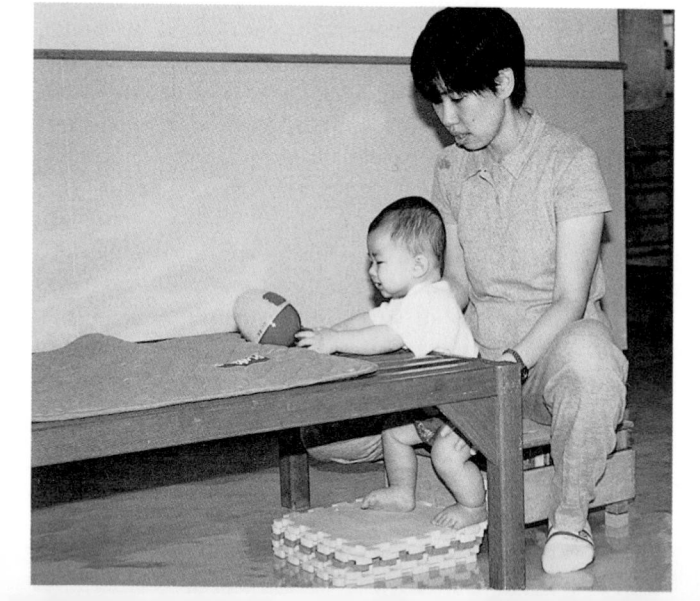

2. Stretch the hands and look at the toy.

Speech/Songs/Rhymes

(Suggested Game: Playing With a Toy)

I Stretch my Hands and Hold on Tight

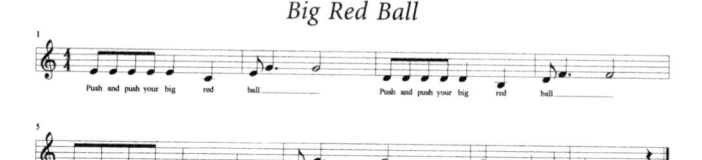

I stretch my hands and hold on tight Hold on tight Hold on tight. My

feet are flat, my bot-tom's pushed back look in the mid-dle I'm sit-ting up-right.

Big Red Ball

Push and push your big red ball⎯ Push and push your big red ball⎯

Push and push your big red ball⎯ la - la la la.

Guidelines

1. The aim of the task is to stimulate the babies to take an interest in their surroundings.

2. The care-giver sits with the baby at the side or behind him and does every step for him.

3. Depending on the ability of the baby, the care-giver may need to refer to the guidelines for sitting at the plinth (see Chapter 10, Task 18, Levels 1–4).

4. It is important from the very beginning to teach him how to sit. Helping him place his feet flat and apart is a preparation for standing and walking training. Helping him grasp and release, stretch his elbows and look at his hands/toy is a preparation for play.

5. Use a toy which will stimulate a response from the baby. A brightly coloured toy, preferably a musical toy, will stimulate him to look in the midline. However, the care-giver's own facial expression and dynamic encouragement is also excellent stimulation.

3. Grasp the toy.

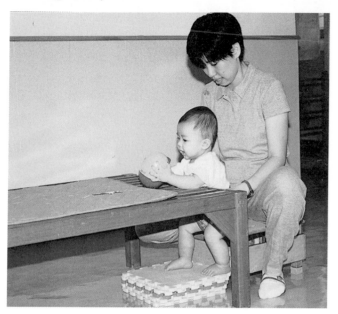

4. Play with the toy.

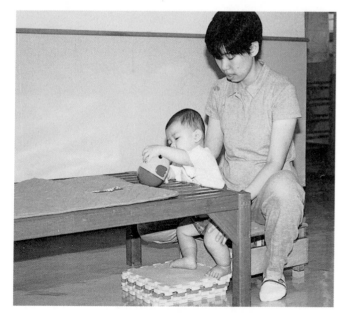

Big Red Ball

Push and push your big red ball _____ Push and push your big red ball _____

Push and push your big red ball _____ la - la la la

Analysis of Motor Task	*Speech/Songs/Rhymes*	*Guidelines*

1. Grasp the plinth and stand up.

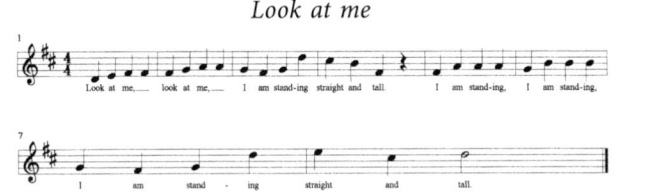

Look at me

Look at me,— look at me,— I am stand-ing straight and tall. I am stand-ing, I am stand-ing,

I am stand - ing straight and tall.

1. This helps the babies experience moving from one position to another and in all the tasks opportunity to practise the basic motor pattern.

2. It is very important from the outset to give the baby this experience. Avoid as far as possible picking him up and putting him sitting on a chair or potty. It is never too early for the baby with cerebral palsy to begin to learn to take an interest in their surroundings and experience normal movement in simple tasks.

3. Depending on the ability of the baby, two care-givers may need to help with this task. One care-giver helps the baby grasp the plinth and keep his head in the midline. The other care-giver helps the baby take weight through the legs.

4. A song with a good rhythm will gradually help the baby accept the standing position.

5. The care-giver's face or brightly coloured musical toy will also help him look in the midline.

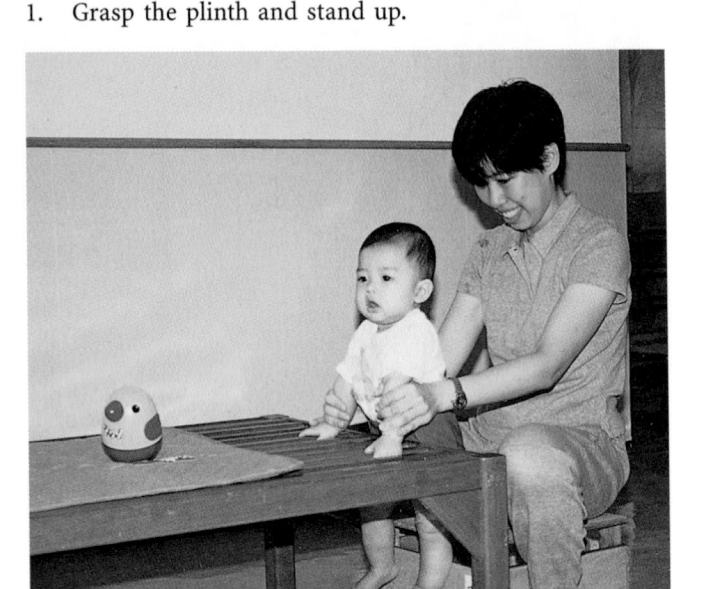

2. Feet flat and apart.

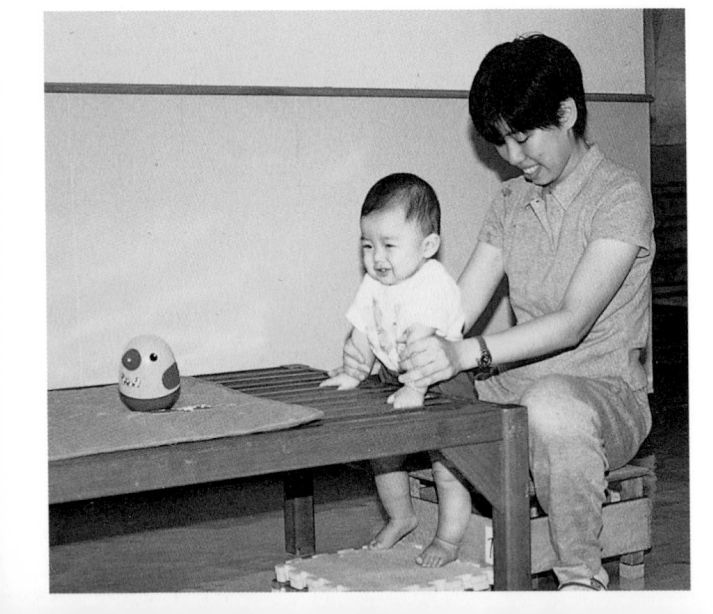

3. Stand straight.

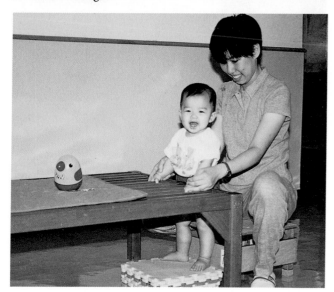

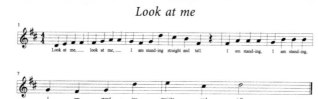

Look at me

Look at me,___ look at me,___ I am stand-ing straight and tall. I am stand-ing, I am stand-ing,

I am stand - ing straight and tall.

Analysis of Motor Task	*Speech/Songs/Rhymes*	*Guidelines*

1. Reach for the toy.

(Suggested game: Follow a Moving Toy)

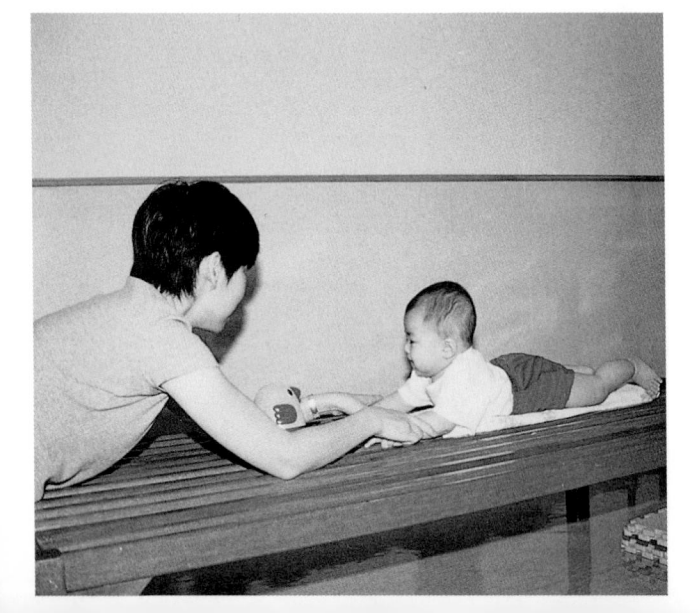

Hold on Tight

[musical notation]

Hold on tight. Pull up right.

Hold on tight. Pull up right.

Reach the toy so shi-ny bright. La la la la la la la la

Reach the toy so shi-ny bright. Hold on tight.

1. This task may also be carried out on a mat on the floor. However, the plinth is very useful as it facilitates the babies experience and learn grasp, stretching their elbows and pulling a little distance. Use a soft towel/small mat under the babies when using the plinth.

2. Encourage the baby to learn to move from one position to another.

3. Many babies do not like the prone position.

4. Give them sufficient time for the task and use all possible stimulation to encourage them to move.

5. Also give them sufficient time to explore the toy.

6. Make sure the baby lifts his head when learning to pull up.

2. Grasp the plinth.

3. Pull up.

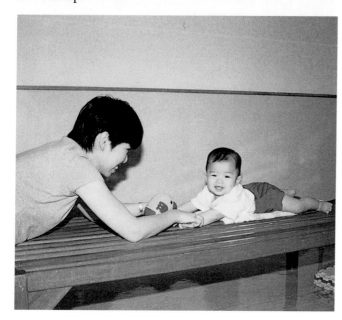

Hold on Tight

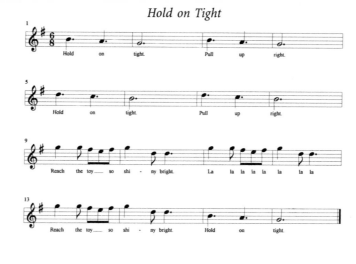

4. Repeat.

Analysis of Motor Task	*Speech/Songs/Rhymes*	*Guidelines*

1. Look at mother's face.

(Suggested Game: Looking at Mother's Face/Musical Toy)

1. This task teaches head control, wrist and hip extension.

2. Depending on the ability of the baby, the care-giver helps him prone on forearms or on extended arms.

3. She will need to help the baby extend the elbows and encourage him to lift his head.

4. Continue this task as long as the baby tolerates it.

5. Make sure the baby's legs are apart.

6. Encourage the more able little ones to release one hand and play with a toy.

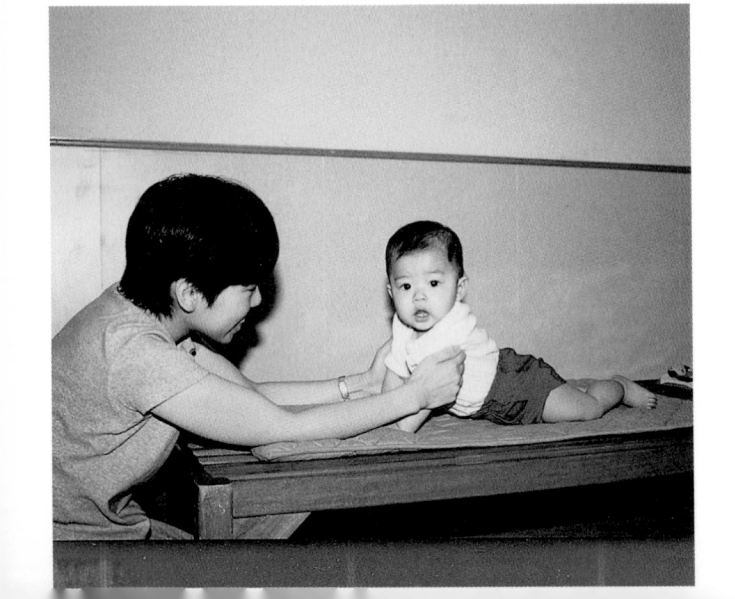

2. Stretch the elbows and lie prone on extended arms.

3. Look up.

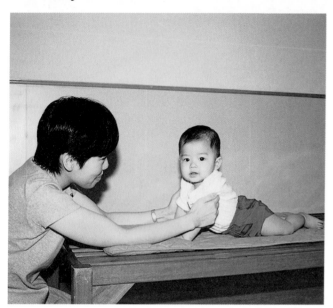

Analysis of Motor Task | *Speech/Songs/Rhymes* | *Guidelines*

1. Look at the toy.

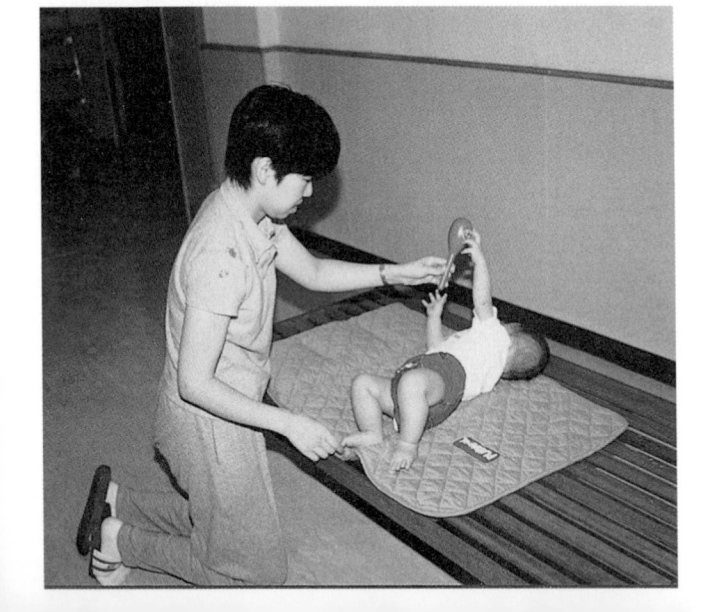

2. Bend the top leg.

Rolling Over

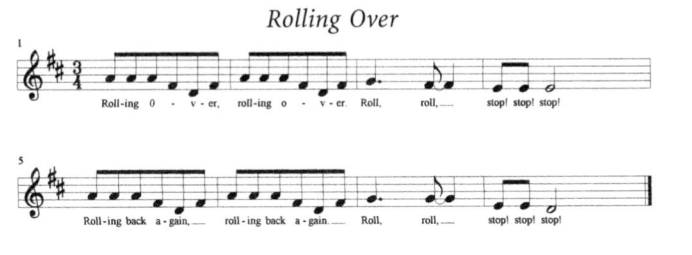

Roll-ing O - v - er, roll-ing o - v - er. Roll, roll,____ stop! stop! stop!

Roll-ing back a - gain, roll - ing back a - gain.____ Roll, roll,____ stop! stop! stop!

1. This task is useful to help the babies learn to move from one position to another. It also prepares them to get in and out of bed at a later stage.

2. The care-giver helps the baby experience every step.

3. Encourage the baby to look towards the side to which he is moving by dangling a brightly coloured/musical toy at that side.

4. The care-giver helps the baby bend the top leg and makes sure the baby moves the head first before rolling over.

5. It is preferable if the care-giver helps the baby raise the hands above the head to facilitate rolling over.

6. The task can be repeated as the care-giver helps the baby roll the length of the plinth or the mat on the floor.

3. Roll over.

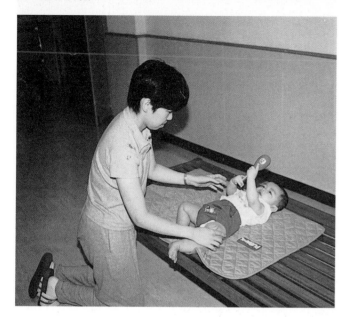

4. Repeat.

Analysis of Motor Task	*Speech/Songs/Rhymes*	*Guidelines*

1. Look at the puppet on the foot.

(Suggested Game: Playing with and Pulling a Puppet off Each Foot)

1. This task helps the babies experience grasp and release, stretching the elbows and knees, bending the hips and dorsi-flexing the feet. This prepares them for sitting, standing, walking training.

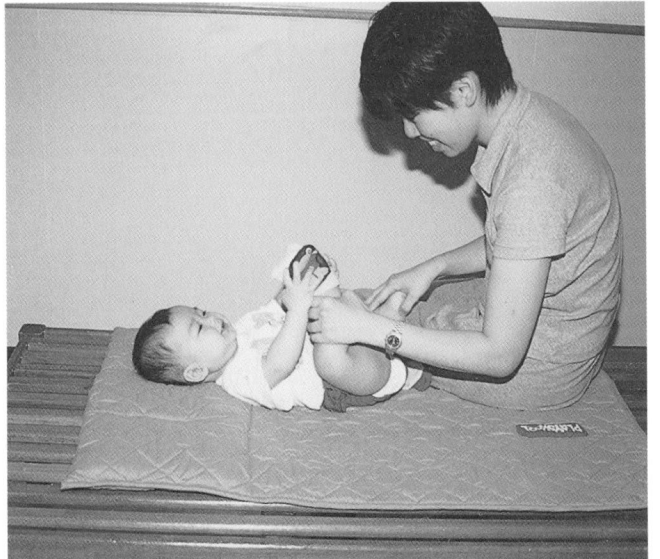

2. The care-giver first shows the puppet to the baby before putting it on his foot. Then she helps him stretch his elbows, grasp the puppet and pull it off.

3. Continue this game while the baby is enjoying it.

4. Make sure the baby keeps his head in the midline.

5. If possible, and when the baby is relaxed, the care-giver may clap the soles of his feet together after "pulling off the puppet" game.

2. Stretch the elbows and grasp the puppet.

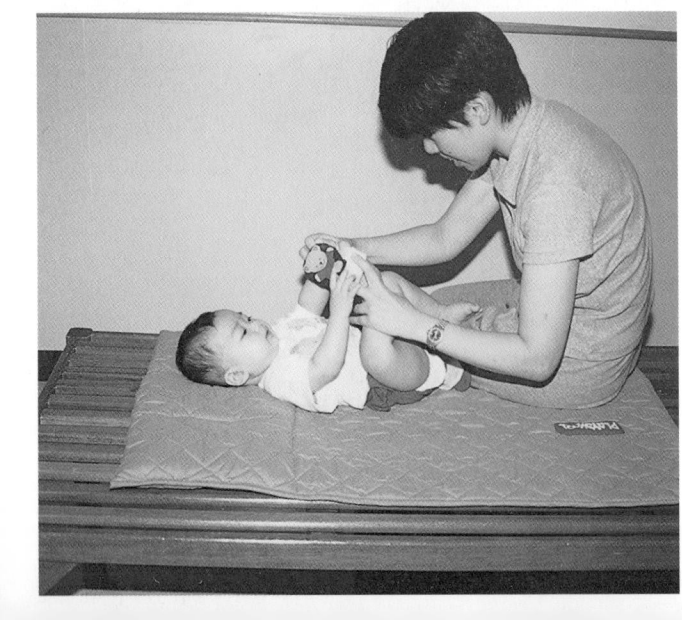

3. Pull off the puppet.

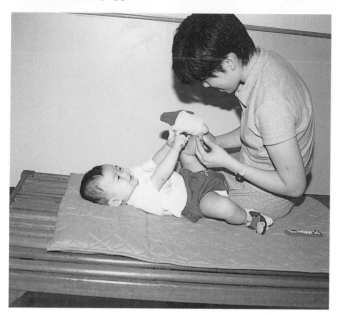

4. Clap the soles of the feet.

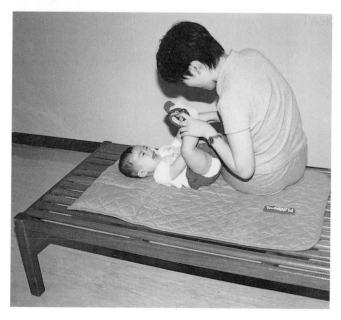

| *Analysis of Motor Task* | *Speech/Songs/Rhymes* | *Guidelines* |

1. Put both feet flat on the plinth.

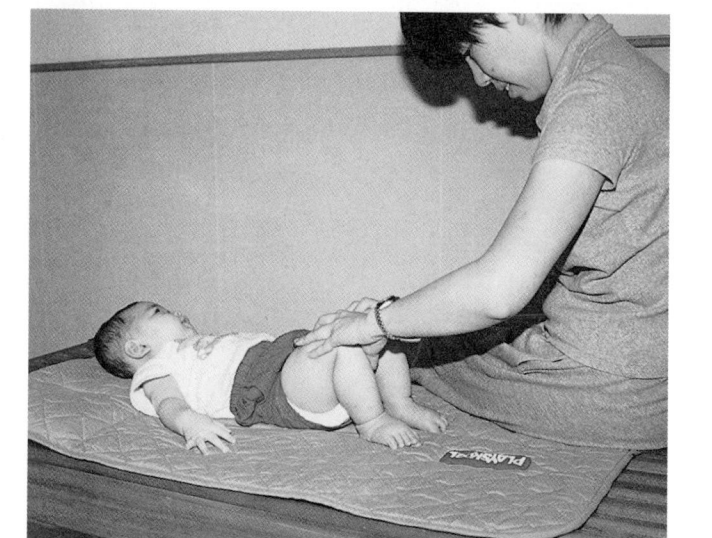

London Bridge is Falling Down

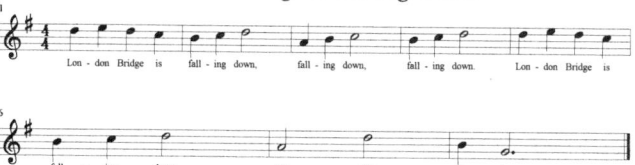

Lon - don Bridge is   fall - ing down,   fall - ing down,   fall - ing down.   Lon - don Bridge is

fall - ing   down,   my   fair   la - dy.

1. This task prepares the babies for nappy changing. It is also a preparation for sitting/standing and walking training as they are experiencing feet flat on the plinth. It also prepares for dressing/undressing.

2. Always use this task when changing the baby's nappy. Gradually the baby will learn to lift up his bottom.

3. Make sure the baby's flat feet are directly under his knees when lifting up his bottom.

4. The care-giver presses gently but firmly on the knees to help the baby lift up his bottom.

5. The care-giver may also need to apply some pressure on the feet if they are constantly moving. The baby must experience fixating the feet flat on the plinth.

6. Do not allow the baby to arch his back when doing this. A small pillow under the head may help prevent arching. Use a squeaky toy to encourage the baby to lift up his bottom.

2. Lift up the bottom.

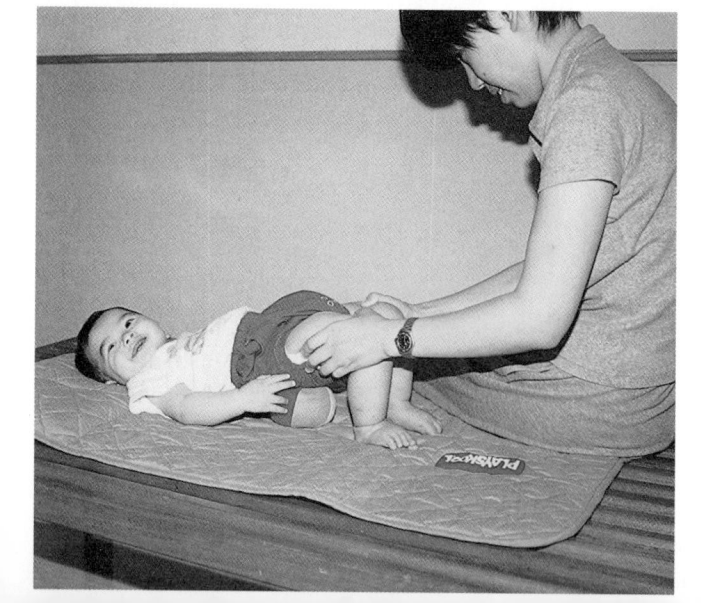

| *Analysis of Motor Task* | *Speech/Songs/Rhymes* | *Guidelines* |

1. Look at toy, reach for it.

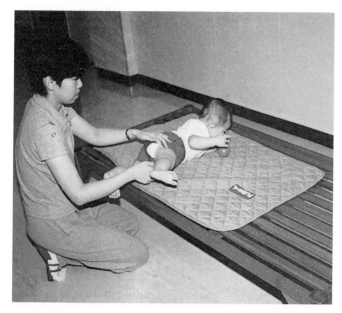

(Suggested Game: Chasing a Rattle)

Rolling Over

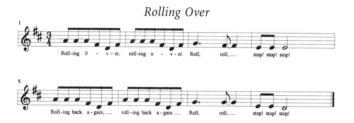

Roll-ing o - v - er, roll-ing o - v - er. Roll, roll, ____ stop! stop! stop!

Roll-ing back a - gain, roll-ing back a - gain. ____ Roll, roll, ____ stop! stop! stop!

1. This task is useful to help the babies learn to move from one position to another. It also prepares them to get in and out of bed at a later stage.

2. The care-giver helps the baby experience every step.

3. She will need to help the baby extend his elbows and encourage him to lift up his head.

4. Continue this task as long as the baby tolerates it.

5. Make sure the baby's legs are apart.

6. Encourage the more able little ones to release one hand and play with a toy.

2. Roll over.

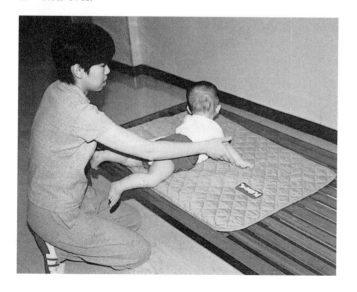

Analysis of Motor Task	*Speech/Songs/Rhymes*	*Guidelines*

1. Hands under the shoulders and legs apart.

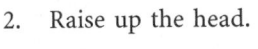

Push off Plinth

We push down the plinth, we push down the plinth. We

lift our head up high. We push down the plinth.

1. This task is useful to help the babies experience straight elbows as they push off the plinth. Gravity and the weight of the body automatically stretches the elbows as they are helped to push off. It also prepares them for getting in and out of bed at a later stage.

2. If the plinth is slightly tilted it is much easier to teach the babies the sensation of the movement. However, be careful when doing this movement.

3. The care-giver helps the baby experience grasping the plinth as he pushes down.

4. As he is helped to push off the plinth onto the floor, the care-giver helps him experience feet flat with heels down on the floor and legs apart.

5. One care-giver helps the baby experience grasping the plinth and keeping his head in the midline. The other care-giver helps him take weight through both legs.

6. Maintain this position as long as the baby can tolerate it. Use a song with a good rhythm.

2. Raise up the head.

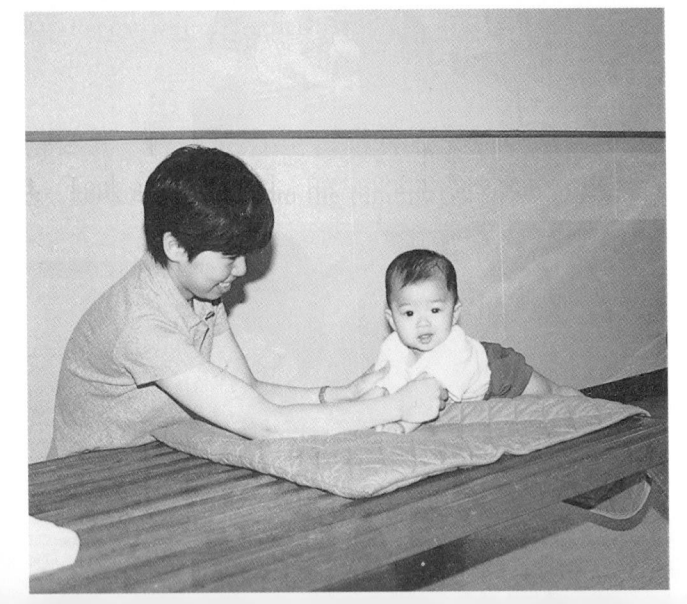

3. Push off.

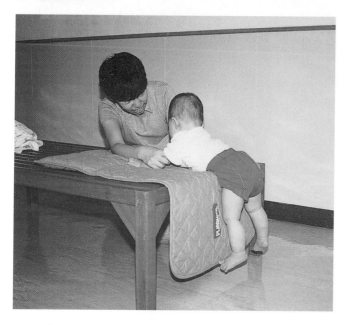

4. Stand straight grasping the plinth.

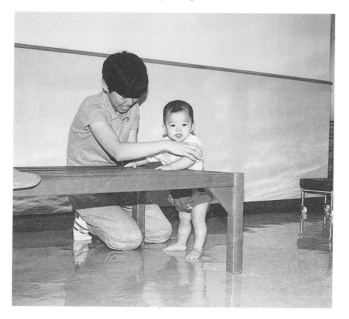

Look at me

Look at me, ___ look at me, ___ I am stand-ing straight and tall. I am stand-ing, I am stand-ing,

I am stand - ing straight and tall.

Analysis of Motor Task	*Speech/Songs/Rhymes*	*Guidelines*

1. Look at the rattle.

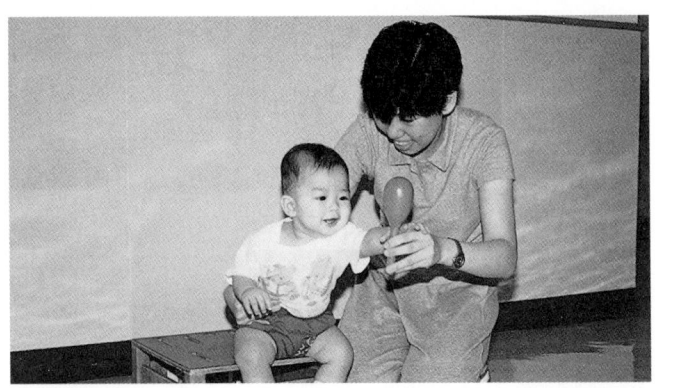

2. Grasp the rattle.

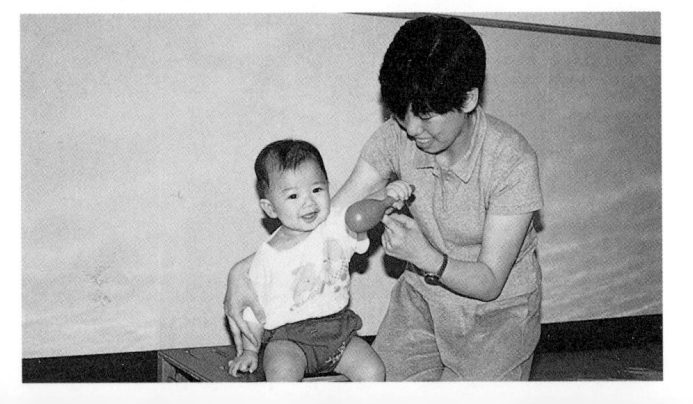

3. Raise up the arm and wave the rattle.

(Suggested Game: "The Trees are Waving")

Up to the Sky

Stretch your hand. Lift up high. Up and down up to the sky. Stretch your hands and lift up high.

Up and down up to the sky. Stretch your hands. Lift up high. Up and down up to the sky.

Stretch your hands and lift up high. Up and down up to the sky.

1. This task helps the babies experience sitting on a low stool with both feet flat and apart.

2. If the baby needs fixation of the lower limbs while using the trunk and upper limbs, the care-giver can press gently on the thighs.

3. It also helps the baby experience fixing one part while moving another part of the body.

4. The care-giver makes sure the baby sits securely while helping him wave the rattle in the air.

5. Make sure the baby learns to keep the feet flat and apart at all times especially when raising the hands.

4. Repeat with the other hand.

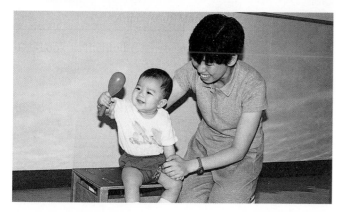

5. Put the rattle in the basket.

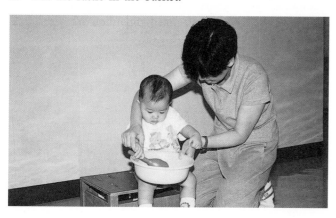

Analysis of Motor Task	*Speech/Songs/Rhymes*	*Guidelines*

1. Look at the mirror.

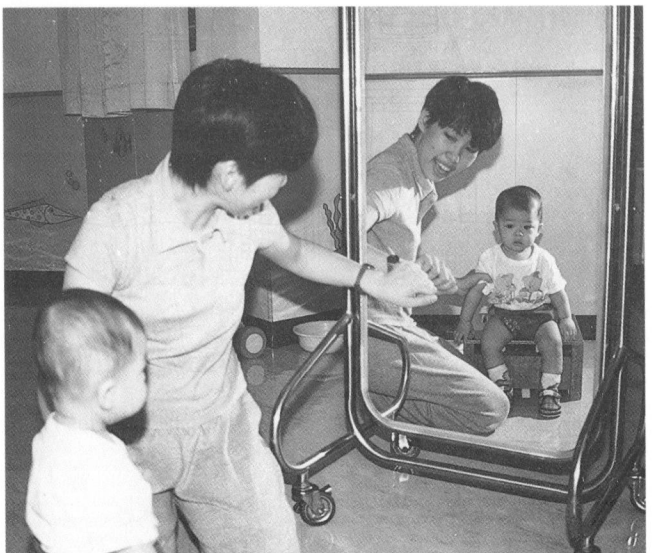

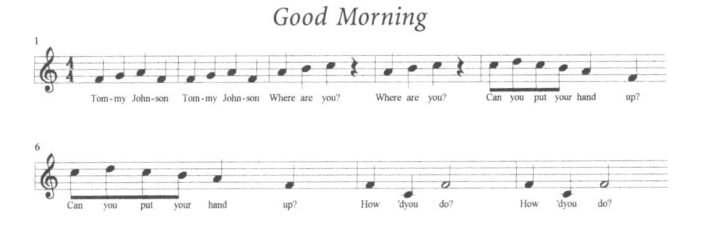

Good Morning

Tom-my John-son Tom-my John-son Where are you? Where are you? Can you put your hand up?

Can you put your hand up? How 'dyou do? How 'dyou do?

1. This task helps the babies experience moving from one position to another. If possible, give them this opportunity at all times.

2. It is important to give the babies the opportunity to learn to stand especially if they are over 12 months and upwards. Standing is essential for the poper development of the hip joints. However, if they stand on tiptoes with the legs crossed hips knees and elbows bent, they are not using a good pattern in standing. They will need help to part the legs, put the feet flat on the floor stretch the elbows and stand up straight.

3. Use a large mirror if available and encourage the baby to look at the mirror.

4. Help him to bring his weight over his feet before helping him to stand up.

2. Stand up.

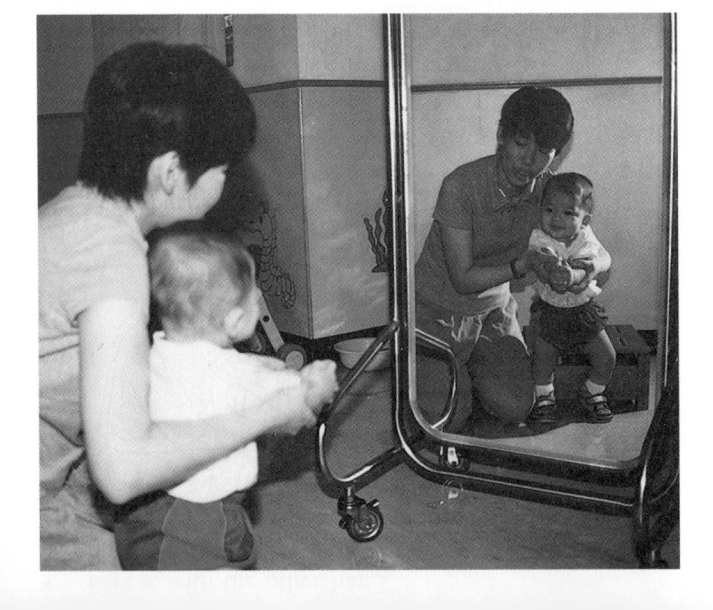

3. Feet flat and apart and stand straight.

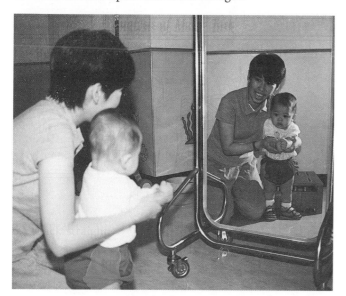

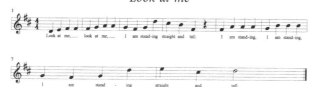

Look at me,___ look at me,___ I am stand-ing straight and tall. I am stand-ing, I am stand-ing,

I am stand - ing straight and tall.

Analysis of Motor Task	*Speech/Songs/Rhymes*	*Guidelines*

1.   Look at the toy on the floor.

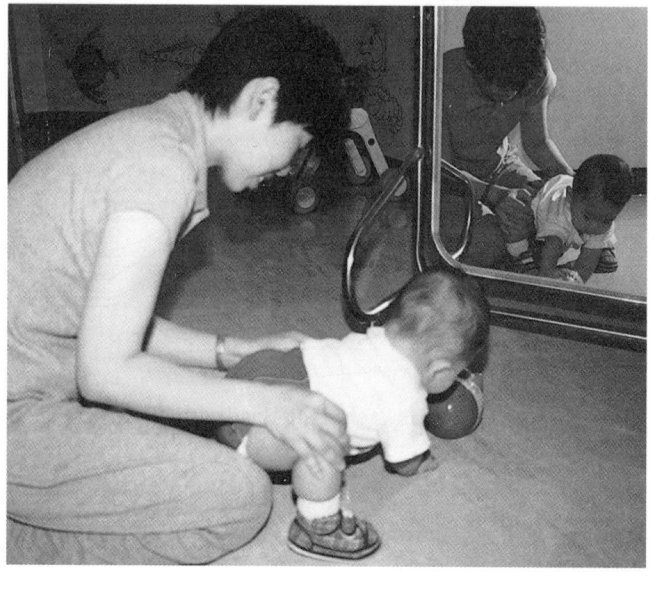

(Suggested Game: Looking/Playing with a Moving Toy in the Squatting Position)

Jack in the Box

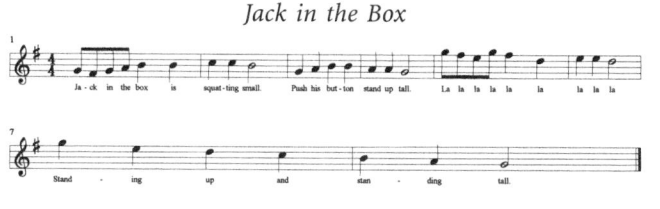

Ja - ck in the box   is   squat - ting small.   Push his but - ton   stand up tall.   La la la la la   la   la la la

Stand - ing   up   and   stan - ding   tall.

1.   This task helps the babies experience moving from one position to another. It prepares them to sit down on the potty and also prepares them for standing and walking training.

2.   A brightly coloured or preferably moving toy helps the baby look down at the toy and facilitates squatting.

3.   Make sure the baby's feet are flat on the floor and the knees are apart in the squatting position.

4.   Help the baby to stand up.

5.   This task may be repeated while the baby tolerates it.

2.   Bend the knees and squat.

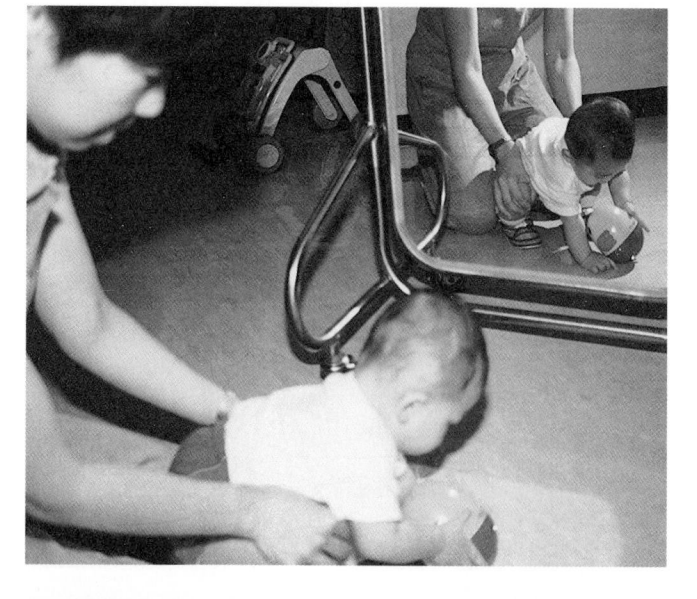

3.   Repeat.

Analysis of Motor Task	*Speech/Songs/Rhymes*	*Guidelines*

1. Grasp the rung of the baby walker/ladderback chair.

Look at me

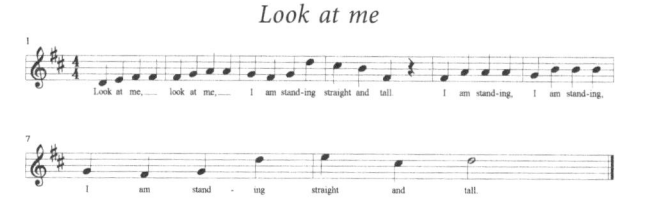

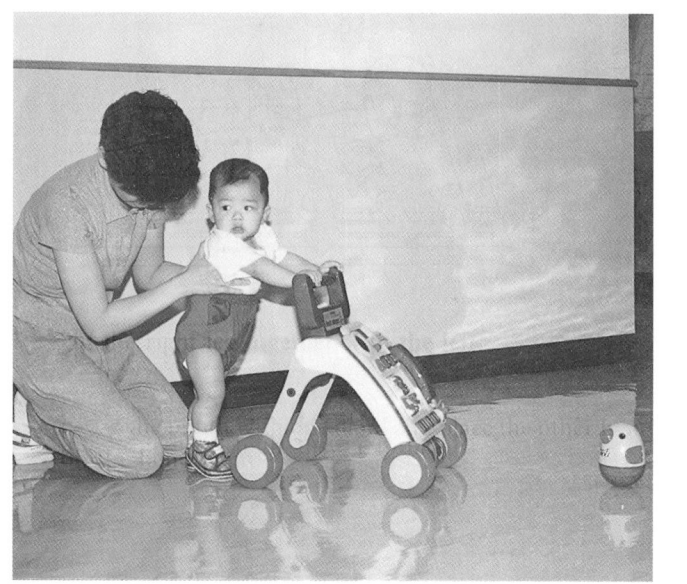

1. If the baby can take weight through both legs encourage him to take some steps by dangling a brightly coloured toy in front of him or encouraging him to use the baby walker/ladderback chair to push a toy along the floor.

2. The care-giver will need to give the baby maximum help to carry out this task.

3. Make sure his feet are flat and apart and help him to bend one knee and keep the other knee straight when learning to take a step.

2. Push the walker/ladderback chair.

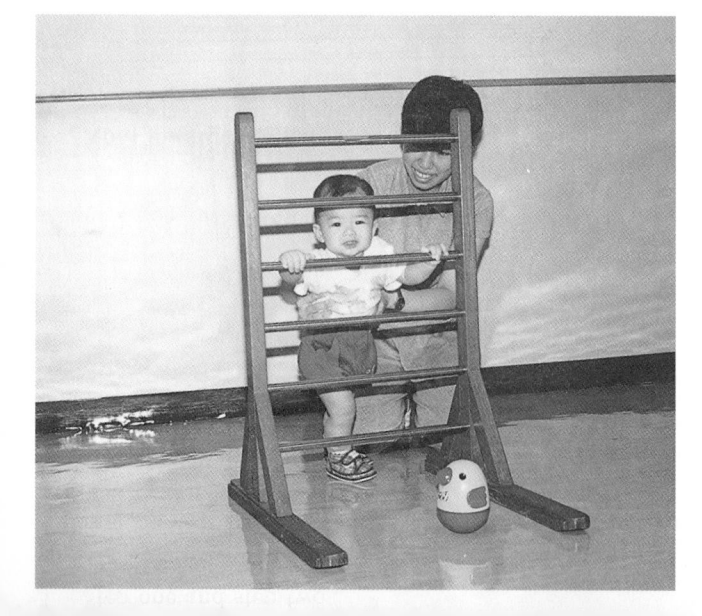

3. Step one and step two.

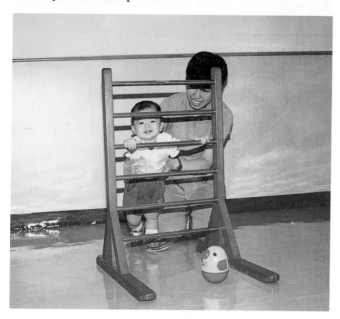

4. Stand straight.

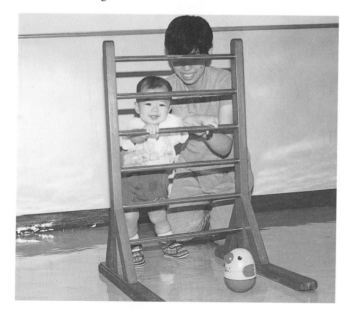

Look at me

Look at me, ... look at me, ... I am stand-ing straight and tall. I am stand-ing, I am stand-ing,

I am stand - ing straight and tall.

Analysis of Motor Task	*Speech/Songs/Rhymes*	*Guidelines*

1. Look at the tambourine.

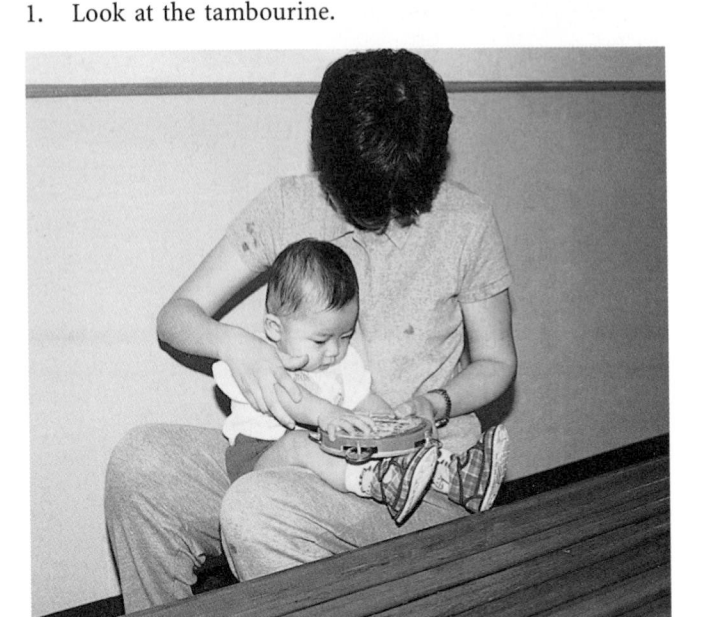

(Suggested Game: Patting Plinth/Table/Tambourine)

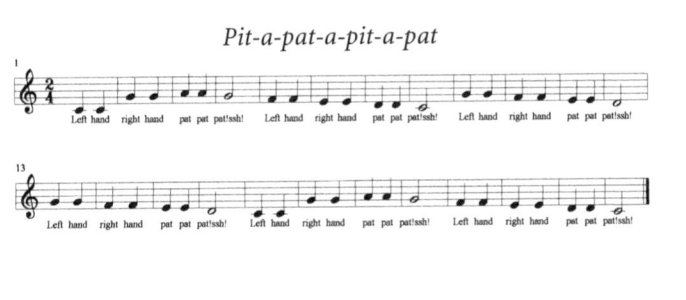

Pit-a-pat-a-pit-a-pat

Left hand   right hand   pat pat pat!ssh!   Left hand   right hand   pat pat pat!ssh!   Left hand   right hand   pat pat pat!ssh!

Left hand   right hand   pat pat pat!ssh!   Left hand   right hand   pat pat pat!ssh!   Left hand   right hand   pat pat pat!ssh!

1. The tasks in this series may also be carried out with the baby sitting on the care-giver's lap or <u>longsitting</u> on the bed/mat on the floor. However the babies should experience sitting at a table/plinth as soon as possible.

2. The task helps the baby experience hands flat on a hard surface and prepares him for play.

3. The care-giver may have to help the baby if he cannot pat on the table/tambourine.

4. Gradually she helps the baby pat to the rhythm of the song.

5. Help the baby to use alternate hands.

6. Remove help as the baby learns to do the task.

7. Make sure the elbows are extended and the hands flat with fingers extended.

8. Use a song with a good rhythm.

2. Put hands flat on the tambourine.

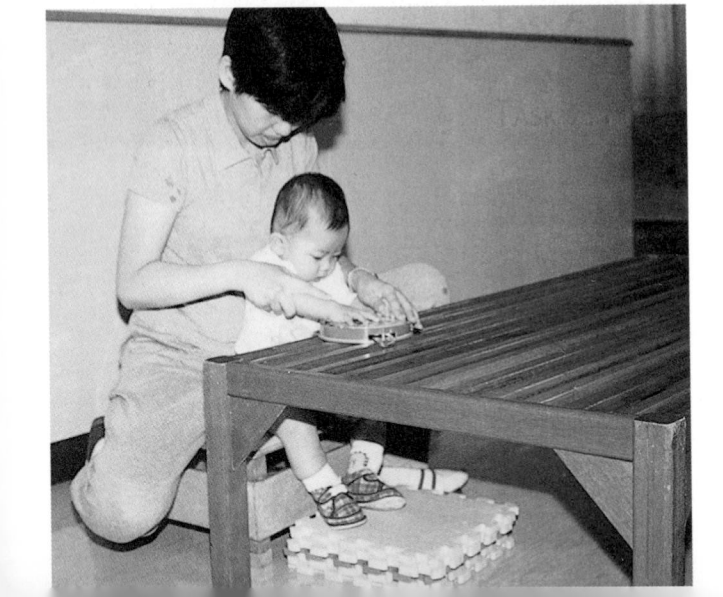

3. Raise one hand and pat.

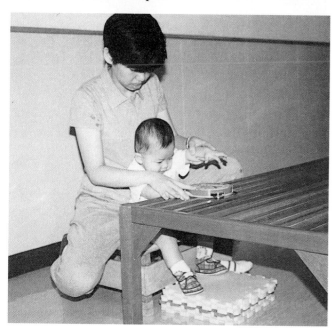

4. Repeat with the other hand.

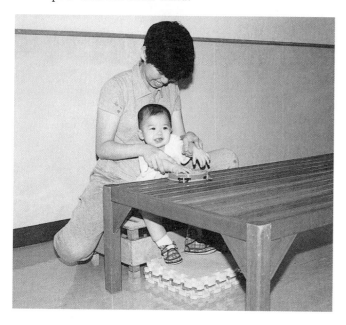

Analysis of Motor Task	*Speech/Songs/Rhymes*	*Guidelines*

Analysis of Motor Task

1. Look at the mirror.

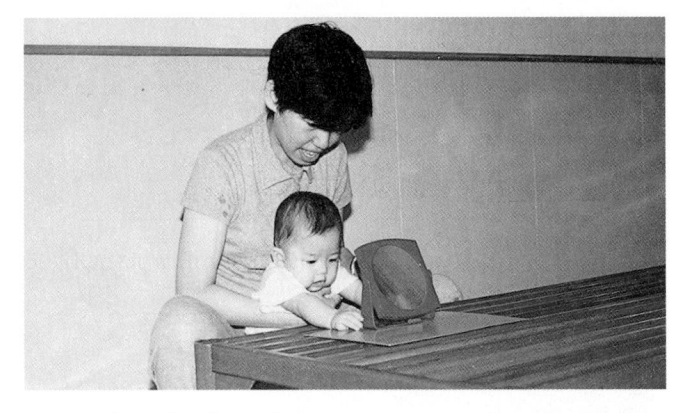

2. Pat the mirror.

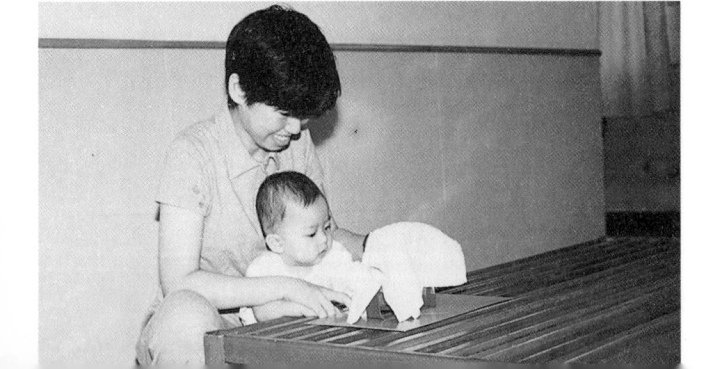

3. Look at the flannel.

Speech/Songs/Rhymes

(Suggested Game: Pat a Cake)

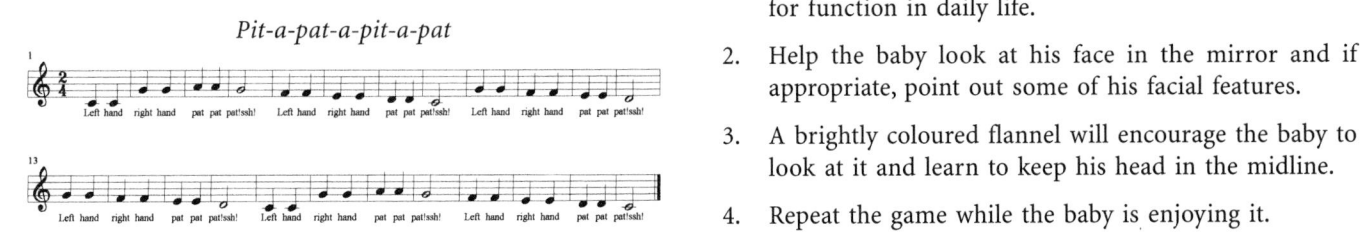

Pit-a-pat-a-pit-a-pat

Guidelines

1. Babies must begin to experience and learn to grasp and release from a very early age. This will help them at a later stage to master their movements and prepare them for function in daily life.

2. Help the baby look at his face in the mirror and if appropriate, point out some of his facial features.

3. A brightly coloured flannel will encourage the baby to look at it and learn to keep his head in the midline.

4. Repeat the game while the baby is enjoying it.

4. Grasp the flannel.

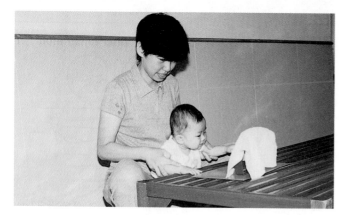

5. Pull off the flannel.

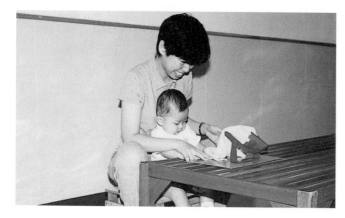

6. Repeat.

Analysis of Motor Task	*Speech/Songs/Rhymes*	*Guidelines*

1.   Look at the rattle and grasp it.

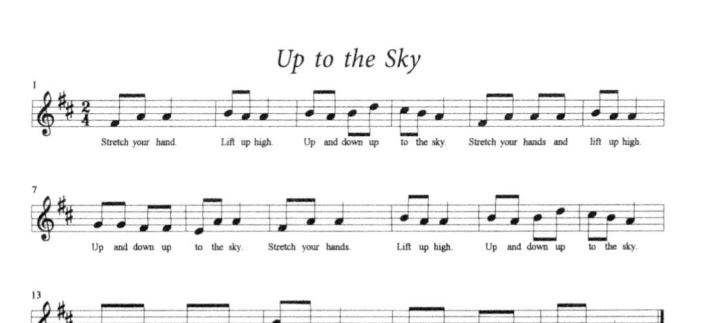

(Suggested Game: Shaking a rattle in the air)

Up to the Sky

1.   This task helps the babies experience grasp and release and extension of the trunk in the sitting position.

2.   Give the baby sufficient time to look at and explore the rattle.

3.   The care-giver helps the baby raise up his hands and shake the rattle. However, remove help if the baby initiates the movement.

4.   Make sure the baby is sitting securely on the chair while doing this task.

5.   Help the baby to release the bells into a basket when finished.

6.   An alternative game is to help the baby put on coloured wrist bands with bells attached. These give positive feedback when the baby is helped to wave them in the air. Make sure the baby does not put the bells in his mouth.

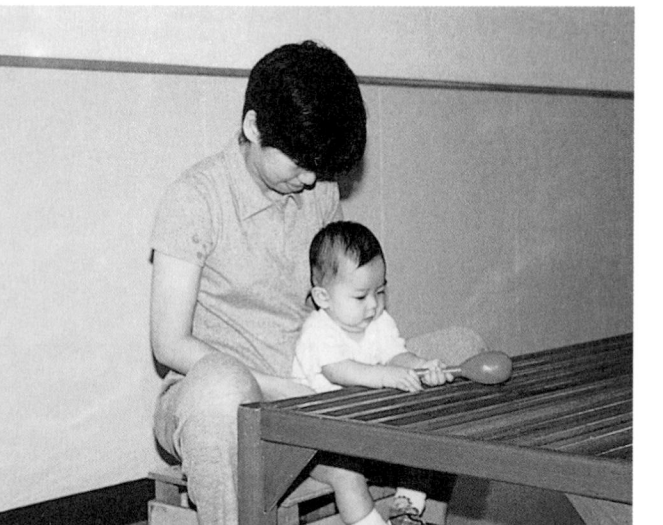

2.   Raise the rattle and shake it.

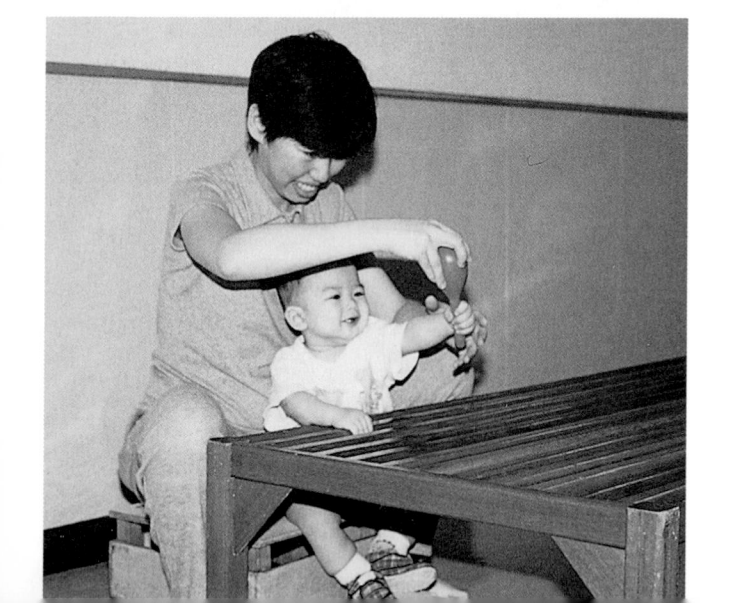

3. Repeat with the other hand.

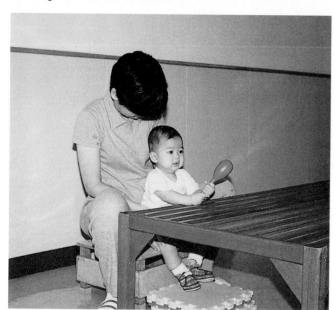

Analysis of Motor Task	*Speech/Songs/Rhymes*	*Guidelines*

1. Squirt cream onto the outstretched palm.

(Suggested Game: Rubbing in Cream)

1. It is important from the beginning for the babies to experience and learn to clasp their hands in the midline position. This is especially important for babies who have asymmetrical tonic neck reflex (ATNR) and also for babies who repeatedly throw themselves backwards.

2. Allow the baby to smell the fragrance of the cream before rubbing it in.

3. Make sure he looks at his hands as the care-giver helps him rub in the cream.

4. If possible, help the baby bring his clasped hands to his face to smell the fragrance of the cream.

5. A baby who has great difficulty bringing his hands together may grasp a doll, make sure he looks at the doll.

6. Extend this task to helping the baby experience clapping his hands.

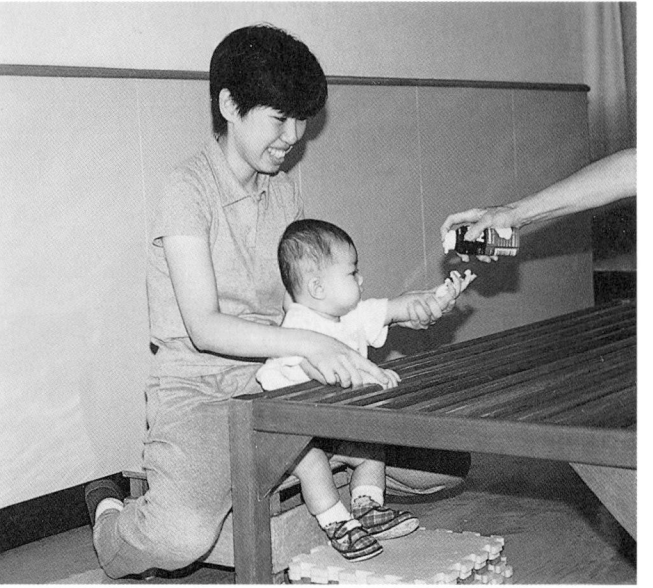

2. Look at the cream.

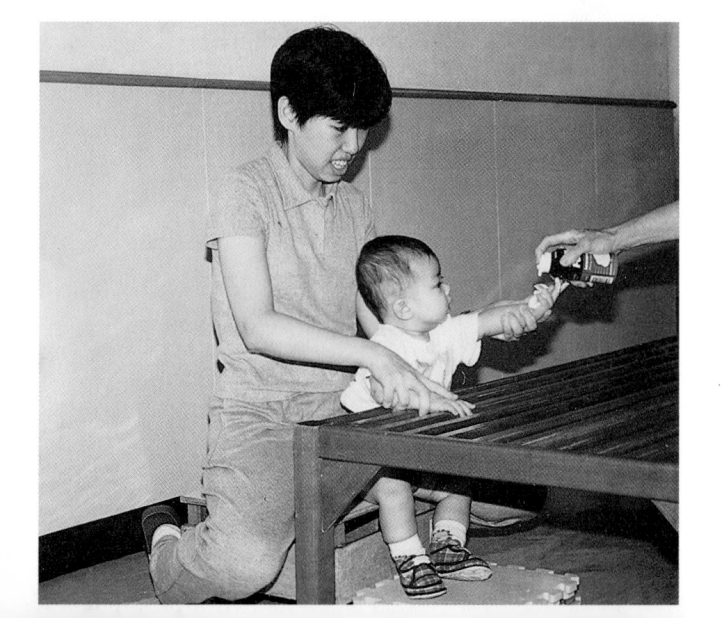

3. Rub in the cream.

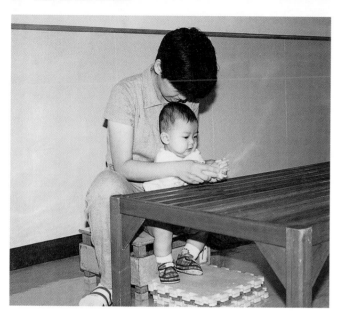

Analysis of Motor Task	*Speech/Songs/Rhymes*	*Guidelines*

1. Look at the doll.

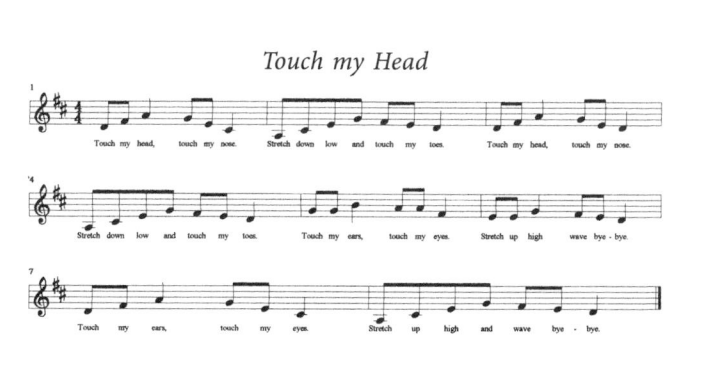

(Suggested Game: Playing with a Doll)

Touch my Head

Touch my head, touch my nose. Stretch down low and touch my toes. Touch my head, touch my nose.

Stretch down low and touch my toes. Touch my ears, touch my eyes. Stretch up high wave bye-bye.

Touch my ears, touch my eyes. Stretch up high and wave bye-bye.

1. The babies should have every opportunity to experience playing with dolls as this prepares them gradually to learn body image. This is crucial for the baby with cerebral palsy to begin the process of learning to function in life.

2. The care-giver helps the baby grasp the doll and explore it, if appropriate, through singing the song.

3. She helps the baby kiss the doll.

4. Make sure the baby is sitting securely for this task.

2. Grasp the doll with both hands.

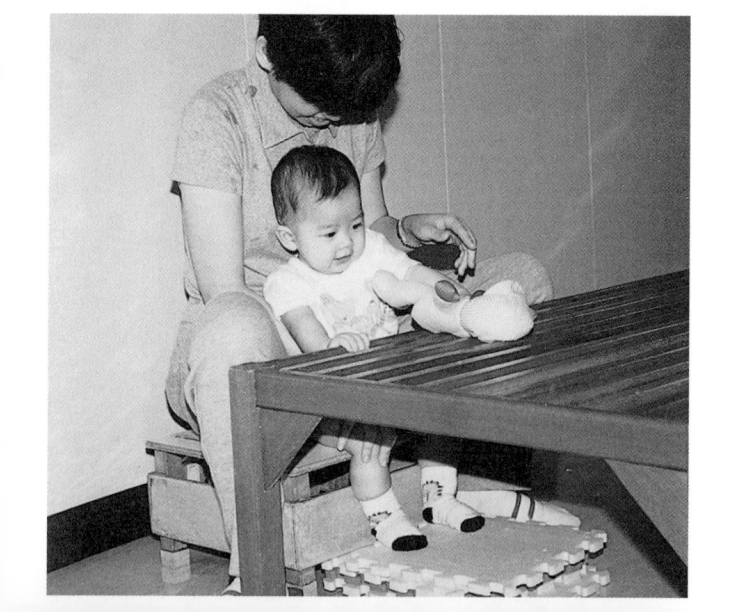

3. Bring the doll to the mouth and kiss it.

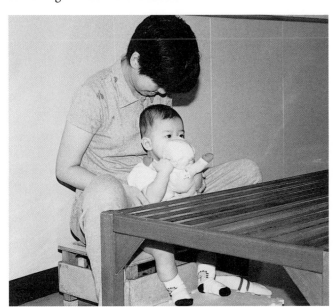

Chapter 15

Groups at Level 1

- LYING TASK SERIES
  (TASKS 1—9)

- SITTING TO STANDING TASK SERIES
  (TASKS 1—5)

- HAND TASK SERIES
  (TASKS 1—5)

TASK 1: SIDE LYING POSITION ON THE PLINTH GRASPING A DOLL/TEDDY BEAR

TASK 2: ROLLING INTO THE SUPINE POSITION FROM SIDE LYING

TASK 3: LYING STRAIGHT IN THE SUPINE POSITION

TASK 4: RAISING BOTH ARMS ABOVE THE HEAD IN THE SUPINE POSITION GRASPING A STICK

TASK 5: BRIDGING IN THE SUPINE POSITION

TASK 6: ROLLING FROM THE SUPINE POSITION TO THE PRONE POSITION

TASK 7: PRONE ON FOREARMS

TASK 8: LYING TASK SERIES

TASK 9: PUSHING OFF PLINTH IN THE PRONE POSITION

Analysis of Motor Task	*Speech/Songs/Rhymes*	*Guidelines*

1. Look at the doll/teddy bear.

I look at doll   look   look   look

2. Grasp the doll/teddy bear.

I grasp doll   grasp   grasp   grasp

3. Stretch the elbows and take the doll/teddy bear to eye level.

I stretch elbows   stretch   stretch   stretch

Guidelines

1. Use a mat on the floor for this task if a plinth is not available.

2. Always count with an even slow tempo and do every step slowly to give the children the experience of each movement and thus help them begin the process of learning.

3. This task is useful to teach the children grasp and release, head in the midline and stretching of the elbows.

4. Children who have difficulty bringing their head into the midline and who cannot stretch their elbows may need gaiters. The children using gaiters can participate in the task by learning to grasp the doll/teddy bear.

5. At this level the use of gaiters to help the children experience straight elbows, head in the midline and stability is necessary for many of them. However, gaiters can be overused and the care-giver should continually monitor when the child is trying to actively initiate a movement and remove the gaiters.

6. The care-giver says every step out loud and if possible encourages the children to speak. She assists them with every step. However, she should decrease assistance if they begin to initiate a movement.

7. Encourage children with visual impairment to participate by asking them to grasp a musical toy.

319

4. Bring the doll/teddy bear to the face and kiss it.   I kiss doll   mm   mm   mm

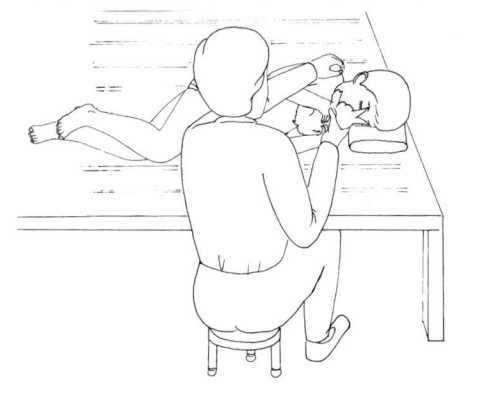

Analysis of Motor Task	*Speech/Songs/Rhymes*	*Guidelines*
1. Bend the top leg.	I bend leg bend bend bend	1. This task helps the children learn to move from one position to another.
		2. The children will need help to bend the top leg and may also need arm gaiters.
		3. Encourage the children to look to the side towards which they are rolling by dangling a toy near the side of the face and making sure they look at it before attempting to roll over.
		4. If some children cannot initiate this movement a slightly tilting surface will encourage them move in the direction of the toy.
2. Look at the toy.	I look at toy look look look	5. The care-giver says every step out loud and if possible encourages the children to speak.
		6. Do not allow the children to release their grasp of the doll/teddy bear while they are rolling over.
3. Roll over.	I roll over roll roll roll	

Stretch your Arms

Stretch your arms and look a-round, look a-round, look a-round.

Stretch your arms and look a-round. Roll right o-ver.

Analysis of Motor Task	Speech/Songs/Rhymes	Guidelines
1. Release the doll/teddy bear.	I release doll 1 2 3 4 5	1. This task helps the children learn to sit/stand/walk straight.

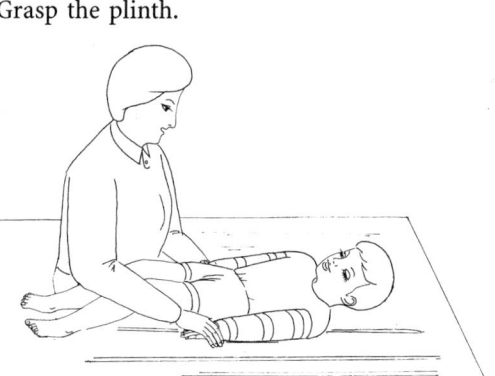

2. It should always be carried out before moving to the next task.

3. If required a small pillow under the head will prevent some children from arching backwards in extension.

4. Encourage the children with asymmetrical tonic neck reflex (ATNR) to bring the head into midline by asking them to look at a toy in the midline position.

5. Always count with an even slow tempo and each step should be carried out slowly giving the children time to experience the movement.

2. Grasp the plinth.

I grasp plinth   grasp grasp grasp

6. The care-giver assists the children who are not using gaiters to stretch their elbows, knees and part their legs.

7. Make sure their toes are pointing outwards and upwards.

8. Children who cannot grasp may need a flexion mitt to help them sustain grasp of the plinth (see Appendix).

3. Part the legs.

I part legs   apart apart apart

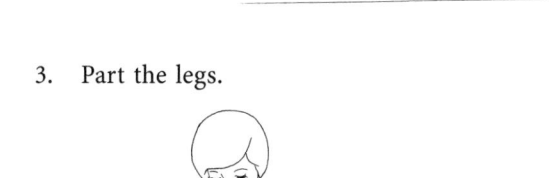

4. Stretch the knees and lie straight.

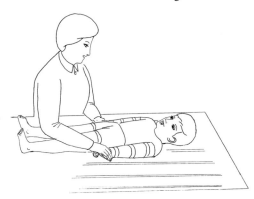

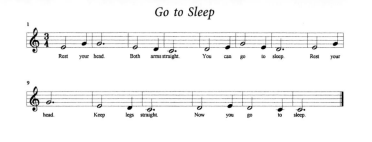

Analysis of Motor Task	*Speech/Songs/Rhymes*	*Guidelines*
1. Look at the stick.	I look at stick look look look	1. This task helps the children learn to stretch at the elbows and shoulder joints.

1. This task helps the children learn to stretch at the elbows and shoulder joints.

2. Motivate them to learn to try and participate by using sticks of different colours. If appropriate invite them to choose a colour.

3. The care-giver assists the child with every step.

4. Always count with an even slow tempo and do every step slowly to give the children the experience of each movement.

5. If some children flex at the hips, allow them to hang their legs over the edge of the plinth with both feet flat on a stool.

2. Grasp the stick.

I grasp stick   grasp grasp grasp

6. Encourage each child to release the stick into the basket when the task is complete.

3. Lower the stick onto the tummy.

Stick on tummy   1 2 3 4 5

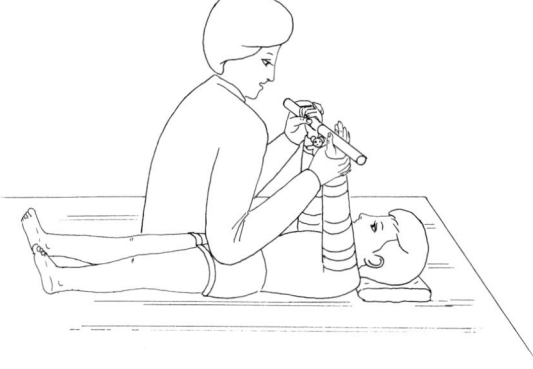

4. Raise the stick.

Stick up   1 2 3 4 5

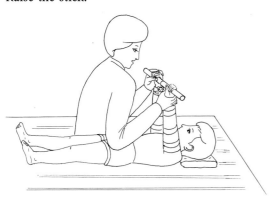

5. Raise the stick above the head. Repeat.

Stick above head   1 2 3 4 5

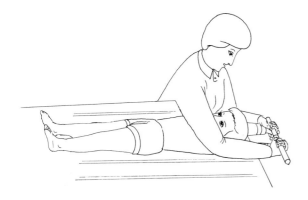

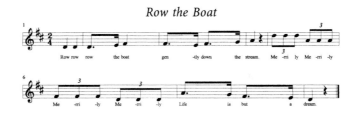

Row the Boat

Row row row the boat gen -tly down the stream. Me -rri ly Me -rri -ly

Me -rri -ly Me -rri -ly Life is but a dream.

6. Release the stick.

I release the stick   release release release

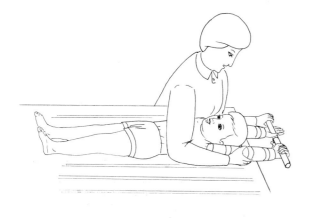

325

Analysis of Motor Task	*Speech/Songs/Rhymes*	*Guidelines*

1. Grasp the plinth.

I grasp plinth   grasp   grasp   grasp

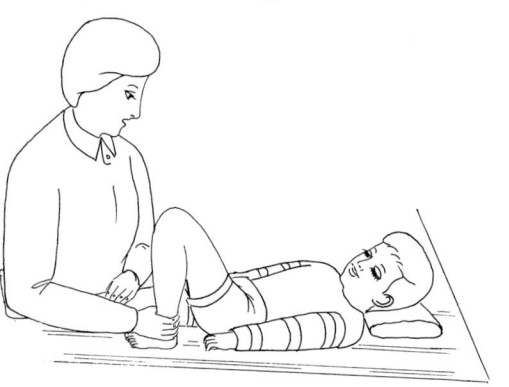

2. Put one foot flat on the plinth.

One foot flat   flat   flat   flat

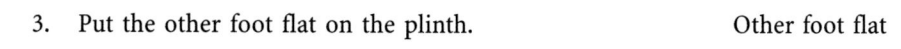

3. Put the other foot flat on the plinth.

Other foot flat   flat   flat   flat

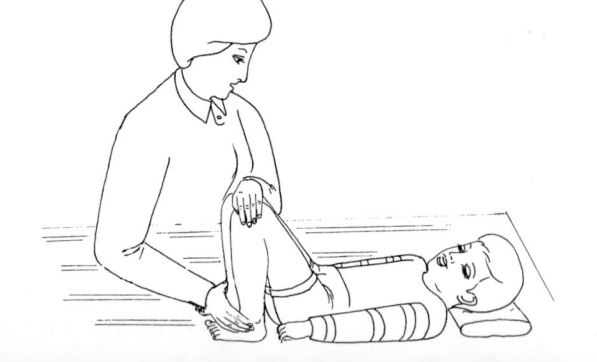

1. This task prepares the children for sitting/standing/ walking training (feet flat) dressing/undressing.

2. The care-giver says every step out loud and if possible encourages them to speak.

3. She will need to assist the child with every step.

4. Make sure the child learns to place his feet directly under his knees. Pressing down gently but firmly on the knees will help the child when attempting to lift up the bottom.

5. Children who cannot grasp the plinth may need flexion mitts to help sustain their grasp (see Appendix).

6. Do not allow the children to arch their back when doing this task.

4. Lift up the bottom.

Lift bottom   up   up   up

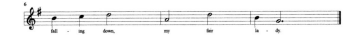

London Bridge is Falling Down

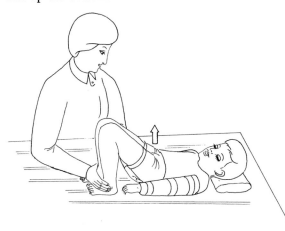

Lon - don Bridge is fall - ing down, fall - ing down, fall - ing down. Lon - don Bridge is

fall - ing down, my fair la - dy.

Analysis of Motor Task	*Speech/Songs/Rhymes*	*Guidelines*

1. Arms above the head.

Hands above head   up up up

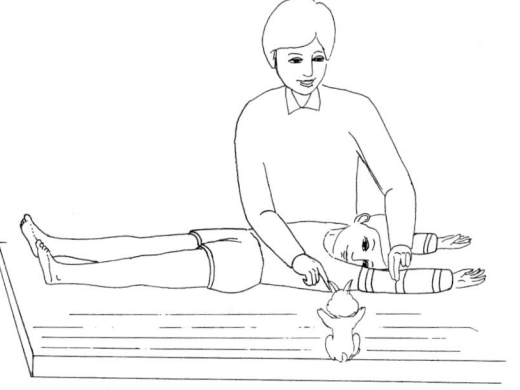

1. This task is important and at this level may be the only means of mobility for the children. They should be given every opportunity to practise it.

2. It helps them learn to move from one position to another and prepares them for getting in and out of bed.

3. They may need arm gaiters to stretch the elbows and raise the arms above the head.

4. They will need help with every step.

5. Make sure that the children turn their heads to look at the toy to facilitate them to roll in that direction.

6. The care-giver says every step out loud and if possible encourages them to speak.

7. To encourage the children learn to roll independently this task can also be practised on a mat on the floor.

8. If a child cannot initiate any movement a slightly tilting surface will encourage him move in the direction of the toy.

2. Look at the toy.

I look at toy   look look look

3. Bend the top leg.

I bend leg   1 2 3 4 5

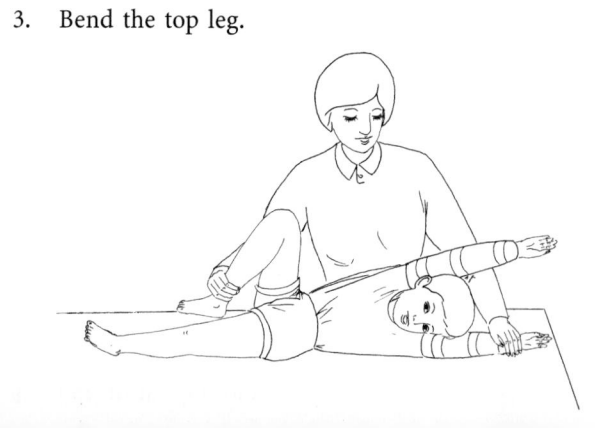

4. Roll over.

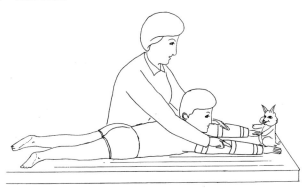

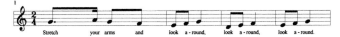

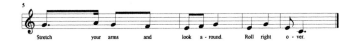

Analysis of Motor Task	*Speech/Songs/Rhymes*	*Guidelines*

1. Put on long leg gaiters (see Appendix) and take off arm gaiters. Grasp the plinth.

I grasp plinth   grasp grasp grasp

1. This task is useful to train head control/hip extension/wrist extension.

2. The care-giver says every step out loud and if possible encourages the children to speak.

3. Children who find it difficult to tolerate the position may need to have a folded towel placed under the chest to help them.

4. During the duration of the task encourage the children to lift up their head. At this level they will need strong stimulation to encourage them to sustain the position.

5. Do not allow the children to excessively extend backwards while in this position.

6. Make sure the childrens' feet are apart. Use a pillow between the knees to help those who cannot keep their feet apart.

2. Push up on hands.

I push up   push push push

3. Lift up the head and look at care-giver/toy.

I look at toy   look look look

Analysis of Motor Task	*Speech/Songs/Rhymes*	*Guidelines*
1. Put on arm gaiters. Look at the toy.	I look at toy look look look	1. This task is important to teach the children learn to move from one point to another. It also prepares them to get in and out of bed.
2. Part the right hand and grasp the plinth.	I part hand, grasp grasp grasp grasp	2. The care-giver says every step out loud and if possible encourages the children to speak. She will have to assist them with every step.
3. Part the left leg.	I part leg apart apart apart	3. Encourage the child to reach out and push the toy/ball a little or push the ball onto the floor. The sound of the ball bouncing off the floor will give him positive feed-back.
		4. Make sure the child raises his head and grasps the plinth before moving his body around on the plinth.

331

4. Put the left hand together with the right and grasp the plinth.

Left hand together   together   together   together

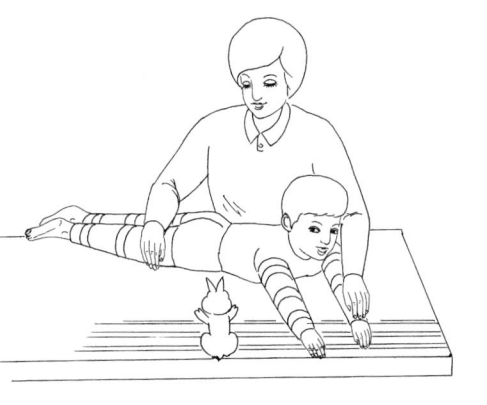

5. Put the right leg together with the left.

Left leg together   together   together   together

Lie on my Tummy

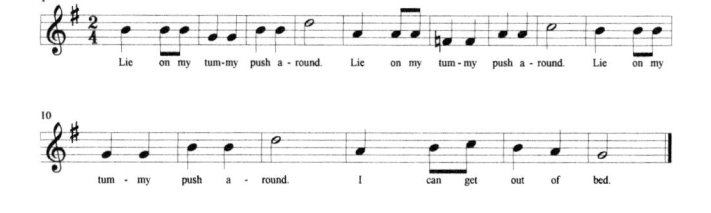

Lie on my tum-my push a - round. Lie on my tum-my push a - round. Lie on my

tum - my push a - round. I can get out of bed.

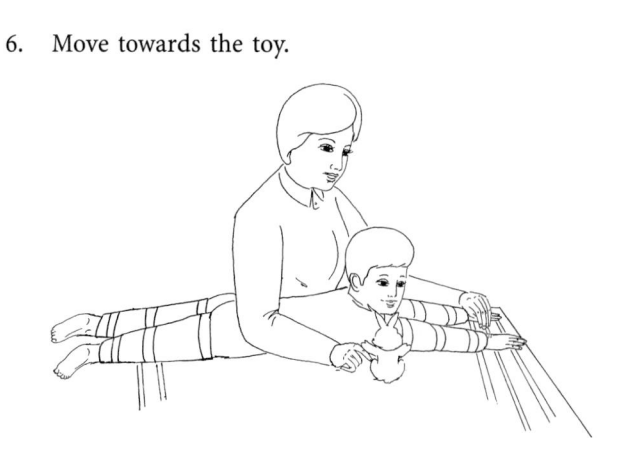

6. Move towards the toy.

I reach for toy   stretch   stretch   stretch

Analysis of Motor Task	*Speech/Songs/Rhymes*	*Guidelines*

1. Take off arm gaiters and put hands under the shoulders.

Hands under shoulders   1 2 3 4 5

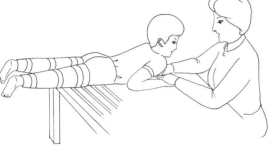

1. This task is useful to facilitate children who cannot stretch their elbows to experience straight elbows. Gravity and the weight of the child's body as he learns to push off the plinth automatically stretches the elbows.

2. This task is also a preparation for standing/walking training as it helps the children learn to put their feet flat on the floor, stretch their knees and part their legs. It also prepares them to push off the bed.

3. The care-giver says every step out loud and if possible encourages them to speak.

4. She assists the children with every step.

2. Grasp the plinth.

I grasp plinth   grasp grasp grasp

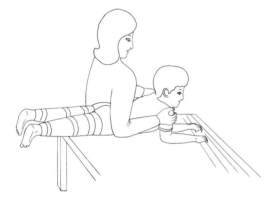

5. Children who have poor weight bearing will need long leg gaiters when standing grasping the plinth. This will also help to extend the knees (see Appendix).

6. Some children may also need arm gaiters to extend the elbows and for stability in the standing position.

7. If a child cannot initiate the movement tilting the plinth slightly will help him learn the sensation of pushing off the plinth. However, be careful when doing this movement.

3. Push off.

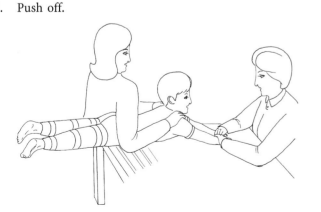

Push of Plinth

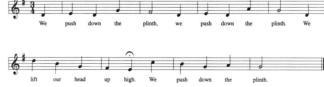

We push down the plinth, we push down the plinth. We

lift our head up high. We push down the plinth.

4. Feet flat on the floor.

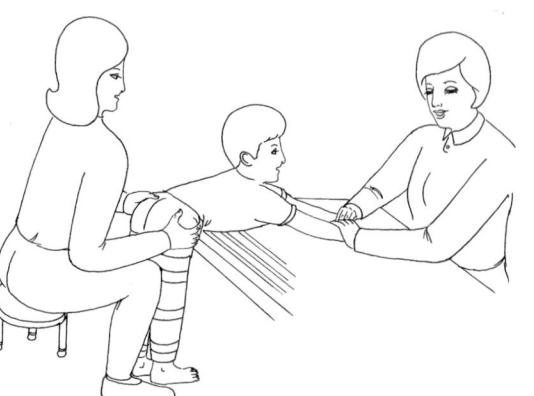

5. Standing task.

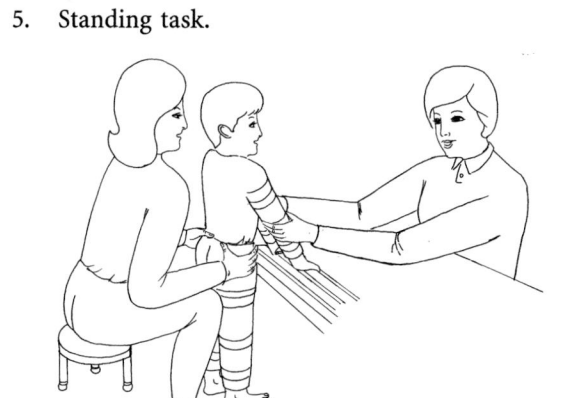

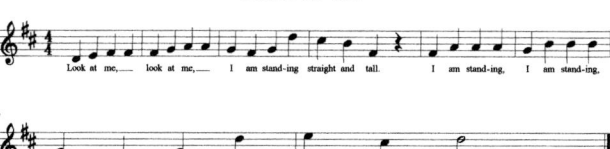

Look at me

Look at me,___ look at me,___ I am stand-ing straight and tall. I am stand-ing, I am stand-ing,

I am stand - ing straight and tall.

TASK 1: SITTING ON STOOL/CHAIR WITH SUPPORT GRASPING THE LADDERBACK CHAIR

TASK 2: SITTING ON STOOL/CHAIR WITH SUPPORT GRASPING THE LADDERBACK CHAIR

TASK 3: CLIMBING UP THE LADDERBACK CHAIR IN THE SITTING POSITION

TASK 4: CLIMBING DOWN THE LADDERBACK CHAIR IN THE SITTING POSITION

TASK 5: TRANSFER FROM SITTING TO STANDING USING THE LADDERBACK CHAIR

Analysis of Motor Task	*Speech/Songs/Rhymes*	*Guidelines*
1. Grasp the rung of the ladderback chair.	I grasp rung grasp grasp grasp	1. In order to clarify the illustrated steps in this task the drawing of the ladderback chair has been simplified.

1. In order to clarify the illustrated steps in this task the drawing of the ladderback chair has been simplified.

2. It is important from the outset the children learn to sit well. They will need this position for many activities of daily living, e.g., play/eating/drinking/grooming/transferring from one position to another/attending class etc.

3. At this level the child may need a chair with sides as well as back supports. The chair/stool should be of a suitable height whereby the child can place his feet firmly on the floor.

3. The child may need gaiters to stretch his elbows and for stability. He may also need ankle straps and thigh straps to help him fixate his feet and thighs, part his knees and give him a good sitting base. The straps will also prevent him pushing himself off the chair at the beginning when he is learning to sit.

4. The care-giver helps the child with every step and at this level may need to help the child sustain his grasp of the rung of the chair. She says every step out loud and if possible encourages the child to speak.

5. Encourage the child to look at the toy to help him learn to sit up straight.

6. If the child is learning to sit on a stool he may still need ankle and thigh straps for fixation.

2. Feet flat.

Feet flat   1   2

3. Feet apart.

Feet apart   apart   apart   apart

4. Push the bottom back.

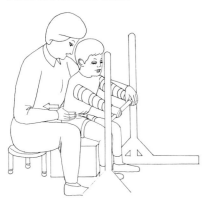

Bottom back   1   2

5. Back straight.

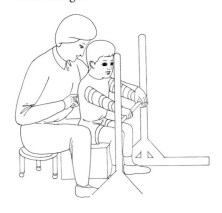

Back straight   straight   straight   straight

6. Sit straight.

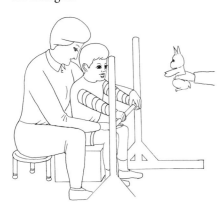

Sit up Straight

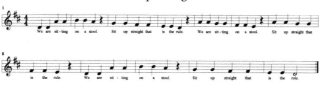

Analysis of Motor Task	*Speech/Songs/Rhymes*	*Guidelines*
1. Look at the toy.	I look at toy look look look	1. This task teaches the children grasp and release, stretching the elbows, moving one part of the body while fixing another part, trunk balance in the sitting position.
		2. Use brightly coloured skittles to encourage the children to look in the midline.
		3. The care-giver says every step out loud and if possible encourages them to speak. She may need to help them with every step.
		4. Some children may need gaiters to stretch the elbows. However do not over use them if possible. The children should actively experience extending and flexing their elbows.
2. Push the ladderback chair forward.	I push chair push push push	5. Children who cannot maintain the sitting position and who push themselves repeatedly out of the chair when doing an activity/game should be fixated with thigh straps and ankle straps (see Part C, Task 15, Level 1).
		6. Give the children sufficient time to experience each step.
3. Pull back the ladderback chair. Repeat.	I pull chair pull pull pull	

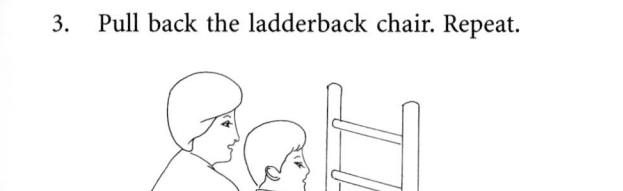

Analysis of Motor Task	*Speech/Songs/Rhymes*	*Guidelines*

1. Both hands climb up the ladderback chair.

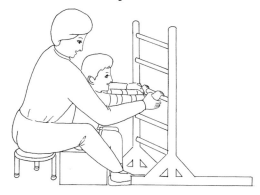

I climb up/down

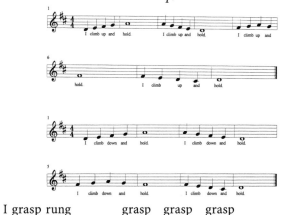

I climb up and hold. I climb up and hold. I climb up and
hold. I climb up and hold.
I climb down and hold. I climb down and hold.
I climb down and hold. I climb down and hold.

2. Grasp the rungs.

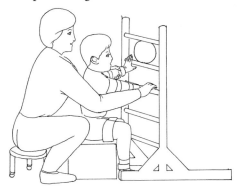

I grasp rung   grasp grasp grasp

3. Release one hand.

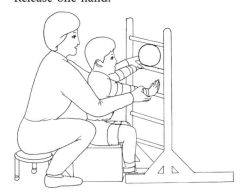

I release hand   release release release

1. This task teaches the children grasp and release stretching the elbows and extension at the wrist.

2. Use a brightly coloured ball to encourage the children bring their head into the midline.

3. Make sure the children are sitting well before attempting this task. Encourage the children in the sitting position to keep their back straight.

4. The care-giver says every step out loud and if possible encourages them to speak. She may also need to help the children with each step.

5. Give the children sufficient time to experience each step, and use a slow even tempo.

6. Make sure the children's hands are open with fingers extended when they are learning to push the ball.

7. Use a musical ball for children who are visually impaired.

8. The sound of the ball bouncing off the floor will give positive feedback to the children and encourage them to repeat the game.

4. Push the ball.

I push ball   push push push

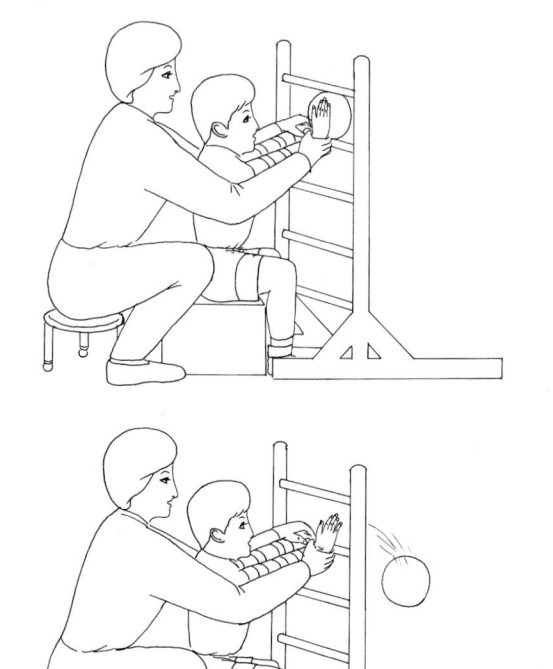

5. Repeat with the other hand.

Analysis of Motor Task	*Speech/Songs/Rhymes*	*Guidelines*

1. Both hands climb down the ladderback chair.

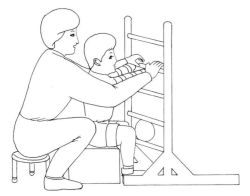

I climb up/down

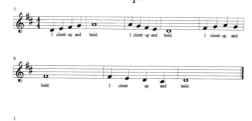

1. This task teaches the children trunk balance in the sitting position. It also helps the children learn to move one part of the body while fixing another part.

2. The care-giver says every step out loud and if possible encourages the children to speak.

3. Give the children sufficient time to experience each step.

4. Make sure the children learn to look at the ball before attempting to push it onto the floor.

5. Help the children push the ball with open hand and extended fingers.

6. Make sure the children maintain good sitting posture while doing the movement.

2. Release one hand.

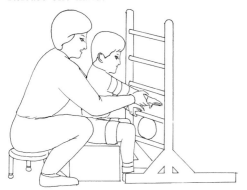

I release hand   release release release

3. Grasp the rung.

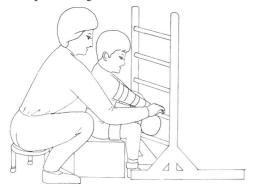

I grasp rung   grasp grasp grasp

4. Push the ball.

I push ball   push push push

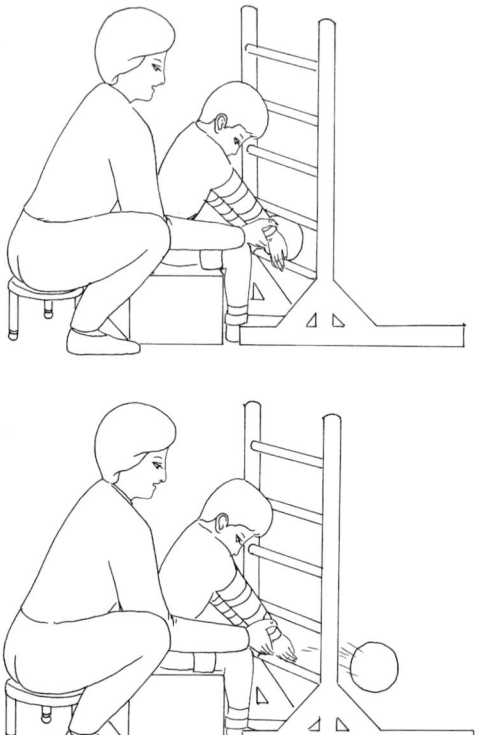

5. Hands climb up to middle rung.

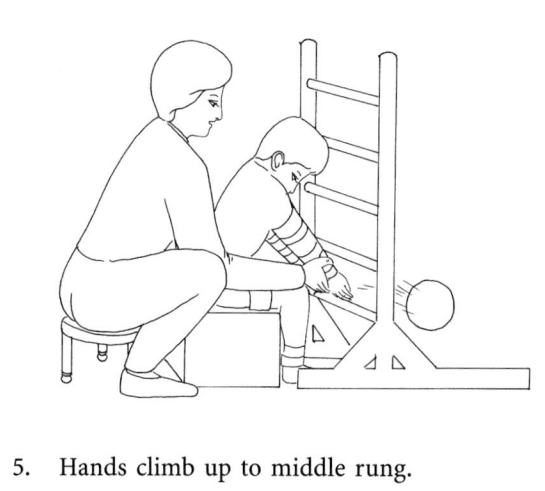

I climb up/down

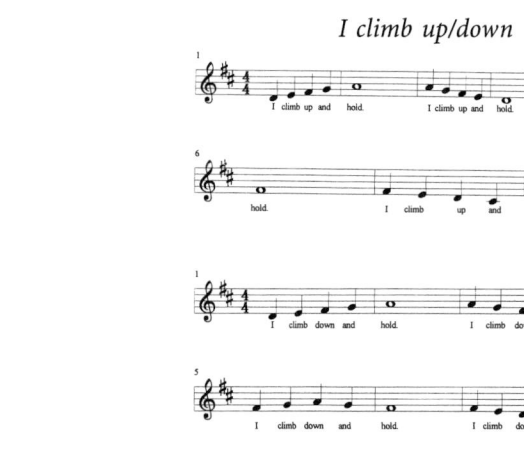

Analysis of Motor Task	*Speech/Songs/Rhymes*	*Guidelines*

1. Grasp the ladderback chair.

I grasp chair   grasp   grasp   grasp

2. Push the ladderback chair forward.

I push chair   push   push   push

3. Look at the feet and stand up slowly.

I stand up   1   2   3   4   5

1. The children should never be picked up from sitting but should be given the opportunity to learn to stand up from sitting to standing.

2. Children at this level will need gaiters to stretch the elbows and for stability.

3. Two care-givers will need to help the child, one care-giver supports the child from behind and helps the child stand up. The second care-giver supports the child in front making sure the child sustains grasp of the rung as they stand up. Depending on the ability of the child she may need to facilitate him at the shoulders/arms for greater stability.

4. Some children may need long leg gaiters to help them learn to weight bear.

5. Make sure the children's body weight is over the feet before they attempt the movement.

6. The care-givers help the children to maintain good standing with feet flat and apart, knees, hips and back straight and head in the midline. Make sure the children's weights fall through their bodies and not behind their feet.

7. To help the children experience the standing position for a period of time the care-giver should engage them in a game/activity to hold their interest and encourage them to look in the midline.

4. Both hands climb up the ladderback chair.

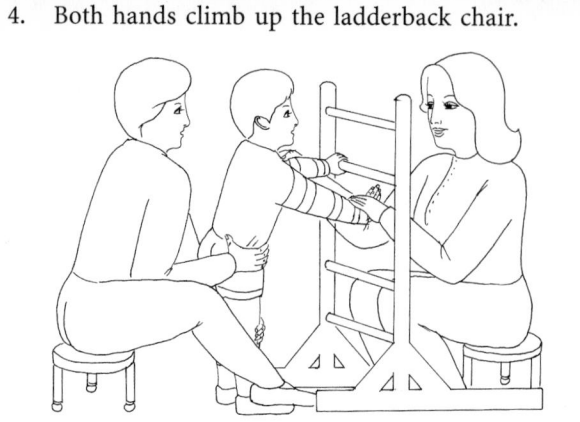

I climb up/down

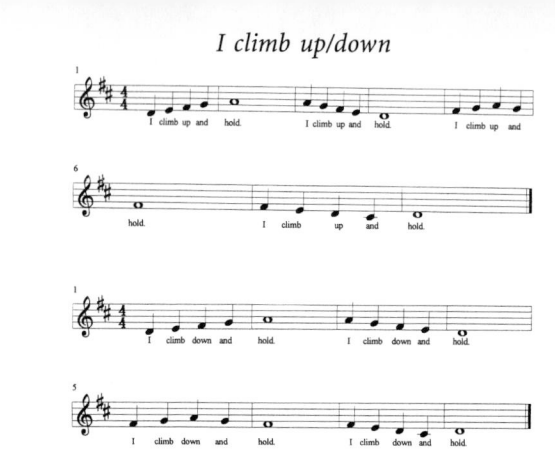

5. Standing task (see Chapter 11, Task 19, Level 1).

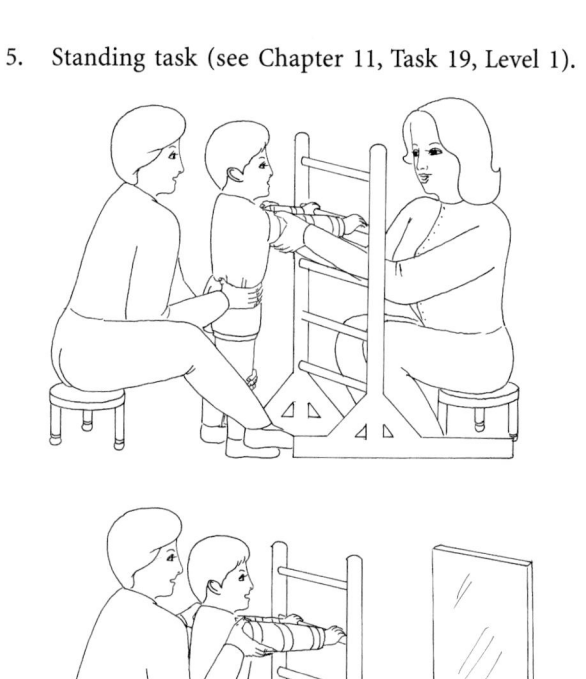

Look at me

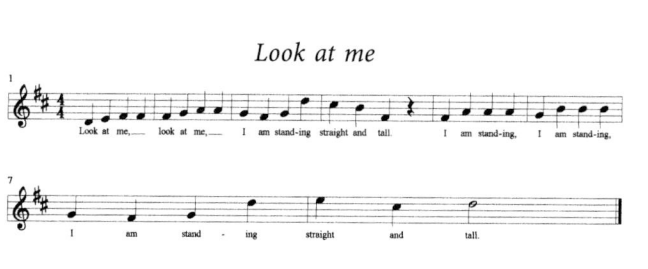

TASK 1: ROLL CALL IN THE SITTING POSITION

TASK 2: FLAT HANDS WITH EXTENDED FINGERS

TASK 3: PUSHING A BALL USING A STICK IN THE SITTING POSITION

TASK 4: RAISING THE ARMS GRASPING A STICK IN THE SITTING POSITION

TASK 5: CLASPING THE HANDS IN THE MIDLINE IN THE SITTING POSITION

Analysis of Motor Task	*Speech/Songs/Rhymes*	*Guidelines*

1. Sitting task (see Chapter 10, Task 18, Level 1).

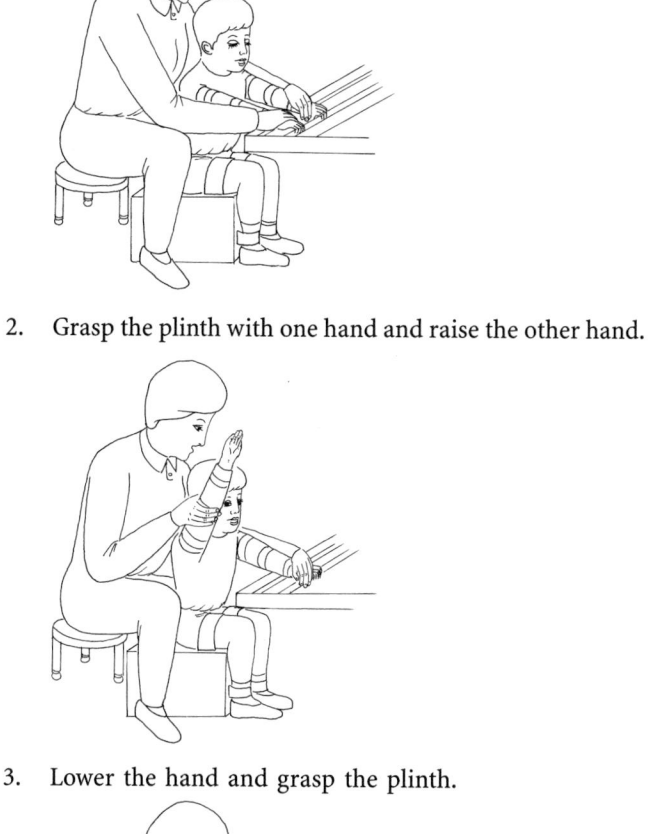

Sit up Straight

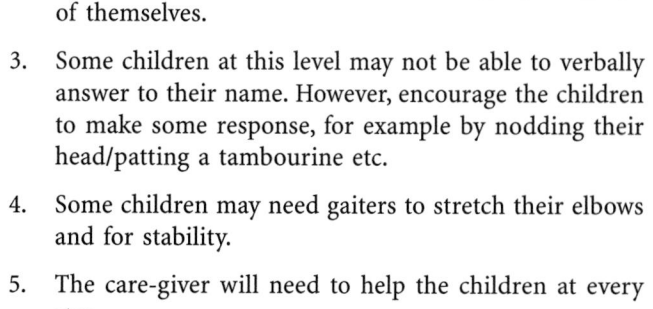

1. This task prepares the children for socialisation and for many activities of daily living as they learn the importance of one hand fixing, one hand moving.

2. Facilitate the children's participation by inviting them to look in the mirror/show them an enlarged photograph of themselves.

3. Some children at this level may not be able to verbally answer to their name. However, encourage the children to make some response, for example by nodding their head/patting a tambourine etc.

4. Some children may need gaiters to stretch their elbows and for stability.

2. Grasp the plinth with one hand and raise the other hand.

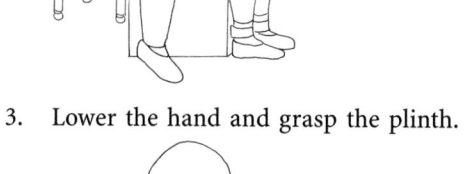

I raise hand   up up up
I am here

5. The care-giver will need to help the children at every step.

6. Give the children sufficient time to try and respond to roll call.

7. Make sure the children are sitting well at all times during the task.

3. Lower the hand and grasp the plinth.

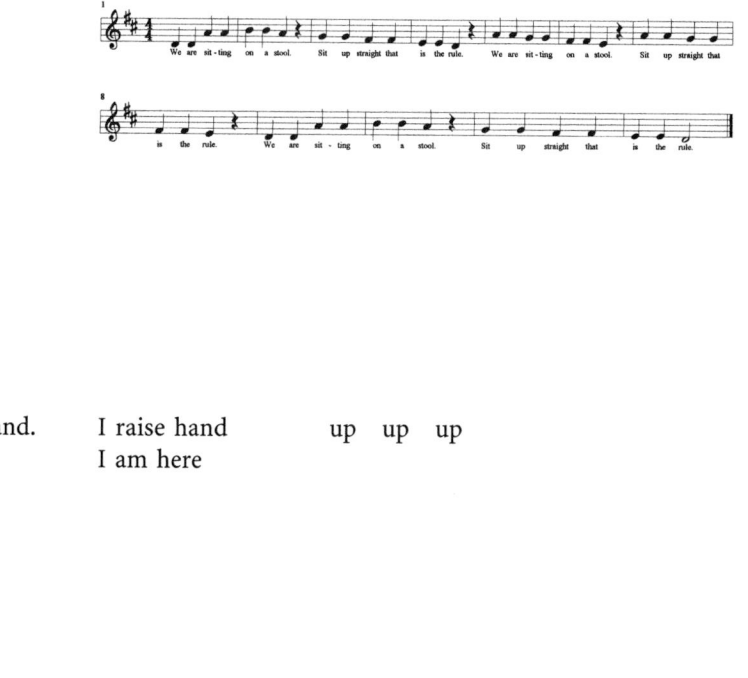

I grasp plinth   grasp grasp grasp

4. Repeat with the other hand.

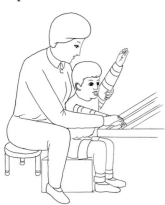

I raise hand   up   up   up
I am here

Analysis of Motor Task	*Speech/Songs/Rhymes*	*Guidelines*

1. Look at the hands.

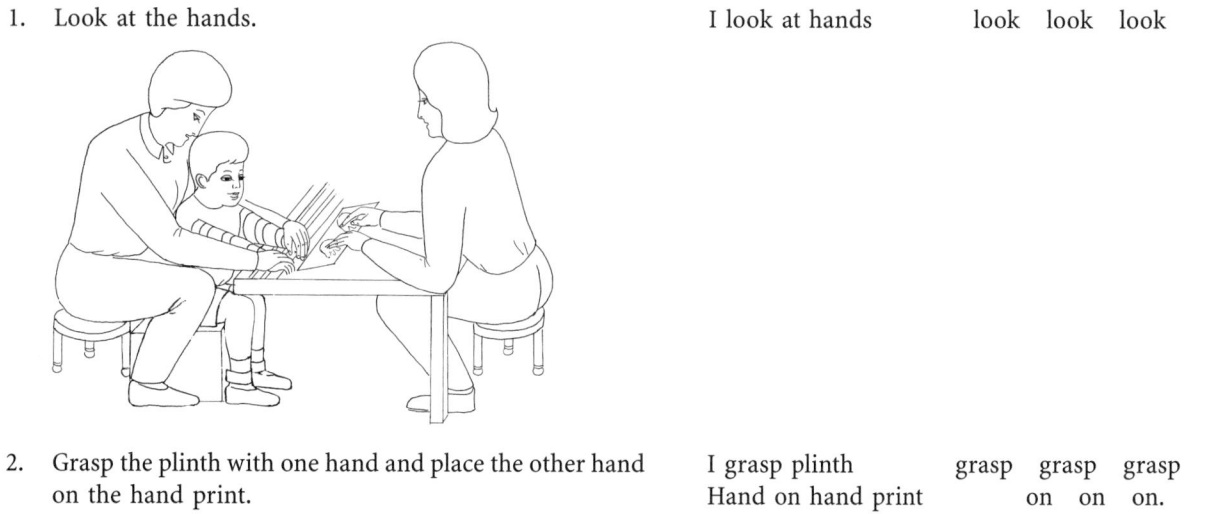

2. Grasp the plinth with one hand and place the other hand on the hand print.

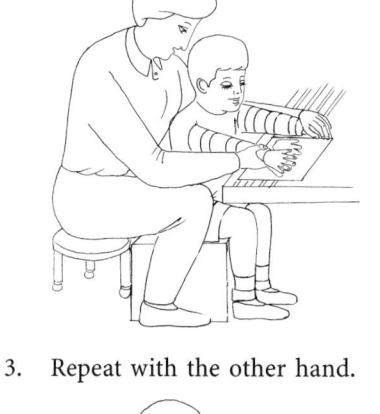

3. Repeat with the other hand.

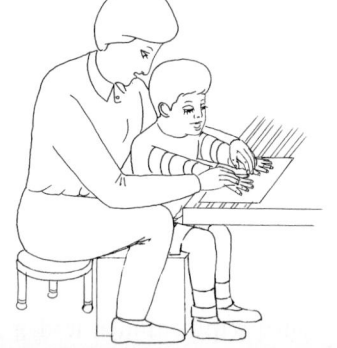

I look at hands   look   look   look

I grasp plinth   grasp   grasp   grasp
Hand on hand print   on   on   on.

Ten Little Fingers

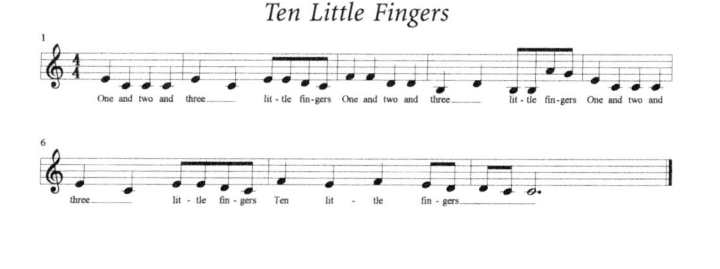

One and two and three___ lit-tle fin-gers One and two and three___ lit-tle fin-gers One and two and

three___ lit-tle fin-gers Ten lit-tle fin-gers

Ten Little Fingers

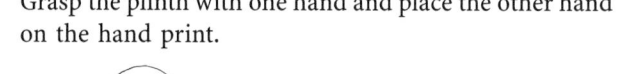

One and two and three___ lit-tle fin-gers One and two and three___ lit-tle fin-gers One and two and

three___ lit-tle fin-gers Ten lit-tle fin-gers___

1. This task is useful to teach the children flat hands, fixing one hand while moving the other, and prepares them for many activities of daily living.

2. Some children may need gaiters to stretch the elbows and for stability. However continually assess the situation and remove the gaiters if the child initiates a movement.

3. Use a song with a strong rhythm for this task.

4. The care-giver will need to help the child with each step and make sure they learn to separate the movement of each hand.

5. Give them sufficient time to do each step.

6. Make sure the children's fingers are extended when patting on the prints/plinth/table.

7. It is important that the children look at what they are doing.

4. Pat on the hand print.

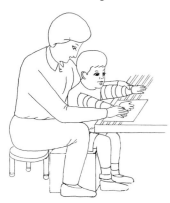

Pit-a-pat-a-pit-a-pat

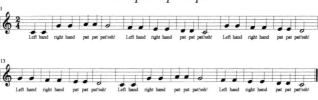

5. Grasp the plinth with one hand.

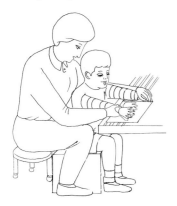

I grasp plinth   grasp grasp grasp

6. Repeat with the other hand.

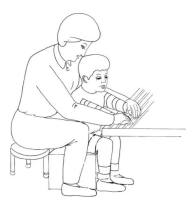

I grasp plinth   grasp grasp grasp

Analysis of Motor Task	*Speech/Songs/Rhymes*	*Guidelines*
1. Look at the stick.	I look at stick look look look	1. This task helps the children learn grasp and release and stretching the elbows. It prepares them for many activities of daily living.

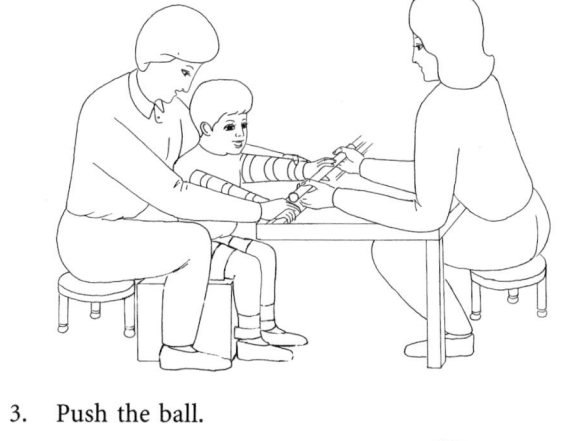

2. Different coloured sticks and brightly coloured balls will encourage the children to try and actively participate. The care-giver invites the children to learn to grasp the stick and take it out of the basket. Use a musical ball for children with visual impairment.

3. Some children may need gaiters to stretch the elbows and for stability.

2. Grasp the stick.

I grasp stick   grasp grasp grasp

4. The care-giver says every step out loud and if possible encourages the children to speak. She may need to help the children with every step.

5. Make sure the thumb is out when the children are grasping the stick.

6. Always make sure the children maintain a good sitting posture when carrying out the task.

3. Push the ball.

I push ball   push push push

4. Repeat.

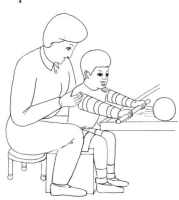

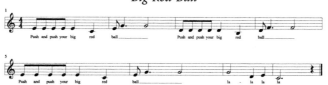

Analysis of Motor Task	*Speech/Songs/Rhymes*	*Guidelines*
1. Look at the stick. 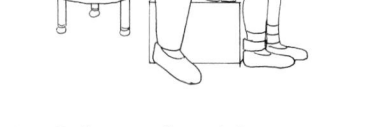	I look at stick look look look	1. This task also helps the children to learn grasp and release and prepares them for many activities of daily living. This task may also improve the children's breathing.
		2. Use different coloured sticks and invite the children to grasp the stick and take it out of the basket.
		3. Some children may need gaiters to stretch the elbows and for stability.
		4. Always use a slow even tempo when doing each step. This helps children with spasticity relax.
		5. The care-giver says every step out loud and if possible encourages them to speak. She may also need to help the child with each step.
2. Grasp the stick.	I grasp stick grasp grasp grasp	6. As the children lower the stick ask them to expel air by saying "aaa/uu".
		7. Make sure the children who are not using gaiters learn to stretch their elbows.
		8. Also make sure the children grasp the stick with the thumb out, when raising the stick.
3. Raise up the stick. 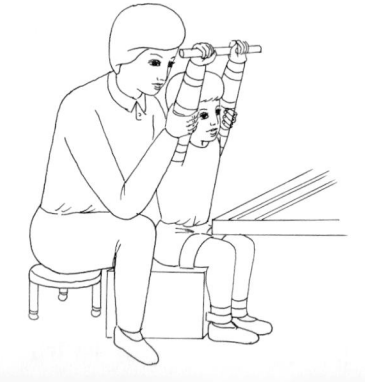	Stick up up up up	

4. Put the stick down on the plinth.

Stick down   down down down

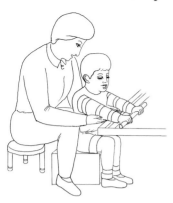

5. Repeat.

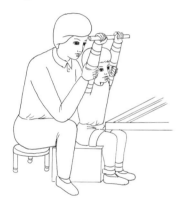

Row the Boat

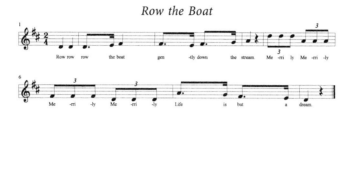

6. Put stick into the basket.

I release stick   release release release

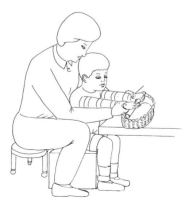

Task 5 Hand Task Series: *Clasping the Hands in the Midline in the Sitting Position (Suggested Game: Rubbing Cream on the Hands)*

Analysis of Motor Task	*Speech/Songs/Rhymes*	*Guidelines*

1. Look at the cream.

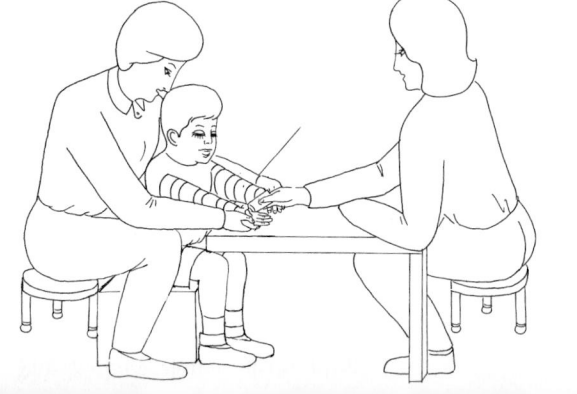

I look at cream   look   look   look

1. This task is useful to teach the children to clasp their hands and helps the children with ATNR to learn to bring the head into the midline.

2. Children who cannot bring their hands to the midline to rub in the cream may hold a doll and look at it.

3. The care-giver says every step out loud and if possible encourages the children to speak.

4. She will need to help the children stretch the elbow with the palm facing upwards.

5. Make sure the children look at their hands as they rub in the cream.

6. Help the children bring the clasped hands to their nose to smell the cream. Learning to bring their hands to their face prepares them for eating/drinking/grooming.

2. Stretch the elbows and hold the hand with the palm up.

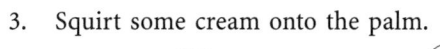

I stretch hand   stretch   stretch   stretch

3. Squirt some cream onto the palm.

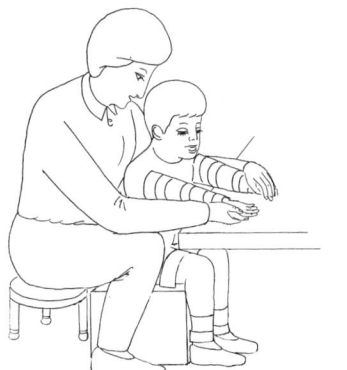

4. Rub in the cream.　　　　　　　　　　　I rub hands　　　rub　rub　rub

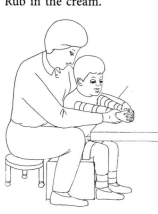

5. Bend the elbows and bring the hands to the nose. Both　　I bend elbows　　bend　bend　bend
   elbows rest on the plinth.

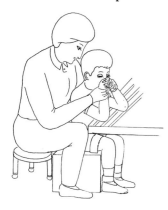

6. Grasp the plinth.　　　　　　　　　　　I grasp plinth　　grasp　grasp　grasp

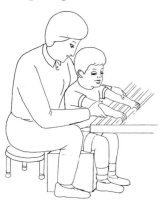

Chapter 16

Groups at Levels 2–4

- LYING TASK SERIES
  (TASKS 1—25)

- SITTING TO STANDING AND WALKING TASK SERIES
  (TASKS 1—19B)

- HAND TASK SERIES
  (TASKS 1—9)

Analysis of Motor Task	*Speech/Songs/Rhymes*	*Guidelines*

1. Both hands grasp the plinth.

I grasp the plinth   1 2 3 4 5

1. Many tasks in this series may be carried out on a mat on the floor, however in order to teach the children functional activities the plinth is a valuable teaching aid.

2. When using speech the care-giver should employ a slow even tempo, this is particularly important for children with spasticity.

3. When doing the steps, children with athethosis should learn to hold, fixate and maintain the position. This is crucial in order to help them function in daily life.

4. If possible and depending on the temperature of the room it is preferable if the children take off their shoes and socks for this task series.

2. Stretch the elbows.

I stretch my elbows   1 2 3 4 5

5. Motivate the children with games and play to encourage them to participate actively.

6. Children at level 2 should try to learn to stretch their elbows without gaiters. However, they may still need ankle straps and thigh straps for fixation while sitting on the stool. Children at level 3 should learn to keep their feet flat and apart with minimal help. Children at level 4 should learn to sit independently.

7. At level 2 the children may need help to stretch their elbows. However, they should be able to grasp the plinth.

8. Always encourage the children to stretch their elbows to facilitate them when learning to sit up straight.

3. Feet flat.

My feet are flat   1 2

9. Give the children sufficient time to do each step and encourage them at all times to use speech to guide their movements.

4. Feet apart.

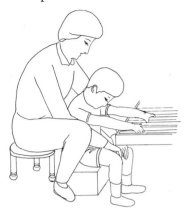

My feet are apart   1 2 3 4 5

5. Bottom back.

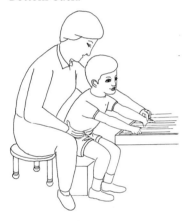

I push my bottom back   1 2

6. Sit up straight.

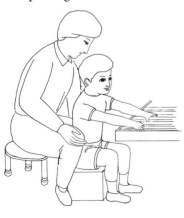

Sit up Straight

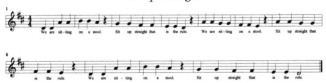

We are sit-ting on a stool. Sit up straight that is the rule. We are sit-ting on a stool. Sit up straight that is the rule. We are sit-ting on a stool. Sit up straight that is the rule.

Analysis of Motor Task	*Speech/Songs/Rhymes*	*Guidelines*

1. Both hands grasp the edge of the plinth.

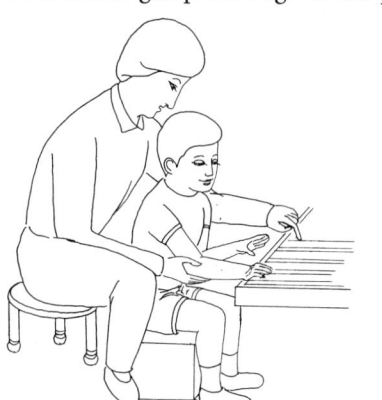

I put my hands at edge of the plinth   1 2 3 4 5

2. Push the plinth forward.

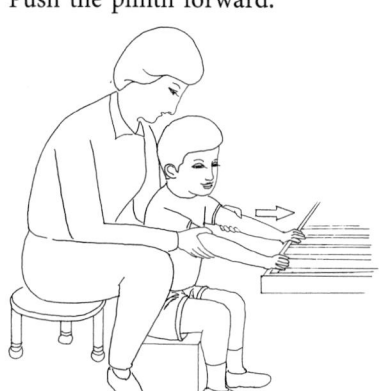

I push the plinth   push   push   push

3. Grasp the slats of the plinth.

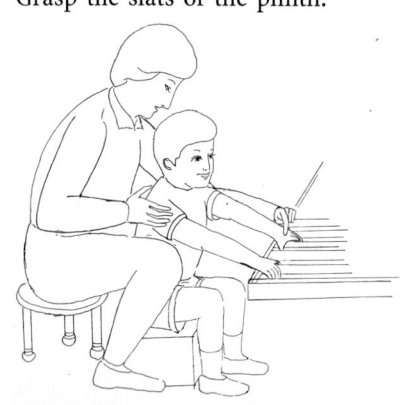

I grasp the slats   1 2 3 4 5

Guidelines

1. Some children may need help to push the plinth forward. Make sure the children's wrists are correctly extended when pushing the plinth. This is important and helps prevent some children from developing wrist deformity at a later stage.

2. Make sure the children's body weight is over their feet before they attempt to stand up.

3. Facilitate children at level 2 who are unable to initiate lifting up their bottom by pressing down firmly on their knees. However, if the child attempts to do the movement remove assistance and encourage them to finish the step.

4. The care-giver may need to help the children at level 2 sustain their grasp as they stand up. She may also need to stabilize the feet by pressing on them gently but firmly with her feet.

5. Children at level 3 may need some help. However, children at level 4 should learn to stand up clasping the hands/quoit/horizontal stick.

4. Look at the feet.

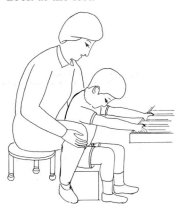

I look at my feet   look look look

5. Lift the bottom up.

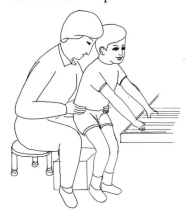

I lift my bottom up   1 2 3 4 5

6. Stand up.

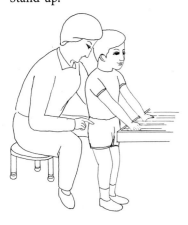

I stand up   1 2 3 4 5

Analysis of Motor Task	*Speech/Songs/Rhymes*	*Guidelines*

1. Grasp the plinth.

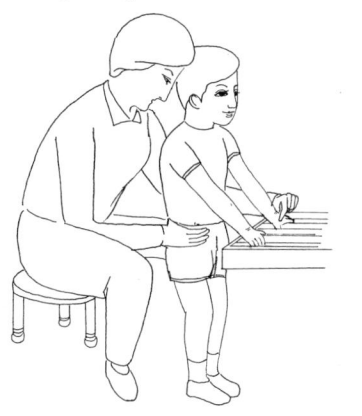

I grasp the plinth   1   2   3   4   5

1. The standing straight task should always be carried out whenever the children move from one position to another where standing is required. The care-giver should encourage the children to stand at every opportunity. This task prepares the children for walking training.

2. Children at level 2 may need gaiters to stretch the elbows and for stability. The gaiters should be put on before the child stands up. They will also need help to stretch the knees and keep the feet flat on the floor.

3. Make sure the children at level 3 and 4 have their heels flat on the floor, legs well parted and knees and back straight. Children at level 3 may need some help to stretch their knees and keep their feet flat. The care-giver may need to fixate the child's feet with her feet. Children at level 4 should learn to do this task independently.

4. Always encourage the children to stretch the elbows in order to learn to stand up straight.

5. Make sure the children's body weight falls through or in front of their feet. Do not allow the children to pull backwards when standing.

6. The plinth should be at the correct height to help the children stand straight (see Appendix).

7. In this position the children are ready to attend roll call.

2. Feet flat.

My feet are flat   1   2

3. Feet apart.

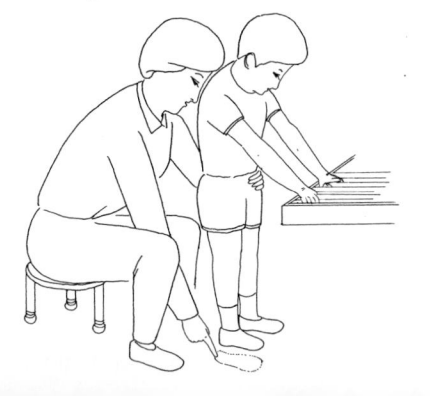

My feet are apart   1   2   3   4   5

4. Stretch the knees.

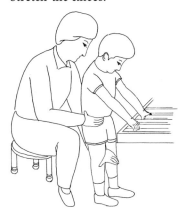

I stretch my knees   1 2 3 4 5

5. Stretch the elbows.

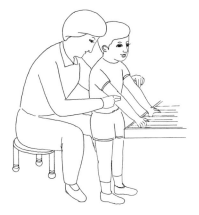

I stretch my elbows   1 2 3 4 5

6. Stand up straight.

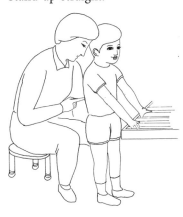

My back is straight   1 2 3 4 5

Stand up Tall

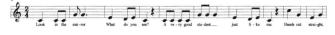

Look in the mir-ror What do you see? A ve-ry good stu-dent___ just li-ke me. Hands out strai-ght,

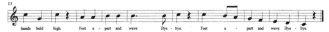

hands held high. Feet a-part and wave Bye-bye. Feet a-part and wave Bye-bye.

Analysis of Motor Task	*Speech/Songs/Rhymes*	*Guidelines*
1. Look at the care-giver.	I look at care-giver　　look　look　look	1. When doing this task the children learn to stretch at the elbows and shoulders and also learn to balance in preparation for free standing and walking training.

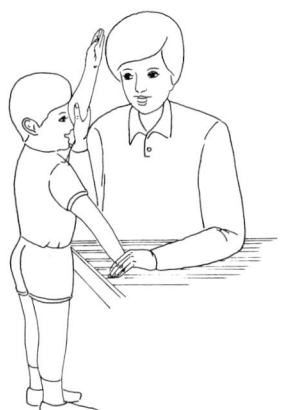

2. Motivate the children to actively participate by inviting them in turn to take roll call. This gives the children the opportunity to become more familiar with one another and learn one another's names.

3. Children at level 2 may need help both to maintain their grasp with one hand while raising the other hand high. Children at level 3 may also need help, children at level 4 should learn to do the task independently.

4. Give the children sufficient time to do the task. Do not over assist them and always ensure correct posture while in the standing position.

2. Raise one hand high answer to name.　　I raise my hand high　　1　2　3　4　5

Analysis of Motor Task	Speech/Songs/Rhymes	Guidelines

1. Slide the hands forward and grasp the plinth.

I slide my hands forward   1   2

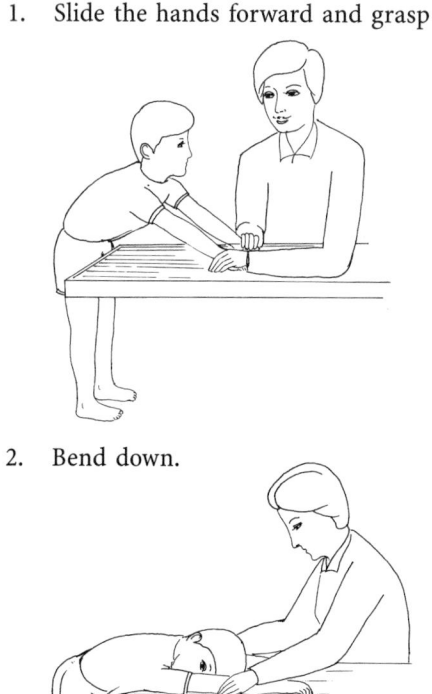

2. Bend down.

I bend down   1   2   3   4   5

3. Lift up the head and look at the toy.

I look at toy   look   look   look

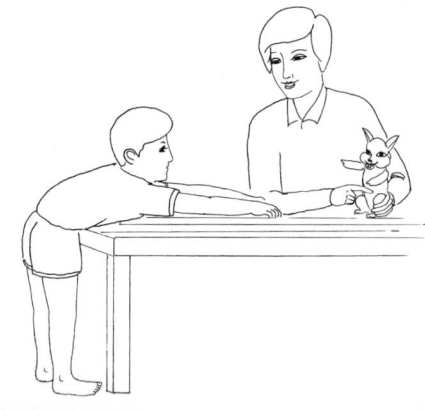

1. Many children do not like the prone position but it is important the children learn to move from one point to another.

2. This task teaches children with hemiplegia to use both hands simultaneously. It also teaches the children mid-line orientation, and how to get into bed.

3. Motivate the children to reach out and move by asking them to reach for their favourite toy. The toy should be brightly coloured and musical if possible. This is necessary for children with visual impairment.

4. Before pulling up allow the children to drop their feet over the edge of the plinth to help them dorsi-flex at the ankles. Gravity will assist this movement.

5. Make sure the children at levels 3 and 4 grasp the plinth with straight elbows before attempting to pull up. Children at levels 2 and 3 will need help to maintain their grasp while pulling up otherwise the exertion the child uses when trying to pull up may pull the shoulders backwards into extension.

6. It is important the children have their head raised and are looking at the goal (toy) when pulling up. Do not allow the children to over-extend when doing this movement.

7. Children at level 2 may need a pillow between the legs to help keep them apart. Children at levels 3 and 4 should learn to actively part their legs when pulling up.

8. Help children who cannot extend their hips by placing a sandbag over the buttocks or use gentle manual pressure. However, encourage the children to gradually learn to extend their hips.

4. Feet apart.

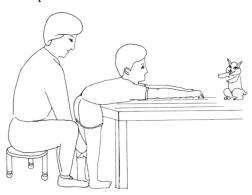

My feet are apart   1 2 3 4 5

5. Pull onto the plinth.

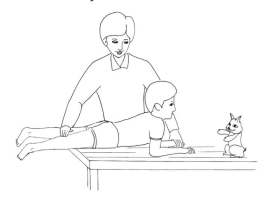

I pull up   1 2 3 4 5

6. Stretch the elbows, grasp the slats and pull up. Repeat.

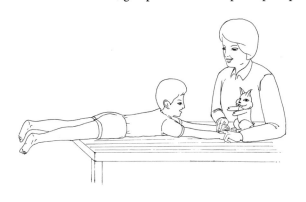

Hold on Tight

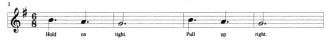

Hold on tight. Pull up right.

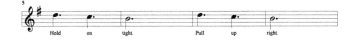

Hold on tight. Pull up right.

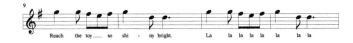

Reach the toy so shi-ny bright. La la la la la la la la

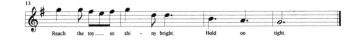

Reach the toy so shi-ny bright. Hold on tight.

Analysis of Motor Task	*Speech/Songs/Rhymes*	*Guidelines*
1. Stretch the elbows.	I stretch my elbows 1 2 3 4 5	1. This task teaches the children to practise shifting weight from one side of body to the other. It is also encourages children with hemiplegia to use the affected hand.

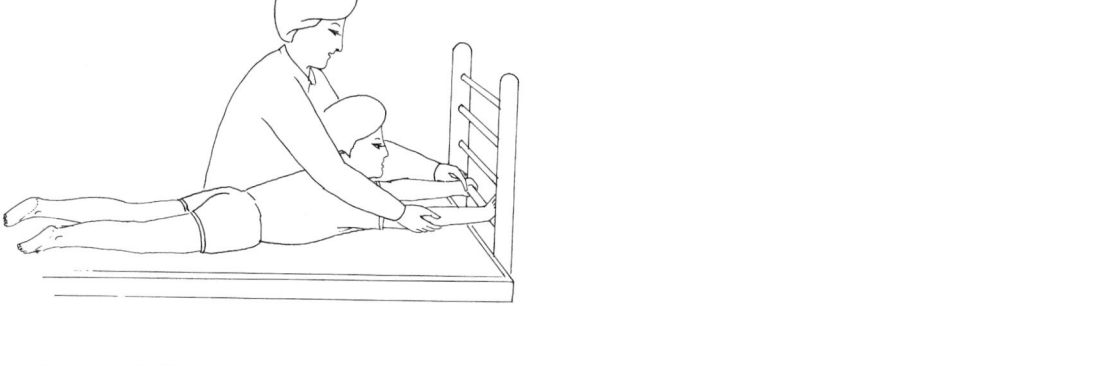

2. Children love playing with balls. A brightly coloured ball that bounces off the floor gives the children excellent feedback and motivates them to become actively involved in the task.

3. Make sure the children lift up their heads and look at the ball while doing the task.

4. Depending on the child he may begin pushing the ball at a lower rung level and gradually aim higher and higher.

2. Grasp the rung.

I grasp the rung   1 2 3 4 5

5. Help children who cannot extend their hips by placing a sandbag over the buttocks or use gentle manual pressure. Children at levels 3 and 4 should be encouraged to actively extend their hips.

6. If the children's legs cross, a pillow or sandbag will help keep the legs apart. However children at levels 3 and 4 should actively learn to keep their feet apart.

3. Look at the ball.

I look at the ball   look look look

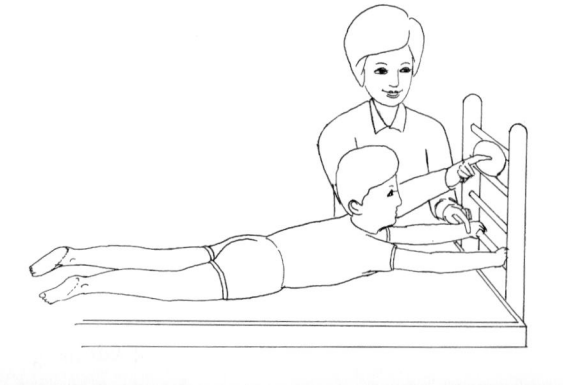

4. Push the ball.

I push the ball   push push push

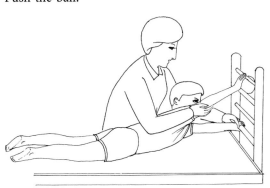

5. Repeat with the other hand.

I push the ball   push push push

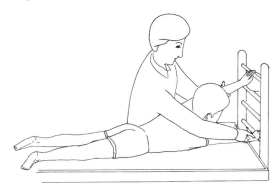

Analysis of Motor Task	*Speech/Songs/Rhymes*	*Guidelines*

1. Both hands straight.

Hands above my head   1 2 3 4 5

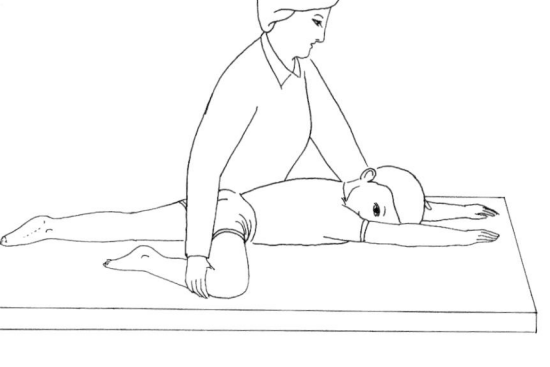

1. Motivate the children to look to the side towards which they are rolling by asking them to look at a toy. Make sure the children learn to move their head first and roll segmentally.

2. Children at level 2 may need help to bend their leg.

3. Children at level 3 may need minimal help. Children at level 4 should try and do it independently.

4. Children at level 4 should learn to roll over with elbows extended and legs well parted.

5. The children may feel afraid when asked to learn to roll over on the plinth. Re-assure them. However it is necessary for the children to experience this task, it helps them develop spatial perception and change of position.

6. Give the children sufficient time to do each step and encourage them to use speech/song to guide their movements.

2. Bend the right leg.

I bend my right leg   1 2 3 4 5

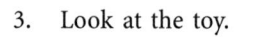

3. Look at the toy.

I look at the toy   look look look

4. Roll over.

I roll over   1   2   3   4   5

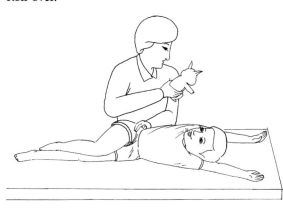

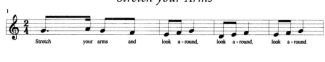

Stretch your Arms

Stretch your arms and look a-round, look a-round, look a-round.

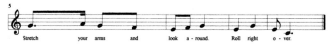

Stretch your arms and look a-round. Roll right o-ver.

Analysis of Motor Task	*Speech/Songs/Rhymes*	*Guidelines*
1. Stretch both elbows.	I stretch my elbows 1 2 3 4 5	1. Use a toy to motivate the children with asymmetrical tonic neck reflex (ATNR) and poor head control bring the head into the midline. Extending the elbows and grasping the plinth is an excellent way to help them bring the head into the midline. Midline orientation is essential for the simplest and most basic functional activity.

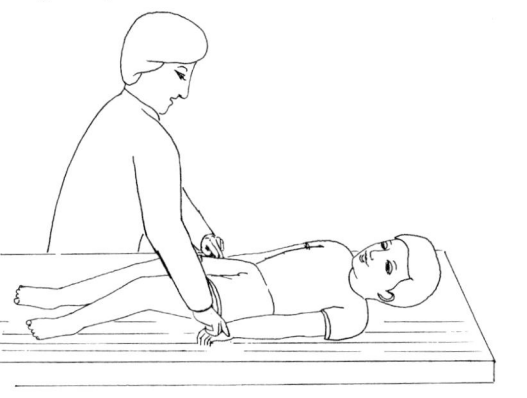

2. Grasp the plinth.

I grasp the plinth   1   2

2. If necessary a small pillow under the head will prevent the children from arching backwards in the extensor pattern.

3. A pillow/sandbag between the legs will help the children at level 2 to keep the legs apart. Children at levels 3 and 4 should learn to part their legs actively.

4. Children at level 2 may need help to stretch their elbows. However they should be able to grasp the plinth.

5. Make sure their toes are pointing outwards and upwards.

6. Encourage the children with athetosis to learn to maintain the "lying straight and still" position on the plinth.

3. Bring the head into the midline position.

My head is in the middle   1   2   3   4   5

4. Stretch the knees, legs straight/back of knees flat on the plinth.

I stretch my knees   1 2 3 4 5

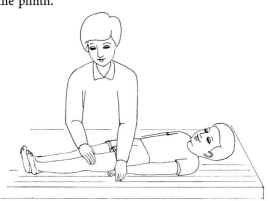

5. Legs apart.

I part my legs   1 2

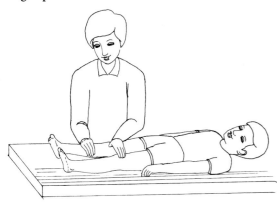

6. Lie straight.

I lie straight   1 2 3 4 5

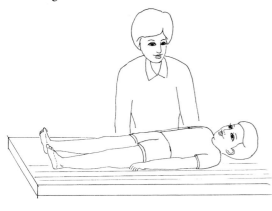

Go to Sleep

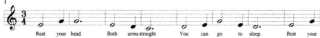

Rest your head. Both arms straight. You can go to sleep. Rest your

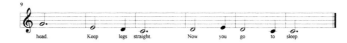

head. Keep legs straight. Now you go to sleep.

Analysis of Motor Task	Speech/Songs/Rhymes	Guidelines
1. Look at the stick.	I look at the stick look look look	1. Motivate the children to actively participate by using sticks painted with different colours. Invite the children to choose a colour. Children at levels 3 and 4 should begin to learn to name the different colours.

1. Motivate the children to actively participate by using sticks painted with different colours. Invite the children to choose a colour. Children at levels 3 and 4 should begin to learn to name the different colours.

2. Children at level 2 will need help to stretch their elbows and raise the stick above their head. Children at level 3 may need minimal help. However children at level 4 should be able to do it independently.

3. Children with poor midline orientation will need strong stimulation to encourage them to keep the head in the midline at all times. Use a musical toy attached to the stick for children with visual impairment.

4. Always count with an even slow tempo when teaching children with spasticity. Do not allow the children to sing the song too quickly.

5. Make sure the children do not flex their hips when doing this task.

6. The care-giver may stand at the top of the plinth behind the children and give them the opportunity for a long stretch by asking them to release the stick and give it to her with the arms above the head.

Analysis of Motor Task

1. Look at the stick.

2. Grasp the stick.

3. Raise up the stick.

Speech/Songs/Rhymes

I look at the stick   look look look

I grasp the stick   1 2 3 4 5

I raise up the stick   1 2 3 4 5

4. Bring the stick up above the head.

The stick above my head   1 2 3 4 5

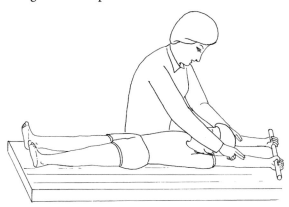

5. Stick on the tummy.

The stick on my tummy   1 2 3 4 5

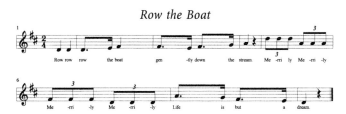

Row the Boat

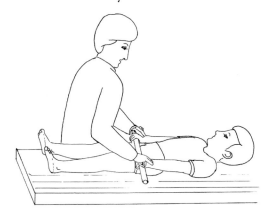

6. Repeat steps 4 and 5.

Analysis of Motor Task	*Speech/Songs/Rhymes*	*Guidelines*

1. Grasp the plinth with one hand.

I grasp the plinth with one hand   1 2 3 4 5

1. The child with cerebral palsy must learn to isolate each movement in order to learn to function.

2. Sticks with bells attached will help the children with visual impairment to target the stick and give them sensory feedback.

3. Make sure the children learn to lie straight at all times and keep their head in the midline. Encourage the children with athetosis learn to sustain their grasp of the stick.

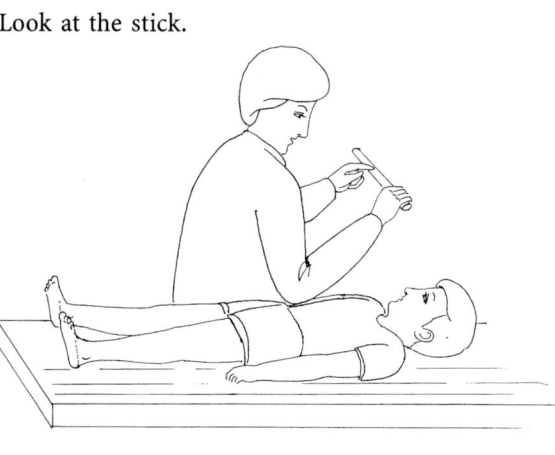

2. Look at the stick.

I look at the stick   look   look   look

4. Children at level 2 will need help to extend the elbows. However the care-giver should be ready to remove help if the child makes an attempt to stretch the elbows. They may also need help to raise their arm above their head.

5. Give the children time to do each step and encourage them to use speech to guide their movements.

3. Grasp the stick with the other hand.

I grasp the stick with other hand   1 2 3 4 5

4. Raise up the stick.

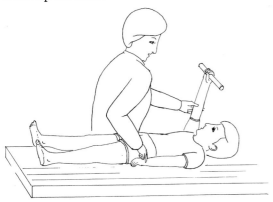

I raise up the stick   1   2   3   4   5

5. Raise the stick above the head.

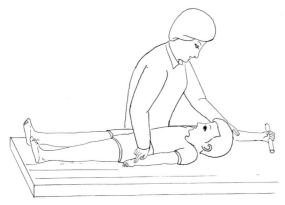

Stick above my head   1   2   3   4   5

6. Bring the stick down to the tummy.

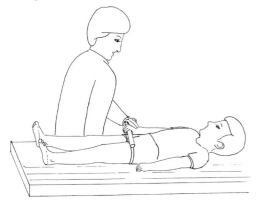

Stick down to my tummy   1   2   3   4   5

Row the Boat

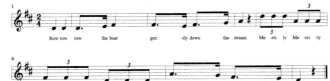

Row row row the boat gen -tly down the stream. Me -rri ly Me -rri -ly

Me -rri -ly Me -rri -ly Life is but a dream.

7. Repeat step 5 and 6.

Analysis of Motor Task	*Speech/Songs/Rhymes*	*Guidelines*

1. Lie straight.

I lie straight   1   2   3   4   5

1. This task is useful for children with unstable hips. It is also a preparation for standing/walking training (flat feet). The task also prepares the children for dressing/undressing.

2. Motivate the children to actively lift up their bottom by telling them a story about a ship passing under the bridge and ask them to lift up to allow the ship to pass.

3. Make sure the children extend their elbows and grasp the plinth while doing the task.

4. The children's feet should be directly under their knees to facilitate them when lifting up the bottom.

5. Do not allow the children to arch their back when attempting to lift up the bottom.

2. Bend the right knee and put the foot flat.

I bend my right knee and put my foot flat   1   2   3   4   5

6. If the children at level 2 cannot lift up the bottom, the care-giver presses gently but firmly on the knees and helps them when lifting up. She may also need to give some assistance to the children at level 3. However, the children at level 4 should learn to do it independently. Make sure the children keep their feet flat on the plinth and the children with athetosis learn to maintain the position.

3. Bend the left knee and put the other foot flat.

I bend my left knee and put my foot flat   1   2   3   4   5

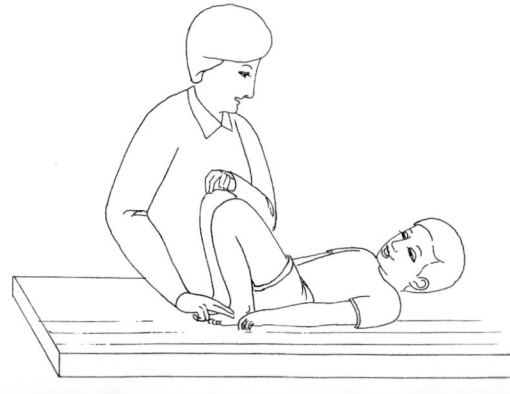

4. Lift up the bottom.

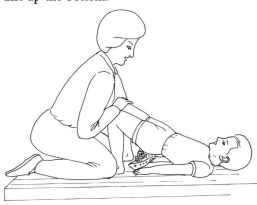

I lift up my bottom   1 2 3 4 5

5. Bottom down on the plinth.

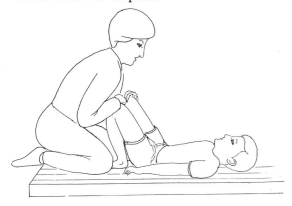

My bottom down   1 2 3 4 5

6. Stretch the right leg. Repeat with the other leg.

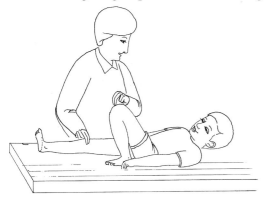

I stretch my right leg   1 2 3 4 5

7. Repeat steps 2 and 3.

Analysis of Motor Task	*Speech/Songs/Rhymes*	*Guidelines*

1. Stretch both elbows and grasp the plinth.

I stretch my elbows and grasp   1 2 3 4 5

1. This movement teaches the children how to fixate themselves distally.

2. Make sure the children learn to sustain their grasp when pulling down the plinth.

3. Children at level 2 will need some help to sustain grasp when moving down. However do not over assist and remove assistance when they attempt to do the step themselves.

4. Children at level 3 may need minimal help, children at level 4 should learn to do it independently.

5. Do not allow the children with athetosis to wriggle when moving down.

2. Pull down to the end of the plinth.

I pull down   1 2 3 4 5

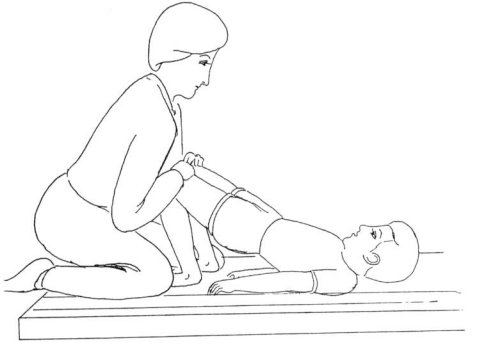

3. Repeat step 2 until both feet are at the end of the plinth.

I pull down   1 2 3 4 5

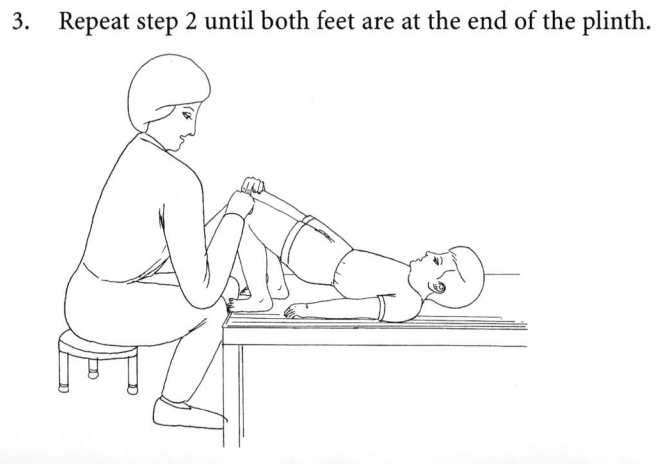

4. Put the right foot flat on the stool.

I put my right foot flat   1   2

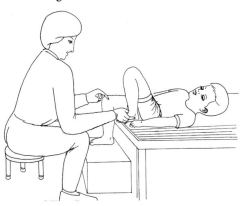

5. Put the left foot flat on the stool.

I put my left foot flat   1   2

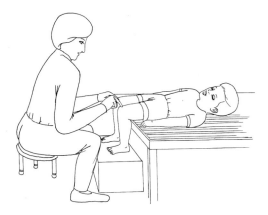

Analysis of Motor Task	*Speech/Songs/Rhymes*	*Guidelines*

1. Lie straight with both feet flat on a stool.

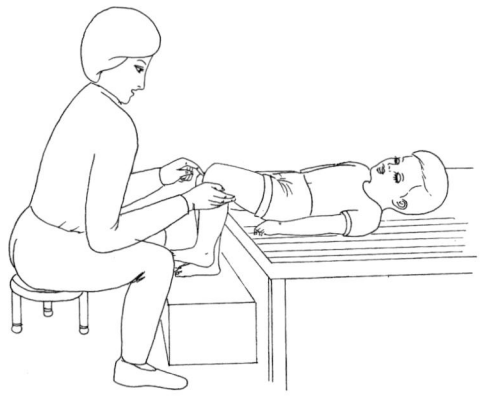

My feet are flat   1 2 3 4 5

1. This movement helps the children learn to isolate the lower limbs, and keep both feet flat which is essential for sitting, standing and walking training.

2. Make sure the children lie straight with elbows extended and head in the midline. Encourage the children to sustain grasp of the plinth as they try to do the steps.

3. Children at level 2 may need some help to extend the elbows. However, remove help if they attempt to do it themselves.

4. Help the children fixate the non-moving leg by pressing gently but firmly on the knee or at the ankle joint.

5. The children may place their feet on different kinds of tactile materials.

2. Lift up the left foot.

I lift up my left foot   1 2 3 4 5

3. Place the left foot flat on the plinth.

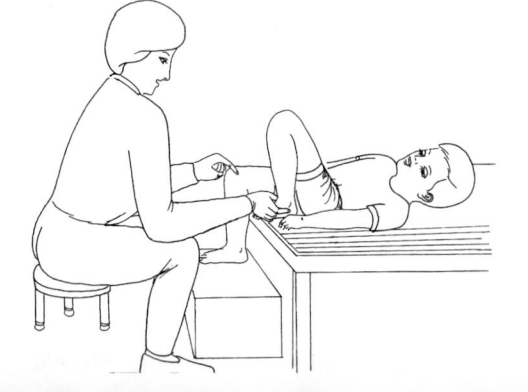

I put my left foot flat   1 2 3 4 5

4. Return left foot to the stool.

I put my left foot on the stool   1 2 3 4 5

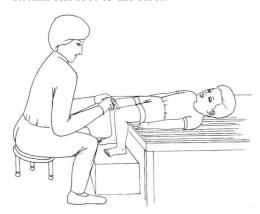

5. Repeat with the right foot.

I lift up my right foot   1 2 3 4 5

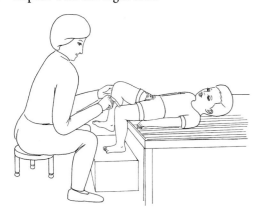

I put my right foot flat   1 2 3 4 5

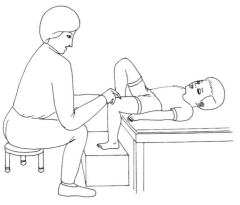

Analysis of Motor Task	*Speech/Songs/Rhymes*	*Guidelines*

1. Put the left foot flat on the plinth.

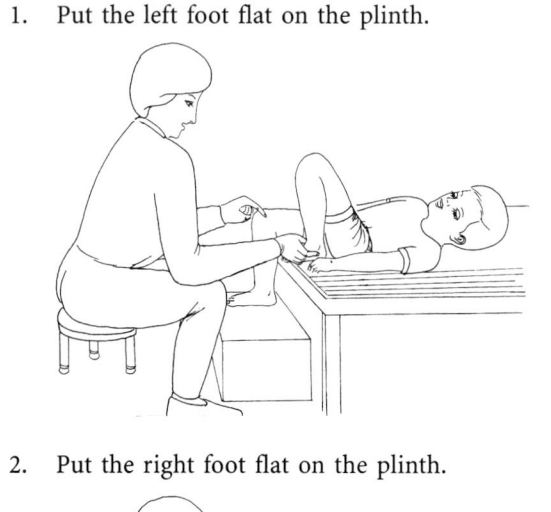

I put my left foot flat   1 2 3 4 5

2. Put the right foot flat on the plinth.

I put my right foot flat   1 2 3 4 5

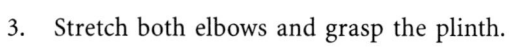

3. Stretch both elbows and grasp the plinth.

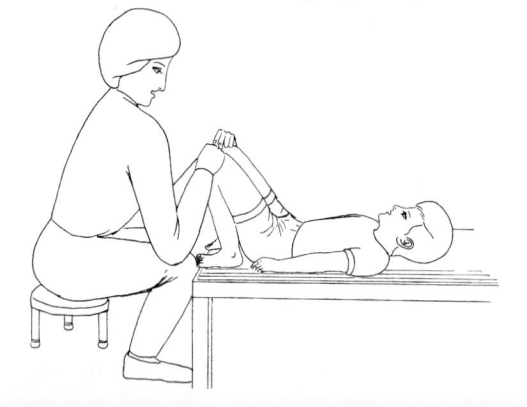

I stretch my elbows and grasp   1 2 3 4 5

1. This task helps the children prepare for sitting, standing and walking training.

2. Make sure the children extend their elbows and sustain grasp of the plinth while doing the steps.

3. The children's feet should be directly under the knees to facilitate them when lifting up the bottom and pushing backwards.

4. Do not allow the children to arch their back when pushing backwards.

5. Help children at level 2 who have difficulty lifting up the bottom by pressing down gently but firmly on both knees to facilitate this step. Ensure they keep both feet flat on the plinth.

6. Encourage children who constantly move to maintain the position of lying straight.

4. Push backwards and extend both knees. Repeat.

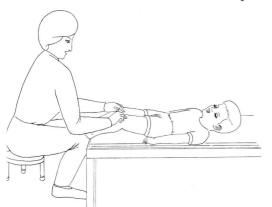

I push backwards   1   2   3   4   5

5. Stretch both arms and grasp the plinth.

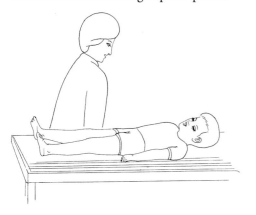

I stretch my elbows   1   2   3   4   5

6. Stretch both knees and lie straight.

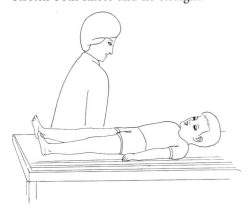

I stretch my knees   1   2   3   4   5

Go to Sleep

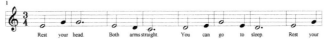

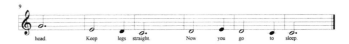

Rest your head. Both arms straight. You can go to sleep. Rest your head. Keep legs straight. Now you go to sleep.

Analysis of Motor Task	*Speech/Songs/Rhymes*	*Guidelines*

1. Put the left leg on the right foot.

I put my left foot on my right foot   1 2 3 4 5

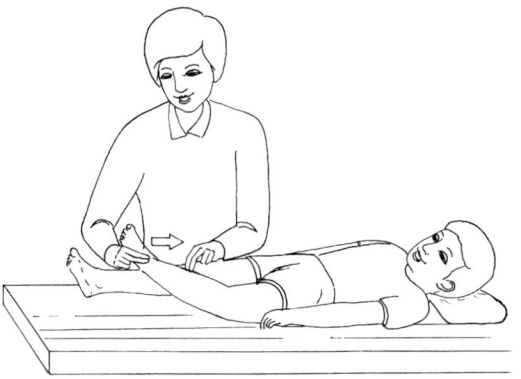

2. Slide the left foot upwards to the right knee.

I slide my left leg up to right knee   1 2 3 4 5

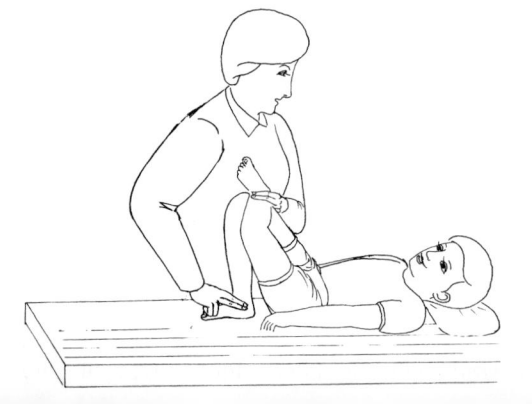

3. Bend the right knee with the right foot flat.

I bend my right knee   1 2 3 4 5

1. This is a useful task to teach the children to actively part their legs. It is also a preparation for removing shoes and socks and for sitting/standing/walking/training (emphasis on feet flat).

2. The following games are excellent to motivate the children to actively participate in the task. Counting the toes/rubbing cream on the toes/foot/taking off a sock/ puppet/coloured elastic ankle band etc.

3. Children with athetosis should learn from the beginning to hold and maintain the position of the foot flat on the plinth.

4. Children at level 2 may need help to slide the foot upwards towards the knee. However some children may not be able to place the foot on the opposite knee. Do not force the movement. The child may put the foot on a low stool.

5. Make sure the child's heel is on his knee and his legs are well parted.

4. Look at the sock/puppet/toes on left foot (care-giver puts sock/puppet on the left toes and asks the child to use the right hand to pull it off).

I put my right foot flat   1   2   3   4   5

I pull off   1   2   3   4   5

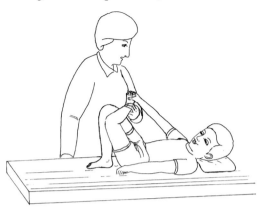

5. Repeat steps 1 to 4 with the other leg.

Analysis of Motor Task	*Speech/Songs/Rhymes*	*Guidelines*

1. Stretch the knees.

    I stretch my knees   1 2 3 4 5

1. This task is suitable for children who cross their legs (scissors gait). Do not use it for children with too much abduction of the legs.

2. The children love this play activity. They enjoy the auditory feedback as the toy bounces off the floor. If a ball is used it should be big with a good bounce on the floor. An excellent toy for the task is a large size soft drinks plastic bottle preferably painted in different colours and containing several small stones.

3. The care-giver fixates the non-moving leg, this makes it easier for the child to part the other leg.

2. Fixate the right leg.

    I fix my right leg   1 2 3 4 5

4. It is important to put the toy in such a position the child can push/kick it. However, as the child improves move the toy to a position that gradually encourages him to increase the space between his legs.

5. Children at level 3 may need minimal help to fixate the non-moving leg. Children at level 4 should learn to fixate the non-moving leg while moving the other leg independently.

3. Part the left leg and kick the toy.

    I kick the toy   kick kick kick

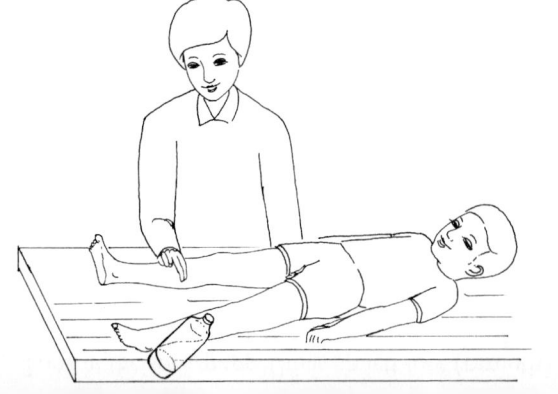

4. Part the other leg and kick the toy. (Repeat this task while the children are enjoying the game).

I kick the toy   kick   kick   kick

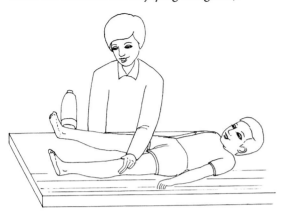

Analysis of Motor Task	*Speech/Songs/Rhymes*	*Guidelines*

1. Look at the toy.

   I look at the toy   look look look

1. This task is essential for activities of the daily routine and the children should be given every opportunity to practise it from left/right side.

2. The children at level 2 will need help in pushing up with both hands. Children at level 3 may also need help to push up into the sitting position. However, children at level 4 should learn to do it independently.

3. Colourful wrist bands with bells can be used to help the children learn right/left hands.

4. Give the children sufficient time to do the task and encourage them to use speech to guide their movements.

5. It may be easier for some children to learn this task on a mat on the floor.

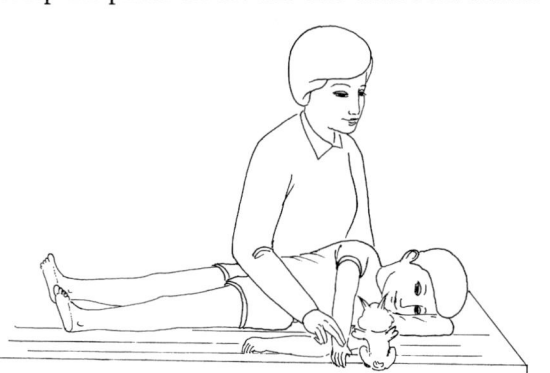

2. Grasp the plinth on the left side with both hands.

   I grasp the plinth on left side   1 2 3 4 5

3. Roll to the left side.

   I roll to left side   1 2 3 4 5

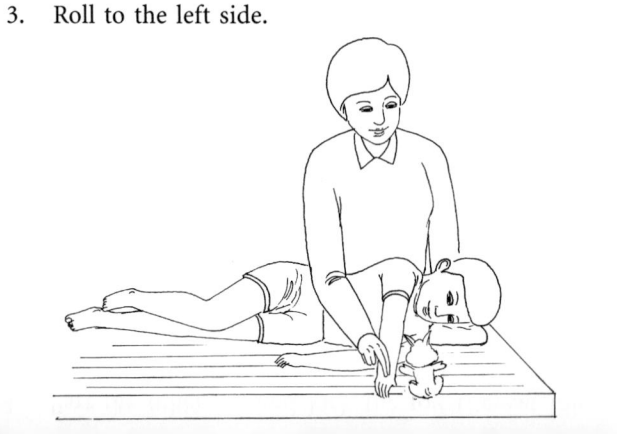

4. Bend both legs.   I bend my legs   1 2 3 4 5

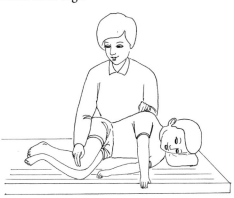

5. Push up on both arms.   I push up on arms   push   push   push

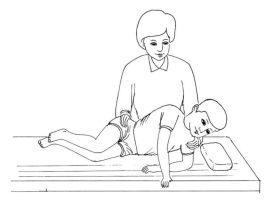

6. Part right arm and grasp the plinth on both sides.   I grasp plinth   1   2   3   4   5

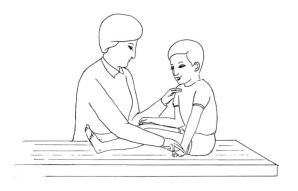

Analysis of Motor Task	*Speech/Songs/Rhymes*	*Guidelines*

1. Grasp the plinth at both sides.

I grasp the plinth   1 2 3 4 5

1. When the children are learning to get up from the supine position to long sitting they may get up through side lying or get up straight from supine.

2. This task is essential for activities of the daily routine and the children should be given every opportunity to practise it.

3. Make sure the children learn to use their abdominal muscles when they are moving from the lying to the sitting position.

4. Children at level 2 will need help to pull up, children at level 3 may also need a little help. However, children at level 4 should learn to do it independently.

2. Look at the toy.

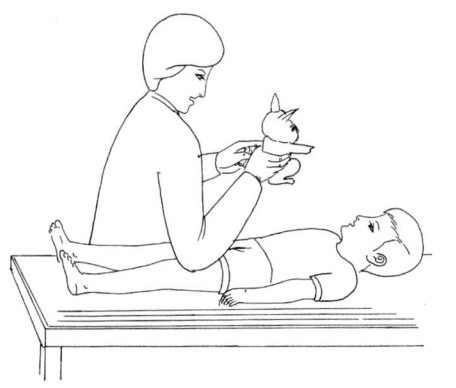

I look at the toy   1 2 3 4 5

5. Give the children sufficient time to do each step and encourage them to use speech to guide their movements.

3. Lift up the head and trunk and pull up with both hands.

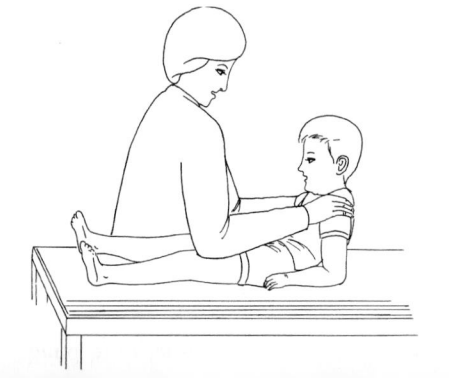

I sit up   1 2 3 4 5

4. Slide both hands forward and bend the hips.   I slide my hands forward   1 2 3 4 5

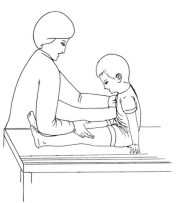

Analysis of Motor Task	Speech/Songs/Rhymes	Guidelines

1. Stretch arms and grasp the plinth between the legs.

I stretch my elbows and grasp the plinth 1 2 3 4 5

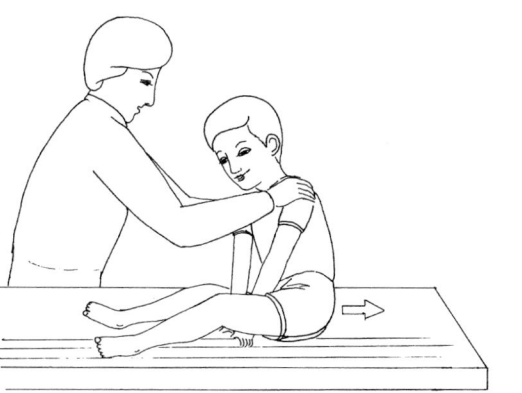

1. This task helps the children learn trunk balance.

2. In this position many children either arch or round their back and cross their legs. Make sure the children learn to push their bottom well back, part their legs and stretch their elbows to help them anchor their bottom on the plinth and sit straight.

3. If their back is too rounded a low stool/thick book (equivalent of a phone book)/sitting downhill on a wedge will help them learn to straighten the back.

4. The care-giver may use this position to teach the children cognitive subjects.

5. Give as much time as possible for the children to remain in this position for play.

2. Push through the hands and push the bottom back.

I push my bottom back 1 2

6. Children at level 2 may need gaiters to stretch their elbows and give them extra stability when learning to sit and grasp the slatted plinths to maintain balance in this position.

7. It is preferable to teach the children to grasp the slats between the knees. In this manner the children are actively learning to part their legs.

8. Children at level 3 should learn to release one hand at a time for play. Children at level 4 should learn to release both hands for play.

9. The more able children use this position for play/dressing and undressing etc.

3. Legs apart.

My legs apart 1 2 3 4 5

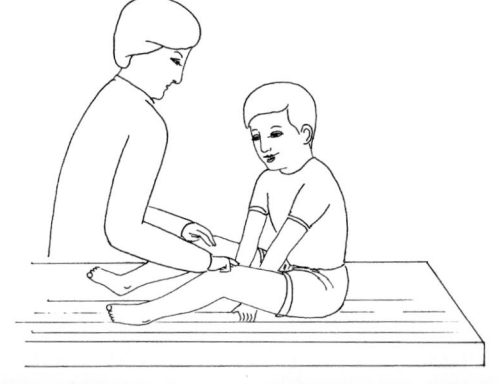

10. For song use knees straight instead of feet flat.

4. Knees straight.

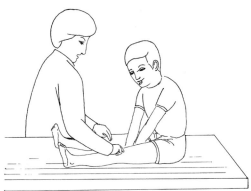

I stretch my knees   1 2 3 4 5

5. Elbows straight.

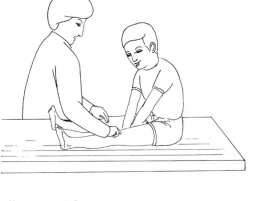

I stretch my elbows   1 2 3 4 5

6. Back straight.

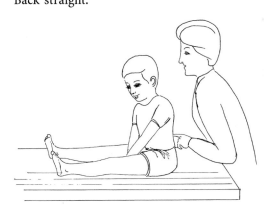

I Stretch my Hands and Hold on Tight

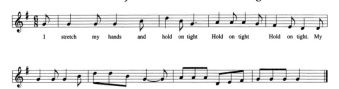

Analysis of Motor Task	*Speech/Songs/Rhymes*	*Guidelines*

1. Hands at sides of the body and grasp the plinth.

I grasp the plinth   1 2 3 4 5

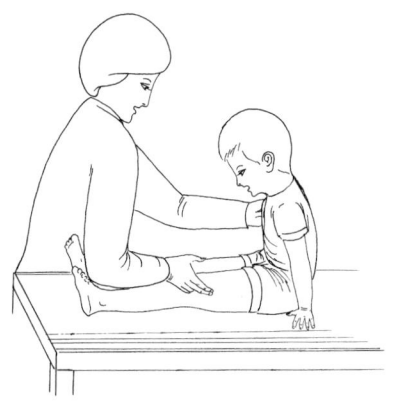

1. This task is essential for activities of the daily routine and the children should be given every opportunity to practise it.

2. Children at level 2 will need help in maintaining the trunk slightly upright when bending the elbows. Children at level 3 may also need help in this position. However, children at level 4 should learn to do it independently.

3. When doing the task, remind the children to keep their chin tucked in to prevent the head falling backwards.

4. Place a pillow under the head to give the children a sense of security/comfort when completing the task.

2. Slide both hands backward and grasp the plinth.

I slide my hands backward   1 2 3 4 5

5. Give the children sufficient time to do the task.

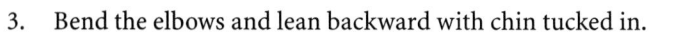

3. Bend the elbows and lean backward with chin tucked in.

I bend my elbows   1 2 3 4 5

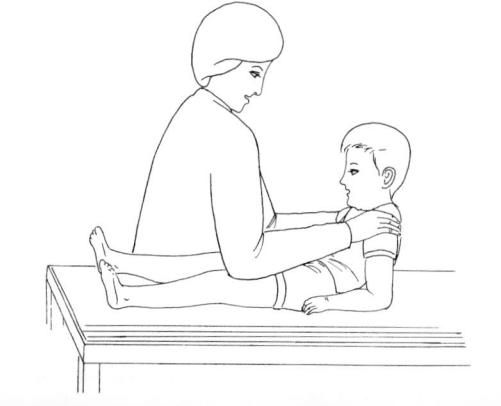

4. Lean backward to lie down with chin tucked in.   I bend my head and lie down   1 2 3 4 5

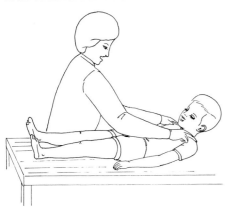

5. Lie straight.   I lie straight   1 2 3 4 5

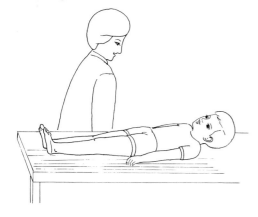

6. Feet apart.   My feet apart   1 2 3 4 5

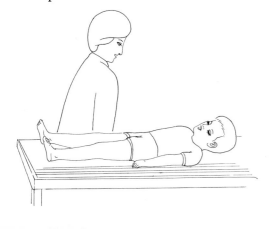

Analysis of Motor Task	*Speech/Songs/Rhymes*	*Guidelines*

1. Hands above the head.

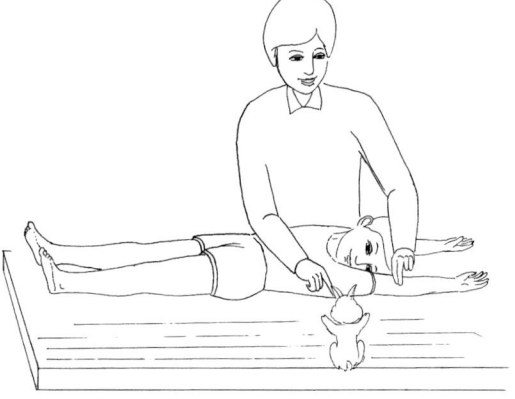

Hands above my head   1 2 3 4 5

1. Children at level 2 may need help to stretch the elbows and raise the hands above the head.

2. Make sure the children turn the head to look at the toy before they begin to roll over. Do not allow the children to arch the back as they roll. Children should learn to roll over segmentally.

3. Children at level 2 may need help to bend the leg.

4. Encourage the children at level 4 to roll over with extended and well parted legs.

5. Children at levels 3 and 4 should learn to respond to the request to roll to right and left side.

2. Look at the toy.

I look at the toy   look   look   look

6. Make sure the children's elbows are straight and the arms are raised above the head when rolling over.

3. Bend one leg.

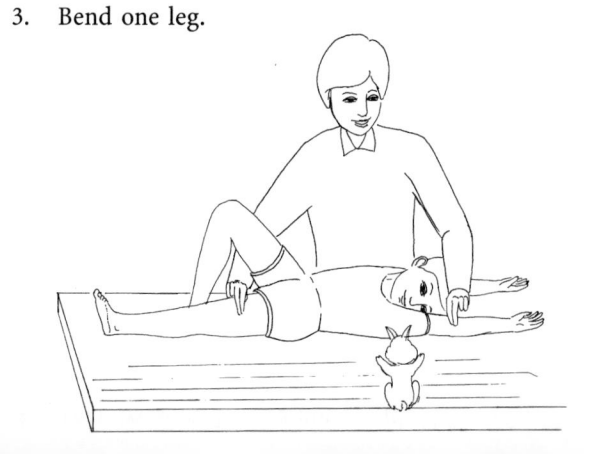

I bend my leg   1 2 3 4 5

4. Roll over and lie straight.

I roll over 　　　1　2　3　4　5

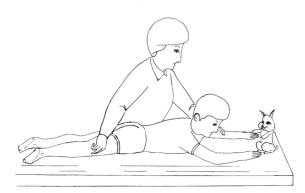

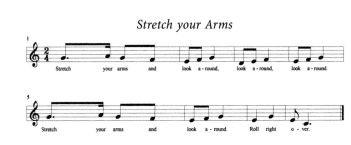

Stretch your Arms

5. Stretch the elbows in front and look at the doll.

I stretch my elbows and lie straight 　　　1　2　3　4　5

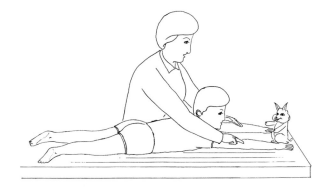

Analysis of Motor Task	*Speech/Songs/Rhymes*	*Guidelines*

1. Look at the toy/care-giver.

I look at the toy   look look look

1. This task helps the children learn head control, wrist extension and hip extension. However do not allow the children to arch backwards in extension while doing the task.

2. Children at levels 2 and 3 will need help to extend the elbows and push up. However the care-giver should decrease the help if the children begin to take weight through the arms.

3. The children at level 2 may need a pillow between the legs to keep them apart. However, encourage the children at levels 3 and 4 to actively learn to part their legs.

4. The care-giver encourages the children to lift up their heads to look in front by asking them to look at toy/ball/musical instrument/playing a tune on the tape recorder etc.

2. Push up on the hands.

I push up on my hands   1   2   3   4   5

3. Look up.

I look up   1   2   3   4   5

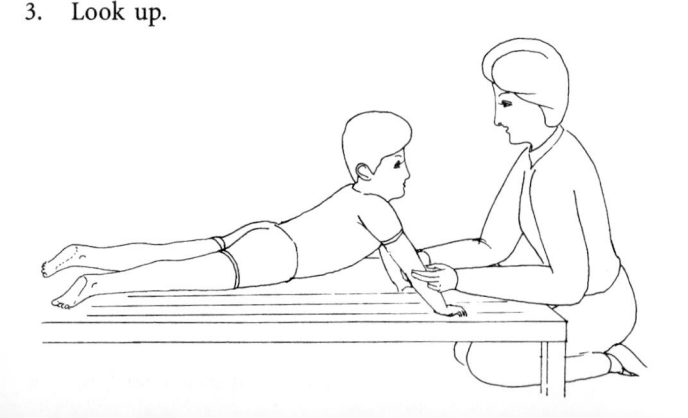

4. Lie down slowly.

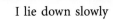

I lie down slowly

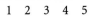   1   2   3   4   5

Analysis of Motor Task	*Speech/Songs/Rhymes*	*Guidelines*
1. Look at the toy.	I look at the toy look look look	1. This task helps the children learn to get in and out of bed. Give the children as many opportunities as possible to practise it.

1. This task helps the children learn to get in and out of bed. Give the children as many opportunities as possible to practise it.

2. Children at level 2 will need help to learn to move around on the plinth. Children at level 3 may also need a little help to learn the movement. However, children at level 4 should try and learn to do it independently.

3. Make sure the children learn to part their legs correctly.

4. Use coloured wrist bands to help them learn to differentiate left and right.

5. Do not allow the children to flex at the hips when doing this task. Use a sandbag/gentle manual pressure to help them keep their hips flat on the plinth. Children at levels 3 and 4 should learn to actively keep their hips flat on the plinth.

6. Encourage the children to learn to actively pivot towards the toy.

7. Give them sufficient time to do the task and encourage them to use speech/song to guide their movements.

2. Part the right hand.

I part my right hand   1 2 3 4 5

3. Part the left leg. The body moves towards the direction of the toy.

I part my left leg   1 2 3 4 5

4. Put the left hand together with the right.

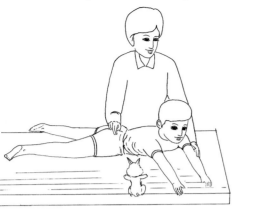

I put my left hand together   1   2   3   4   5

5. Put the right leg together with the left.

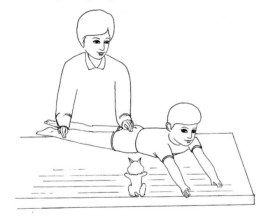

I put my right leg together   1   2   3   4   5

6. Repeat steps 1 to 5 until the child has pivoted 180°.

Lie on my Tummy

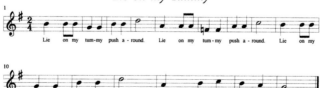

403

Analysis of Motor Task	*Speech/Songs/Rhymes*	*Guidelines*

1. Put the right hand under the shoulder. (Repeat with the other hand).

Right hand under my shoulder   1 2 3 4 5
Left hand under my shoulder   1 2 3 4 5

1. This task facilitates children who have difficulty stretching the elbows to experience straight elbows. Gravity and the weight of the child's body as he pushes off the plinth automatically stretches the elbows.

2. This task is also a preparation for standing/walking training as it helps the children learn to put their feet flat on the floor, stretch their knees and part their legs. It also prepares the child to push off the bed.

3. When facilitating the children to push off make sure they sustain their grasp of the slats. Children at levels 2 and 3 will need some help to grasp. Children at level 4 should try and learn to do it independently.

4. Make sure the children have their legs well parted when pushing off the plinth and also when standing.

5. When pushing off the plinth gravity pulls the legs down and bends the hips. Gravity also overcomes extensor spasticity facilitating parting of the legs and dorsi-flexion in an natural manner.

2. Lift up the head.

I lift up my head   1 2 3 4 5

3. Push off the plinth.

I push off   push push push

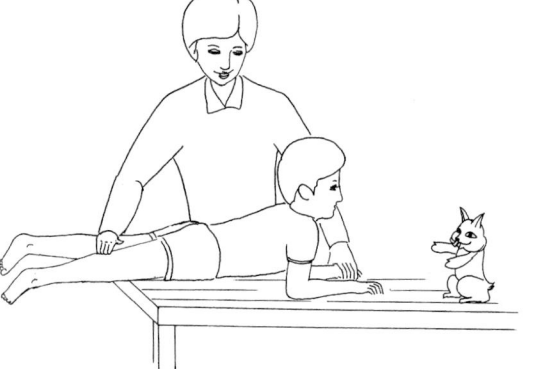

4. Repeat steps 1 to 3 until the child has the feet flat on the floor and both legs parted.

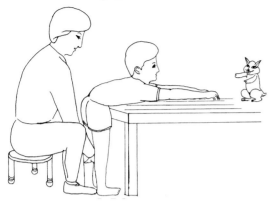

Push off Plinth

We push down the plinth, we push down the plinth. We lift our head up high. We push down the plinth.

5. Slide the hands backwards and grasp the plinth to stand up.

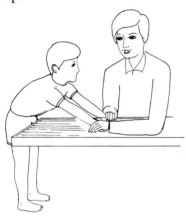

I push up   1   2   3   4   5

Analysis of Motor Task	*Speech/Songs/Rhymes*	*Guidelines*

1. Grasp the slats.

I grasp the slats   1 2 3 4 5

1. Having pushed off the plinth onto the floor facilitates the children when learning to stand straight.

2. Grasping the plinth gives the children with poor balance a greater feeling of stability.

3. Children at level 2 may need gaiters to stretch their elbows and for stability in the standing position. The care-giver will need to help the child at level 2 keep his feet flat and apart, the knees and back straight and his head in the midline.

4. Children at level 4 should learn to stand independently by clasping the hands. If required they may hold a horizontal stick/quoit.

2. Feet flat.

My feet are flat   1 2

5. Make sure the children learn to keep their weight over their feet and do not allow them to pull backwards in extension.

6. Always insist on feet flat and apart, knees and elbows straight and back upright.

7. Encourage the children to stand tall by asking them to look at the mirror or play "tall policeman" game.

8. Give the children every opportunity to stand e.g. learning songs/rhymes/listening to stories.

9. Children practising standing balance may at other times stand against the wall for greater security. However gradually wean them from using the wall as a support.

3. Feet apart.

My feet are apart   1 2

4. Knees straight.

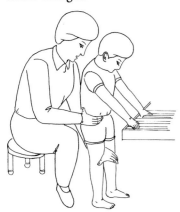

I stretch my knees   1 2 3 4 5

5. Elbows straight.

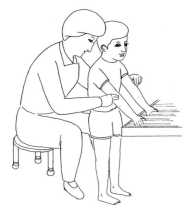

I stretch my elbows   1 2 3 4 5

6. Back straight.

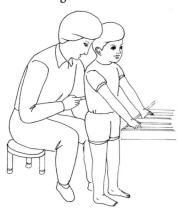

My back is straight   1 2 3 4 5

Look at me

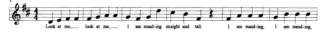

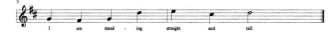

Analysis of Motor Task	*Speech/Songs/Rhymes*	*Guidelines*

1. Grasp the plinth with one hand.

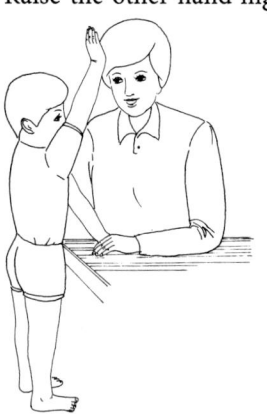

2. Raise the other hand high.

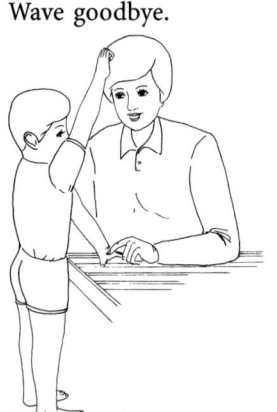

3. Wave goodbye.

I grasp the plinth with one hand   1   2   3   4   5

I raise up my other hand   1   2   3   4   5

Now we are Going to Say Goodbye

Now we are go-ing to   say good-bye,   bye-bye bye-bye   bye!

Now we are go-ing to   say good-bye,   bye-bye bye-bye   bye!

1. Never omit this task as it is the beginning of training balance and prepares the children for walking training. The children enjoy it as all children love saying "goodbye" and facilitates their active participation. The song/rhyme may be repeated many times while the children are enjoying it.

2. Children at level 2 may need gaiters to stretch the elbows and for stability. They may also need help to raise the hand. Children at level 4 should learn to stand independently. If required they may hold a horizontal stick/quoit.

3. Make sure the children weight bear on the correct side while raising the hand high.

4. This task encourages children with hemiplegia to use the affected hand.

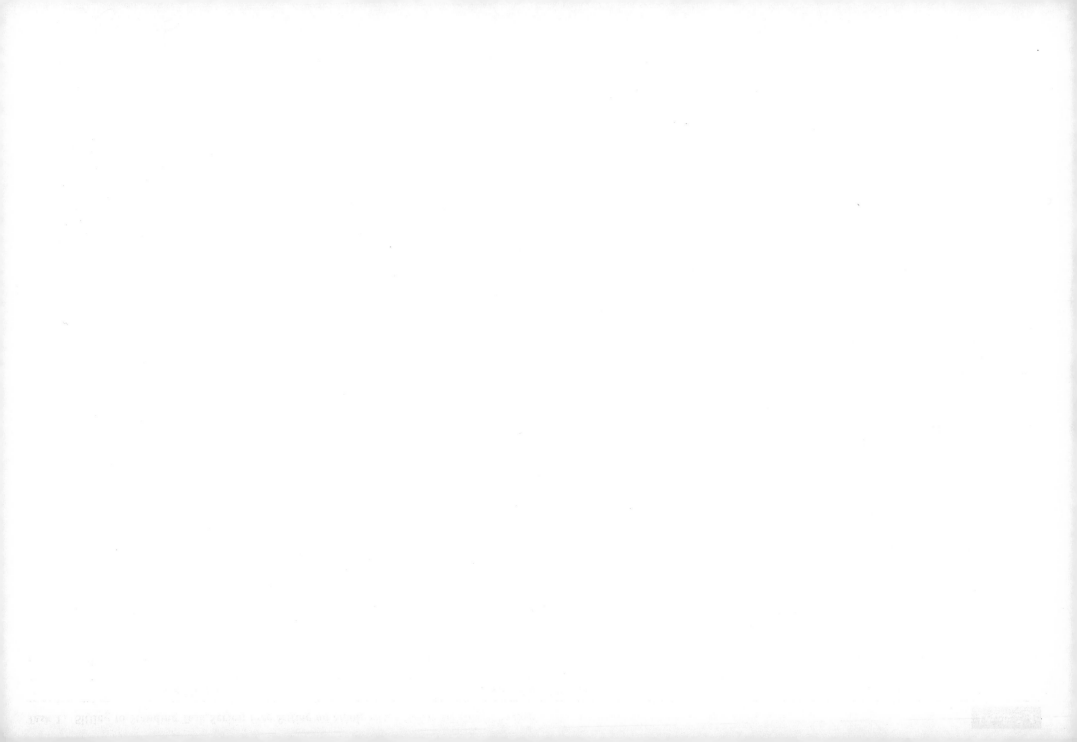

Analysis of Motor Task	*Speech/Songs/Rhymes*	*Guidelines*

1. Grasp the stool.

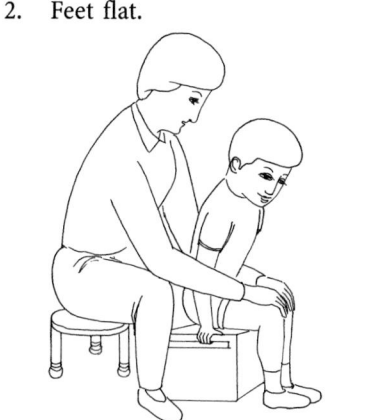

I grasp the stool   1   2   3   4   5

1. When using speech the care-giver should employ a slow even tempo, this is particularly important for children with spasticity.

2. When doing the steps children with athetosis should learn to hold, fixate and maintain the position. This is crucial in order to help them function in daily life.

3. Children at level 2 may need gaiters to stretch the elbows and for stability. They may also need ankle and thigh straps for fixation and security when learning to sit freely on a stool. However, assess the child regularly to determine if it is possible to remove the straps gradually (see Appendix).

2. Feet flat.

My feet are flat   1   2

4. Children at level 3 may need minimal help, it may be sufficient to stabilise their feet. Children at level 4 should learn to sit freely on the stool.

5. When the children are learning to free their hands for activities it is preferable to manually fixate the children at the pelvis/thighs. This gives more security and stability to the child and allows him to use his trunk and upper limbs.

6. Give sufficient time for the children to do each step and encourage them to use speech/song to guide their movements.

3. Feet apart.

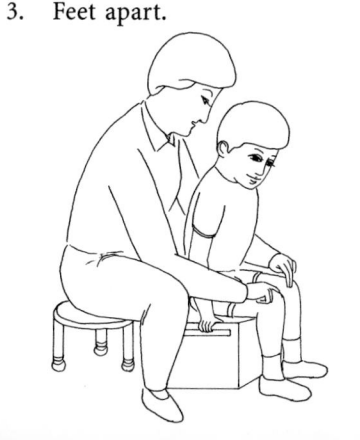

My feet are apart   1   2

4. Bottom back.

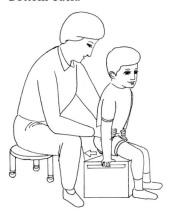

I push my bottom back   1   2

5. Stretch the elbows.

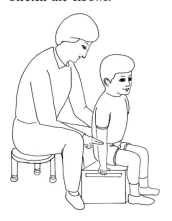

I stretch my elbows   1 2 3 4 5

6. Sit straight.

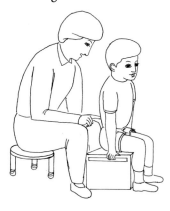

Sit up Straight

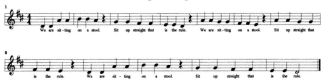

Analysis of Motor Task	*Speech/Songs/Rhymes*	*Guidelines*

1. Look at the care-giver.

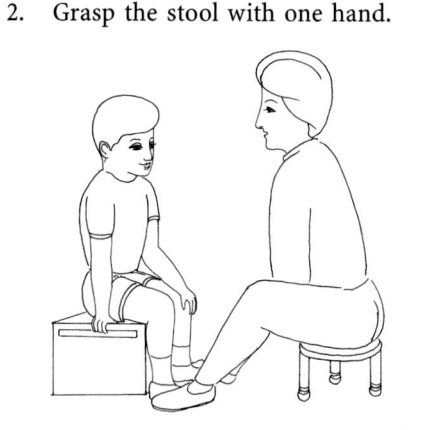

2. Grasp the stool with one hand.

3. Raise up the other hand.

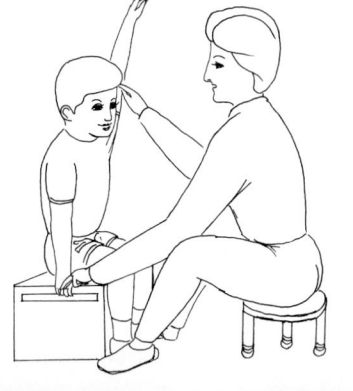

I look at the care-giver   look   look   look

I grasp the stool   1   2   3   4   5

I raise my hand   1   2   3   4   5

I am here

1. The care-giver may invite one child in the group to take roll call. This helps the children become familiar with and interact with one another.

2. Children at level 2 may need gaiters to extend their elbows and for stability when learning to sit freely on a stool. They will also need help to raise the hand to answer to their name.

3. Children at levels 3 and 4 may feel insecure when they raise the hand high. The care-giver facilitates them and gives them a feeling of security by gently but firmly placing her feet on the children's feet for fixation.

4. Do not over assist the children and remove help as soon as the children begin to learn to do it independently.

5. Give the children sufficient time to do the task.

Analysis of Motor Task	*Speech/Songs/Rhymes*	*Guidelines*
1. Release one hand. 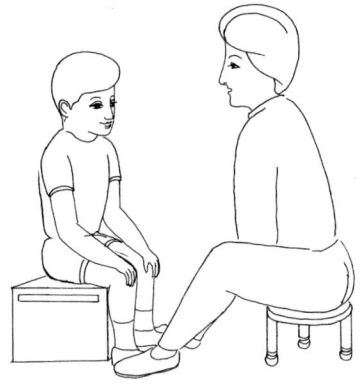	I release one hand 1 2	1. This task teaches the children to shift weight from one side to the other. It encourages children with hemiplegia to shift weight onto the affected side. 2. The game/song should motivate the children to raise their hands and wave from side to side. It is important the children are encouraged to forget their insecurity and learn to participate. 3. Children at level 2 will need help to raise their hands. The care-giver fixates the child's feet with her foot while helping him to raise the hands. 4. Children at level 3 may also need fixation at the feet. 5. Children at level 4 should learn to do it independently. 6. Make sure the children are learning to actively shift weight from one side to the other. 7. Do not allow the children to sing too fast.
2. Release the other hand. 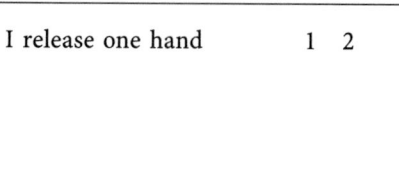	I release the other hand 1 2	
3. Raise both hands up high. 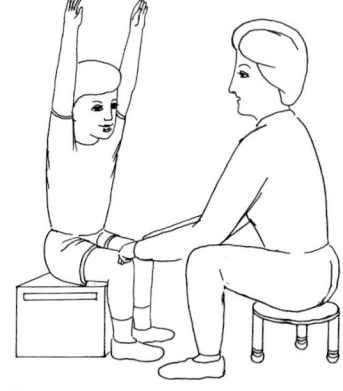	I raise up my hands 1 2 3 4 5	

4. Wave from side to side. (Repeat the game while the children are enjoying it)

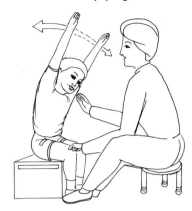

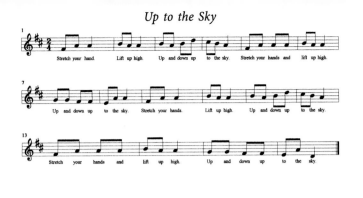

Up to the Sky

Analysis of Motor Task	*Speech/Songs/Rhymes*	*Guidelines*

1. Release one hand.

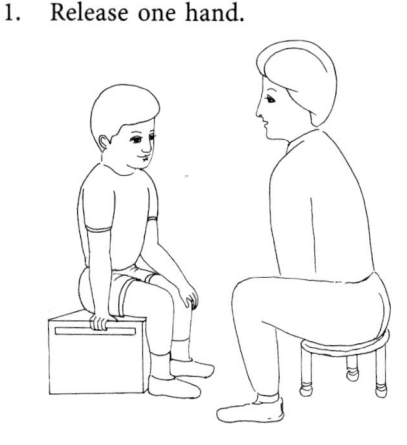

I release my hand   1   2

1. This task is useful for teaching trunk balance/hip flexion/protective extension/body parts.

2. The care-giver should sing the song slowly, clearly and with a good rhythm miming each action.

3. Children at level 2 will need help. Children at level 3 may also need a little help. However, children at level 4 should learn to do it independently.

4. Fixate the children at the pelvis/thighs and feet to allow them freedom at the trunk and upper limbs to do the actions.

2. Release the other hand.

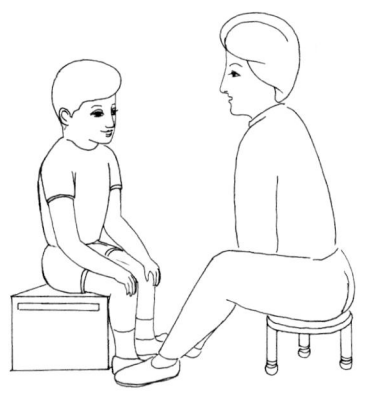

I release the other hand   1   2

3. Put both hands on the head.

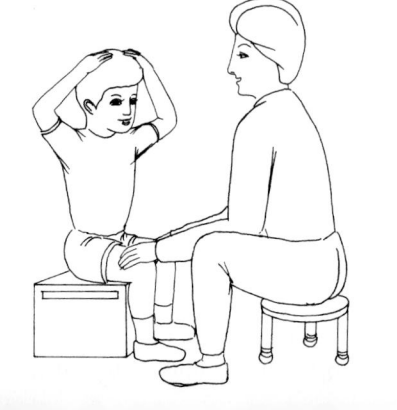

I put my hands on my head   1   2   3   4   5

Touch my Head

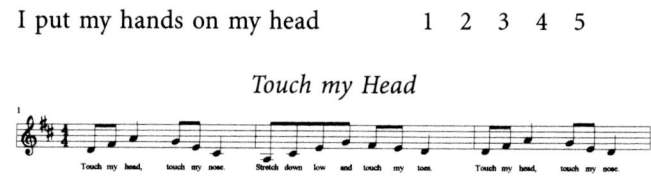

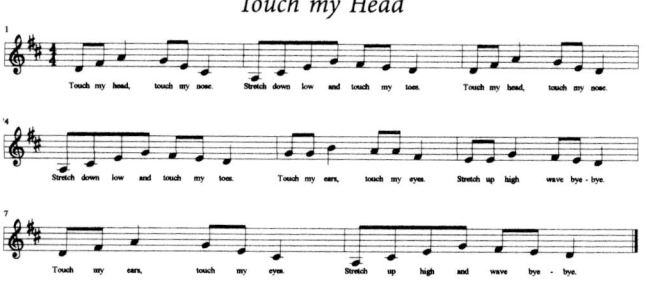

Analysis of Motor Task	*Speech/Songs/Rhymes*	*Guidelines*

1. Look at the ball.

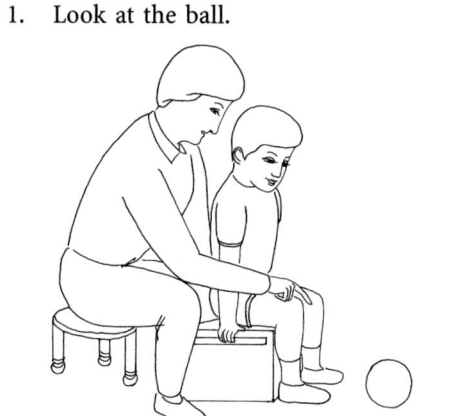

I look at the ball   look look look

1. This task teaches the children trunk balance/protective extension/weight shifting/parting the legs/socialisation.

2. If skittles are not available, use large brightly coloured plastic soft drinks bottles.

3. The task motivates the children to actively participate. All children enjoy the positive feedback from the ball bouncing and knocking the skittles. Aiming at and hitting the target is a great source of fun for them. They forget their insecurity in the free sitting position.

4. Children at level 2 will need help to grasp the ball and throw it. Make sure they are sitting well before they participate. Children at level 3 may also need some help. Children at level four should try and learn to do it independently.

2. Bend down.

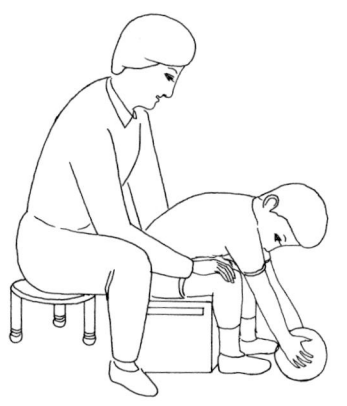

I bend down   1 2 3 4 5

5. Place the ball between the feet as this encourages the children to part their legs. Make sure the children place their hands between their knees when bending down to grasp the ball.

6. In the act of throwing the ball some children may feel insecure, fixate them at the pelvis/thighs and feet rather than at the trunk if possible.

7. Make sure the children learn to grasp the ball with hands open and fingers extended.

8. Place the skittles/bottles in such a way it is possible for the children to hit the target.

3. Pick up the ball.

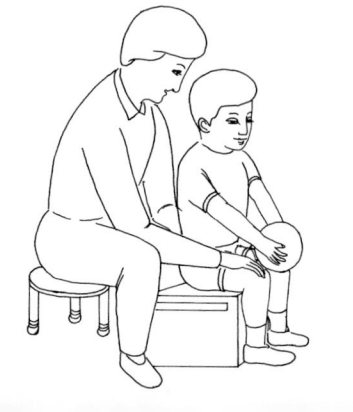

I pick up the ball   1 2 3 4 5

4. Raise the ball up high.

I raise up the ball   1 2 3 4 5

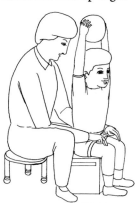

5. Throw the ball.

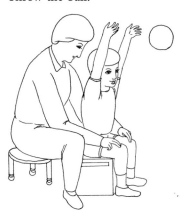

Analysis of Motor Task	*Speech/Songs/Rhymes*	*Guidelines*

1. Grasp the ball with both hands.

I grasp the ball   1 2 3 4 5

2. Look at the friend.

I look at my friend   look look look

3. Pass the ball to the friend.

I pass you the ball   1 2 3 4 5

1. This task teaches the children to move the trunk and upper limbs from side to side while fixating the pelvis on the stool.

2. Motivate the children to actively participate by using brightly coloured balls.

3. The care-giver invites the children to pass along *x* number of balls and then return them to the sender. The children sit in a straight row and pass the balls along to one another.

4. Children at level 2 will need help to grasp the ball and deliver it safely to their friend. They may need fixation in sitting using ankle and thigh straps.

5. Children at level 3 may also need some fixation at the pelvis thighs. However, encourage them to grasp the ball with thumb and fingers extended.

6. Children at level 4 should learn to try and do it independently.

7. Make sure children with hemiplegia learn to open their affected hand and extend the thumb and fingers.

8. This game introduces an element of competition as the children try to prevent the ball from falling on the floor while they are passing it to their friend.

4. Sit straight. (Repeat the game).

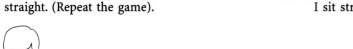

I sit straight   1 2 3 4 5

Analysis of Motor Task	*Speech/Songs/Rhymes*	*Guidelines*
1. Look at the friend.	I look at my friend look look look	1. This task trains weight shifting/parting the legs/socialisation and is useful for children who cross their legs (scissors gait).
		2. Motivate the children to move actively through games, e.g., placing a toy behind the stool and asking the children to pick it up and place it in a basket/pivoting to shake hands with little friend.
		3. Give the children sufficient time to learn to move around on the stool while doing the task.
		4. Children at level 2 will need help to part the legs. The care-giver fixates one leg while the child moves the other leg.
2. Part the right hand.	I part my right hand 1 2 3 4 5	5. Children at level 3 may need a little help to actively move their bottom as they pivot. Children at level 4 should learn to try and do it independently.
		6. Always make sure the children fixate one leg with the foot flat while moving the other leg.
3. Part the right leg.	I part my right leg 1 2 3 4 5	

4. Put the left leg together with the right leg.

My left leg together   1   2   3   4   5

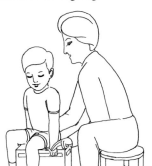

5. Put the left hand together and say "hello". (Repeat and go back to the original position).

My left hand together   1   2   3   4   5

Apart and Together

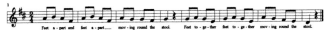

Feet a - part and feet a - part..... mov - ing round the stool. Feet to - ge - ther feet to - ge - ther mov - ing round the stool.

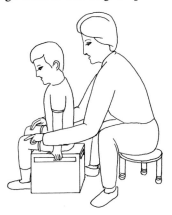

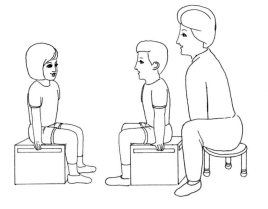

Analysis of Motor Task	*Speech/Songs/Rhymes*	*Guidelines*
1. Put the left ankle on the right foot. 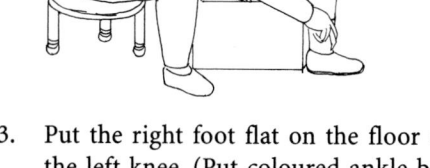	Left ankle on right foot 1 2 3 4 5	1. This task teaches the children to part their legs/prepares for dressing/undressing pants/socks and shoes. 2. Children at level 2 will need help to fixate their pelvis on the stool while doing the task. Children at level 3 may also need some help with fixation on the stool. However, children at level 4 should learn to try and do the task independently. 3. Make sure the children keep their heels on the floor when they stretch their knees. 4. Use a low stool for children who are unable to bring the heel to the knee. Gradually encourage them to slide it higher and higher up towards the knee.
2. Slide the left foot up to the right knee.	I slide my foot to my knee 1 2 3 4 5	5. Fixate the children at the pelvis to free their trunk and upper limbs to pull the coloured ankle bands over their feet. 6. Encourage the children to learn the colours of the ankle bands.
3. Put the right foot flat on the floor and push down on the left knee. (Put coloured ankle bands on left foot). 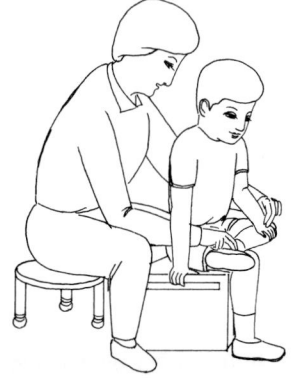	I put my right foot flat 1 2 3 4 5	

4. Slide the left foot down and place it flat on the floor.   I put my left foot flat   1 2 3 4 5

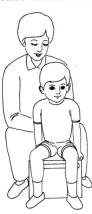

5. Repeat with the other leg.

Analysis of Motor Task	*Speech/Songs/Rhymes*	*Guidelines*
1. Feet flat. 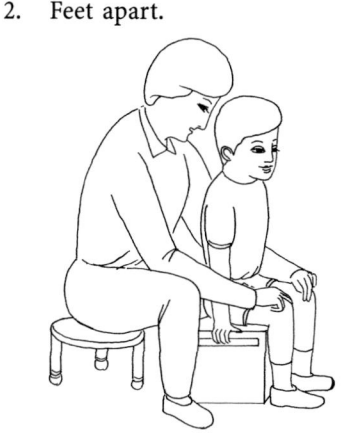	My feet are flat 1 2	1. Children at level 2 may need gaiters to extend the elbows and for stability. They may also need a little help to push the chair forward. The care-giver may have to facilitate them to initiate standing up by pressing down gently but firmly on their knees. Do not allow them to climb up the ladderback chair and pull up to stand.
2. Feet apart.	My feet are apart 1 2	2. Children who cannot keep their feet flat on the floor will need the care-giver to fixate them with her feet. However children at levels 3 and 4 should learn to actively fixate the feet.
3. Grasp the ladderback chair. 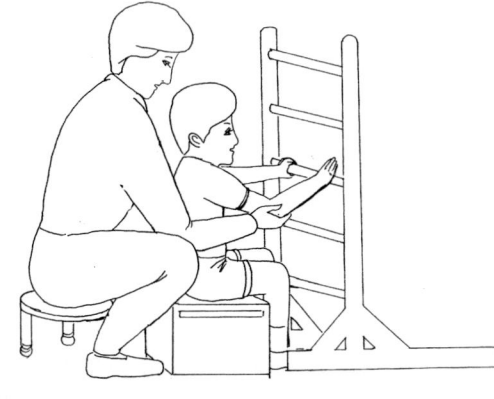	I grasp the chair 1 2 3 4 5	3. Children at level 4 should learn to stand up independently. If they feel insecure they may grasp a horizontal/stick quoit.

4. Make sure the children's weight is well over their feet before they stand up. |

4. Push the ladderback chair forward.

I push the chair   1 2 3 4 5

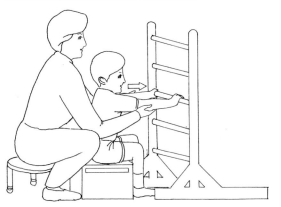

5. Lift up the bottom and stand up.

I lift my bottom and stand up   1 2 3 4 5

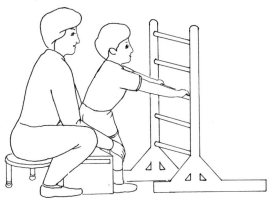

6. Climb up the ladderback chair with both hands and stand straight.

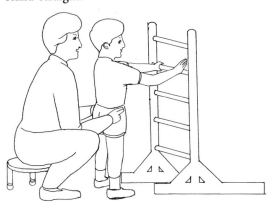

I climb up/down

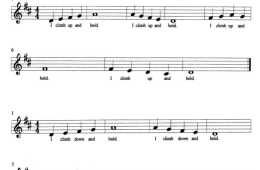

Analysis of Motor Task	*Speech/Songs/Rhymes*	*Guidelines*

1. Look at the toy.

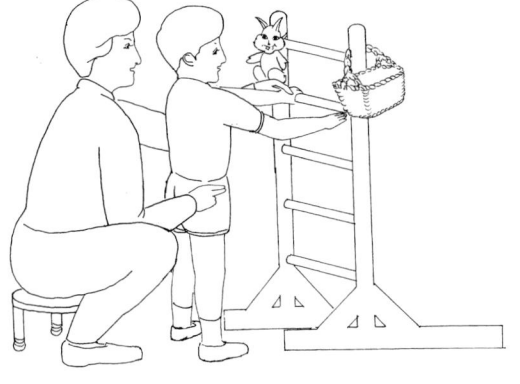

I look at toy   look look look

2. Release one hand.

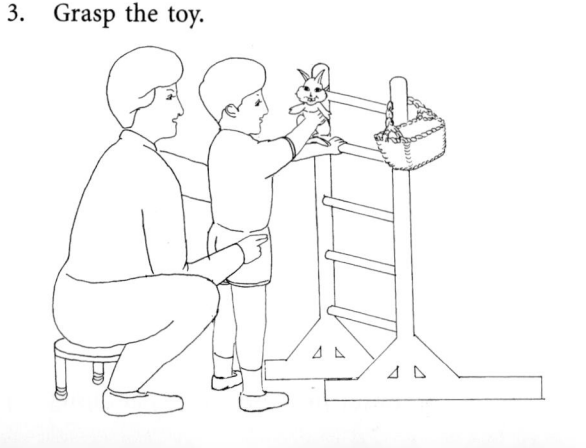

I release my hand   1   2

3. Grasp the toy.

I grasp the toy   1   2   3   4   5

Guidelines

1. Standing is necessary for many activities of daily living. The children should be given every opportunity to practise this task.

2. Children at level 3 may need help to extend the elbows and stand straight. Child at level 4 should learn to stand grasping a horizontal stick/quoit.

3. Make sure the children's weight fall through their bodies and not behind their feet. Remind them to stretch their elbows to help them to stand straight. Insist on feet flat and apart and knees straight.

4. While standing, children at level 3 should begin to learn to release both hands and clap.

4. Put the toy in the basket.

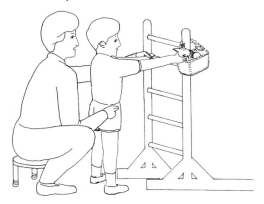

I put the toy in the basket   1   2   3   4   5

5. Grasp the rung.

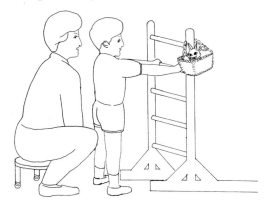

I grasp the rung   1   2   3   4   5

I put the toy in the basket   1   2   3   4   5

Analysis of Motor Task	*Speech/Songs/Rhymes*	*Guidelines*
1. Put the right leg on the rung. 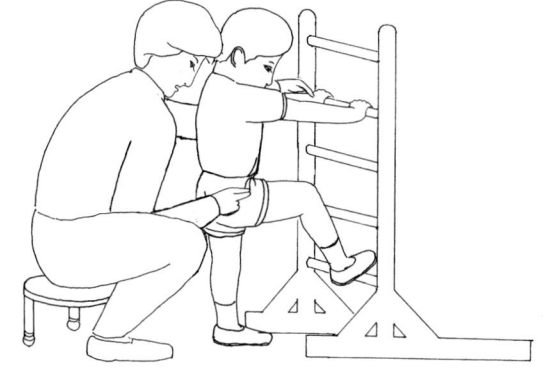	I put my right leg on the rung 1 2 3 4 5	1. Motivate the children to participate actively by inviting them to kick a ball placed between the rung of the chair.
2. Stretch the left knee. 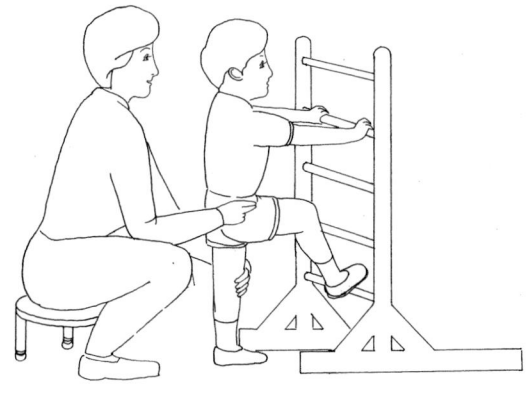	I stretch my left knee 1 2 3 4 5	2. Children at level 2 may need help to fixate the left leg on the floor while the right leg is moving onto the rung of the chair. They may also need a little help to place the leg on the rung.
3. Stand straight. 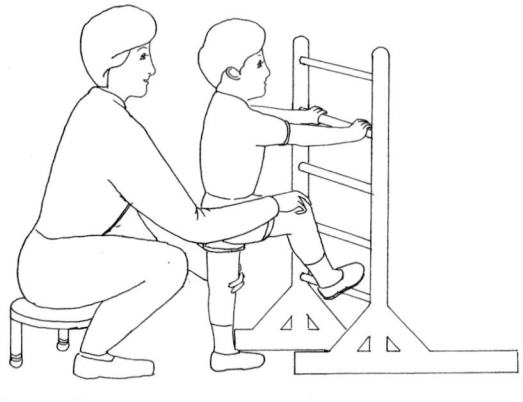		3. Encourage the children to point the leg resting on the rung of the chair outwards. Make sure they keep the other knee straight and the foot flat on the floor.

2. Children at level 2 may need help to fixate the left leg on the floor while the right leg is moving onto the rung of the chair. They may also need a little help to place the leg on the rung.

3. Encourage the children to point the leg resting on the rung of the chair outwards. Make sure they keep the other knee straight and the foot flat on the floor.

4. Use a two inch block for children to step on at level 4 intead of a ladderback chair.

5. Always encourage the children to stretch their elbows to help them stand straight.

6. Continue the game as long as the children are enjoying it.

Look at me

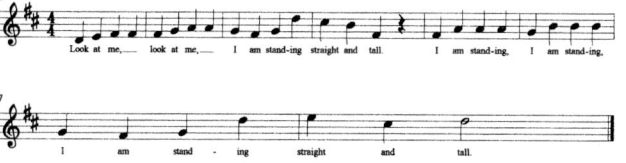

Look at me,____ look at me,____ I am stand-ing straight and tall.   I am stand-ing. I am stand-ing.

I   am   stand - ing   straight   and   tall.

4. Put the right leg on the floor. (Repeat step 1 to step 4 with the other leg).

I put my right leg on the floor   1   2   3   4   5

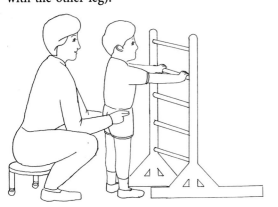

Analysis of Motor Task	*Speech/Songs/Rhymes*	*Guidelines*

1. Feet flat.

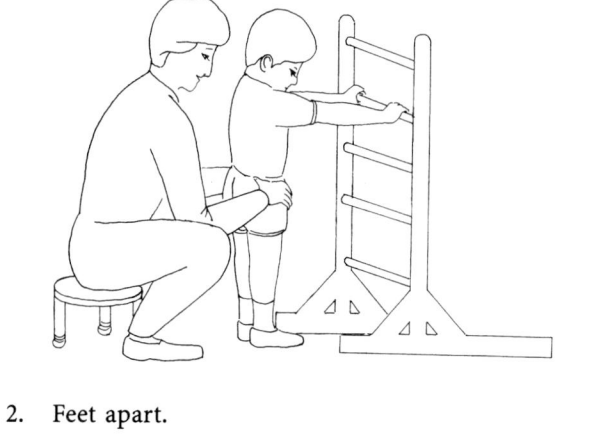

My feet are flat   1 2

1. This task is useful for children with hyperextension at the knees/unstable hips/preparing to sit down on the potty.

2. Motivate the children to actively participate by singing/asking them to pick up a toy from the floor.

3. Children at level 2 will need help to sustain their grasp of the rung as they squat down. They will also need help to learn to keep their feet flat and apart in the squatting position.

4. Encourage children at level 3 to maintain a good position while squatting.

5. Children at level 4 should learn to do it independently.

2. Feet apart.

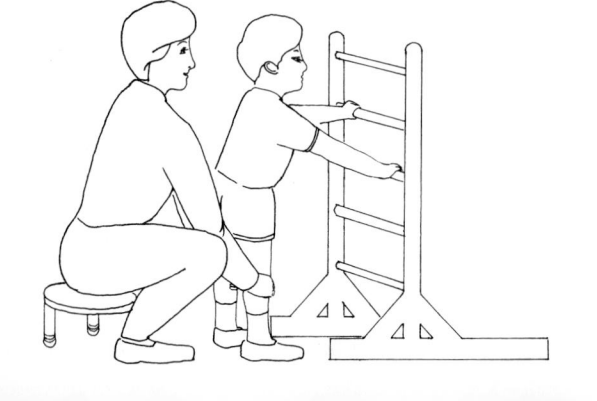

My feet are apart   1 2

3. Hands climb down to the middle of the chair.

I climb up/down

I climb up and hold.   I climb up and hold.   I climb up and

hold.   I climb   up   and   hold.

I   climb down and   hold.   I climb down and   hold.

I   climb down and   hold.   I climb down and   hold.

4. Squat.

I squat down   1 2 3 4 5

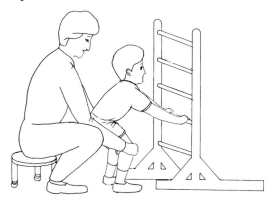

5. Feet flat and knees apart.

My feet are flat   1 2

My knees are apart   1 2

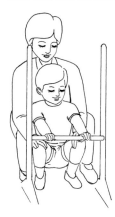

Analysis of Motor Task	*Speech/Songs/Rhymes*	*Guidelines*

1. Push the ladderback chair forward.

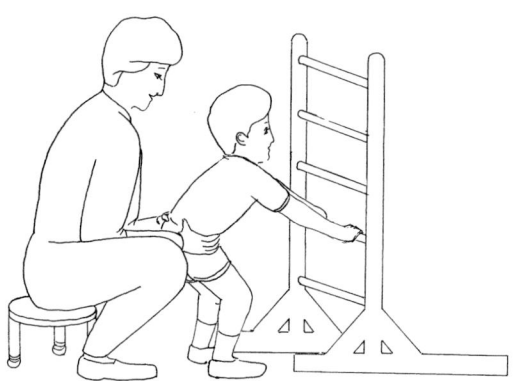

I push the chair   push push push

1. This task is useful for children with hyperextension at the knees and unstable hips.

2. Children at level 2 will need help to sustain their grasp of the rung as they stand up. When getting from squatting to standing, the care-giver may need to help them initiate standing up by pressing down gently but firmly on their knees. However, do not over assist them and encourage them to try and do it themselves.

3. Children at level 3 may also need some help, however children at level 4 should learn to stand up independently.

2. Stand up.

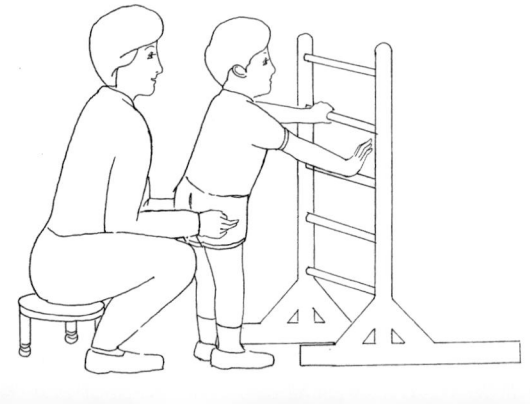

I stand up   1 2 3 4 5

Jack in the Box

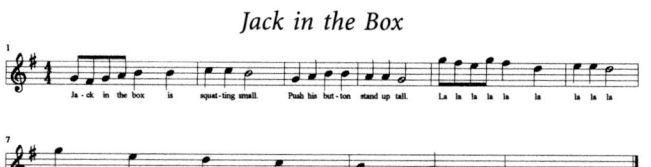

Jack in the box is squatting small. Push his button stand up tall. La la la la la la la la la

Standing up and standing tall.

3. Climb up the ladderback chair.

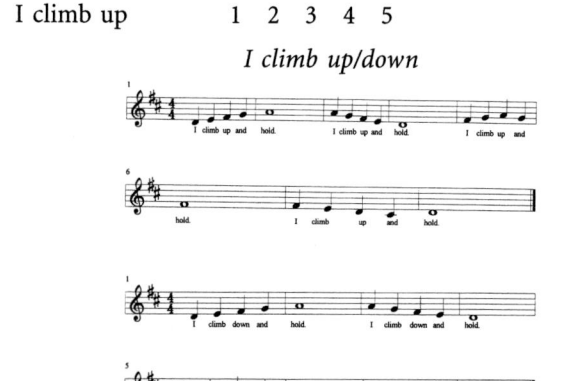

I climb up   1 2 3 4 5

I climb up/down

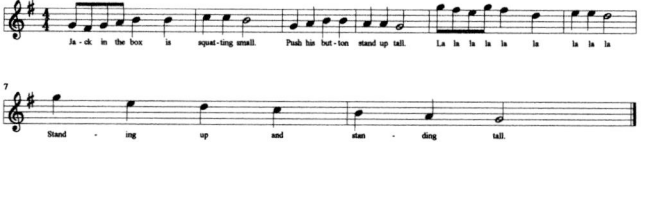

I climb up and hold. I climb up and hold. I climb up and hold.

hold. I climb up and hold.

I climb down and hold. I climb down and hold.

I climb down and hold. I climb down and hold.

4. Stand straight.

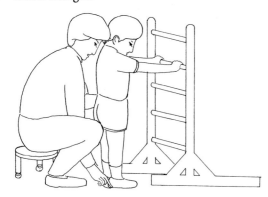

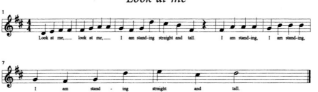

Look at me

Look at me,— look at me,— I am stand-ing straight and tall. I am stand-ing, I am stand-ing,

I am stand - ing straight and tall.

Analysis of Motor Task	*Speech/Songs/Rhymes*	*Guidelines*

1. Climb down the ladderback chair.

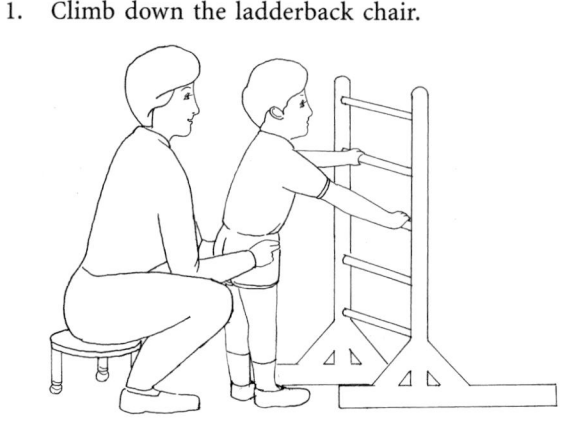

I climb up/down

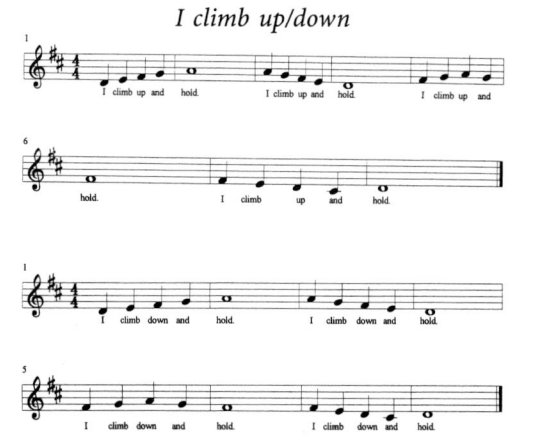

1. This task teaches the children to get down onto the floor and is necessary for activities on the floor.

2. Children at level 2 will need help to sustain their grasp on the rung of the chair as they kneel down. They will also need help to kneel up straight.

3. Children at level 4 should learn to kneel down with minimal manual help.

4. Encourage the children to stretch their elbows and kneel up straight.

5. Do not allow the children to sit back between the heels.

6. The children may kneel on a mat or piece of carpet.

2. Bend the right knee and kneel down.

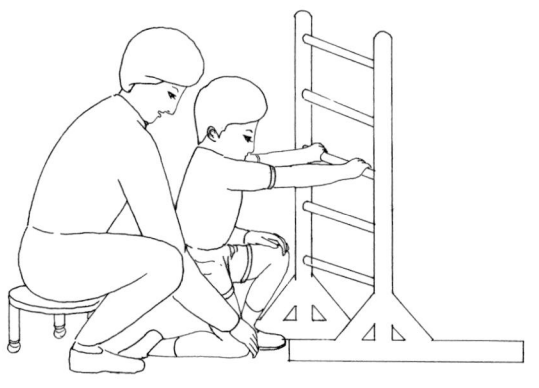

I bend my right knee and kneel down　　1　2　3　4　5

3. Left foot flat.

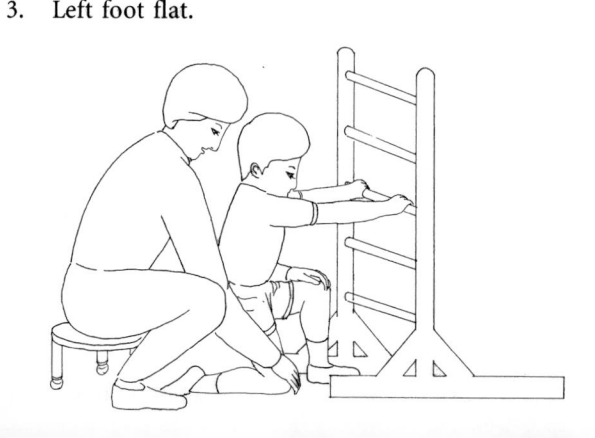

My left foot is flat　　　　flat　flat　flat

4. **Bottom straight.**

My bottom is straight   1   2   3   4   5

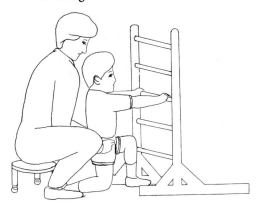

5. **Look at the toy.**

I look at the toy   look   look   look

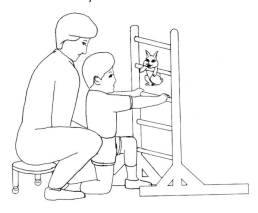

6. **Kneel straight.**

I kneel straight   1   2   3   4   5

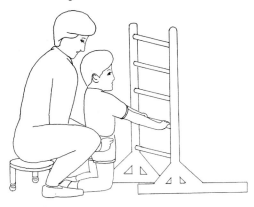

437

Analysis of Motor Task	*Speech/Songs/Rhymes*	*Guidelines*
1. Push the ladderback chair forward.	I push the chair push push push	1. This task teaches the children to transfer from kneeling on the floor to standing up.
		2. Children at level 2 may need gaiters to extend their elbows and for stability in standing.
		3. Children at level 3 may also need a little help to extend the elbows in standing. Children at level 4 should learn to do it independently.

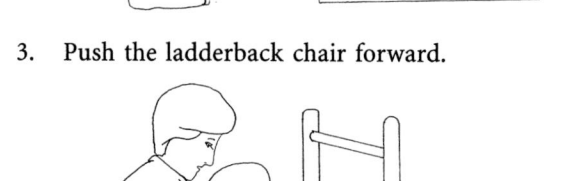

2. Put the left foot flat.   I put my left foot flat   1 2 3 4 5

3. Push the ladderback chair forward.   I push the chair   push push push

4. Stand up and climb up the chair with both hands.

I stand up   1 2 3 4 5

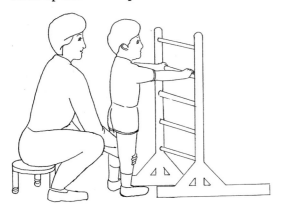

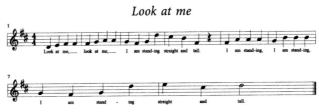

Analysis of Motor Task	*Speech/Songs/Rhymes*	*Guidelines*

1. Climb down the ladderback chair.

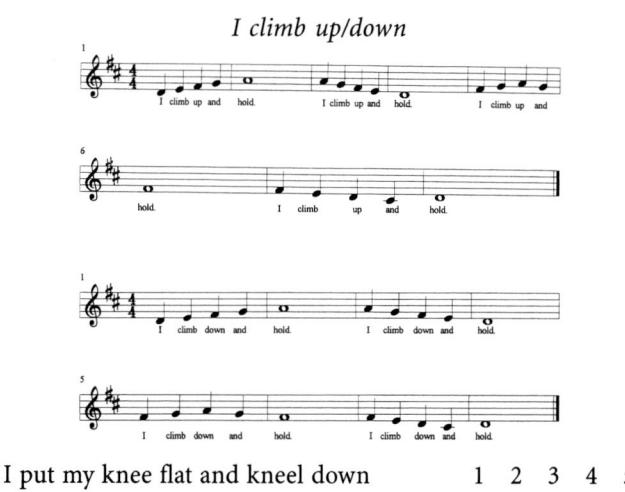

I climb up/down

1. This task teaches the children to transfer from standing to getting onto the floor for floor activities.

2. Children at level 2 may need gaiters to extend the elbows and kneel correctly.

3. Children at level 3 may also need a little help to extend the elbows in order to kneel well. Children at level 4 should learn to do it independently.

4. Do not allow the children sit back between their heels.

5. The children may kneel on a mat or piece of carpet.

2. Put one knee flat on the floor to half kneeling and kneel down.

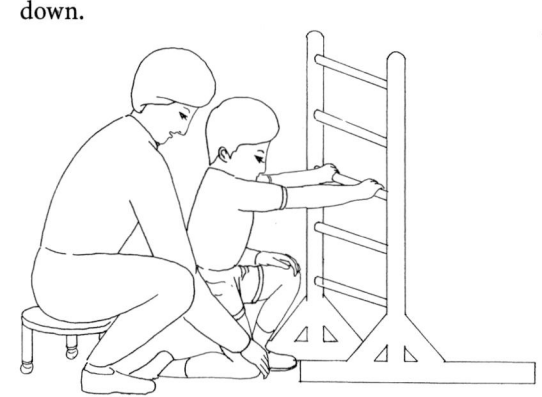

I put my knee flat and kneel down   1 2 3 4 5

3. Bottom straight.

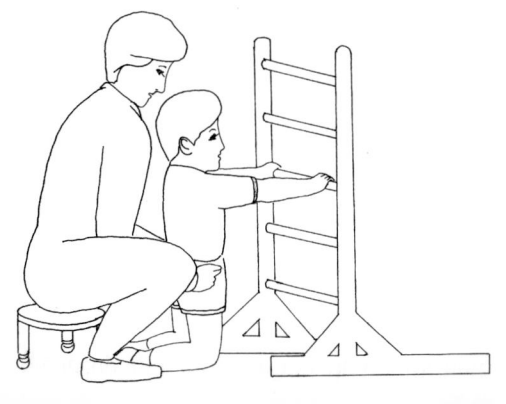

My bottom is straight   1 2 3 4 5

4. Push the ladderback chair forward.

I push the chair   push push push

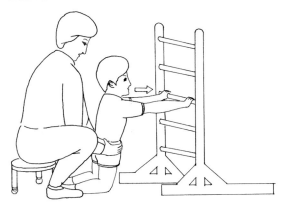

5. Put the right hand on the floor.

My right hand flat   1 2 3 4 5

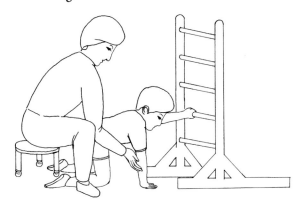

6. Put the left hand on the floor and straighten the elbows.

My left hand flat   1 2 3 4 5

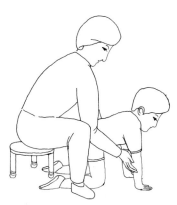

Puppy/Kitten

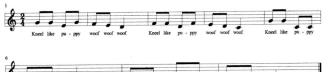

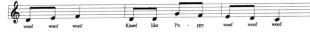

Kneel like pu - ppy woof woof woof. Kneel like pu - ppy woof woof woof. Kneel like pu - ppy

woof woof woof. Kneel like Pu - ppy woof woof woof.

Analysis of Motor Task	*Speech/Songs/Rhymes*	*Guidelines*

1. Sit to the left side.

I sit to my left side   1 2 3 4 5

2. Put the right hand to the right side.

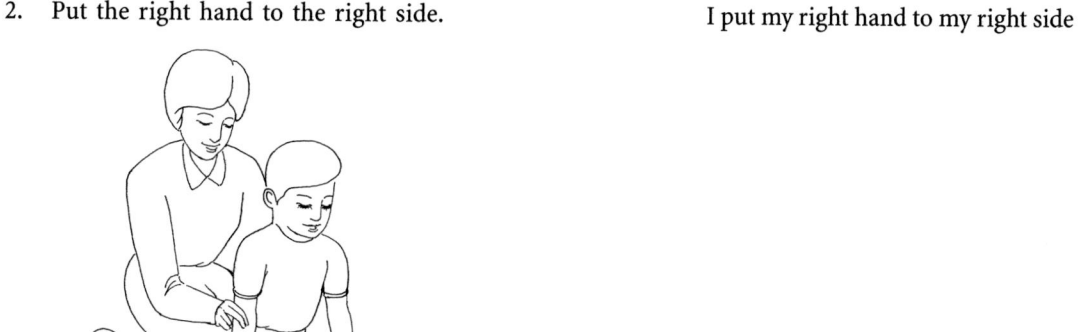

I put my right hand to my right side   1 2 3 4 5

3. Stretch the left knee.

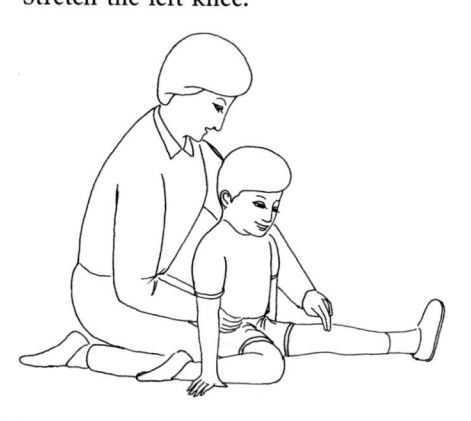

I stretch my left knee   1 2 3 4 5

1. This task is necessary for activities on the floor and for dressing/undressing.

2. Give the children every opportunity to practise it.

3. Children at level 2 will need help to do this task. Children at level 3 may also need a little help. However, children at level 4 should learn to do it independently.

4. It is important the children learn to push through their hands and push their bottom well back. They also need to learn to part their legs to help them achieve a good sitting base and anchor their bottom on the floor.

5. They need to feel secure sitting on the floor before they can engage in any activities. Some children may feel more secure sitting against the wall/furniture when they are learning this task.

6. Use a low stool/thick book (equivalent of a telephone directory)/sitting downhill on a wedge for children who have rounded backs to help them learn to straighten the back.

7. Children should practise sitting on both sides.

8. Give the children sufficient time to do each step and encourage them to use speech to guide their movements.

4. Stretch the right knee.

I stretch my right knee   1   2   3   4   5

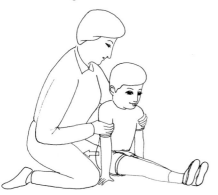

5. Hands flat on the floor push through the hands and push the bottom back.

My hands flat   1   2   3   4   5

I push my bottom back   1   2   3   4   5

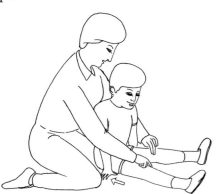

6. Sit up straight.

I sit up straight   1   2   3   4   5

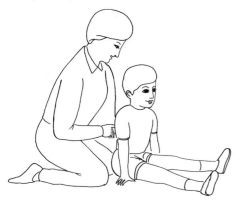

Analysis of Motor Task	*Speech/Songs/Rhymes*	*Guidelines*
1. Right hand to the left side. 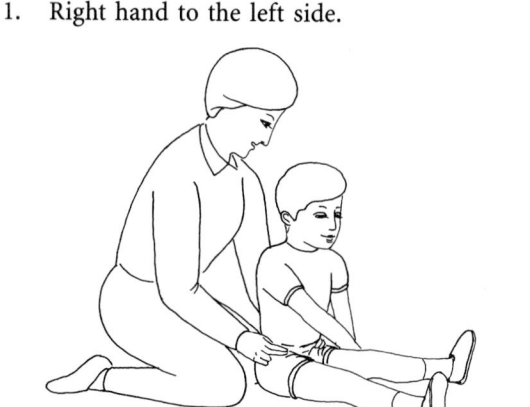	My right hand to left side　　1　2　3　4　5	1. This task teaches the children to transfer from one position to another. 2. Children at level 2 will need help to stretch the elbows in order to kneel correctly. 3. Children at level 3 may need a little help. However, children at level 4 should learn to do it independently. 4. Always encourage the children to stretch the elbows in order to kneel correctly. 5. Encourage the children to move backwards, forwards, and sideways when singing the song. Give the children sufficient time to do each step and encourage them to use language to guide their movements. 6. It is not recommended that children especially those with spasticity spend undue time in the four-point kneeling position.
2. Lean to the left side. 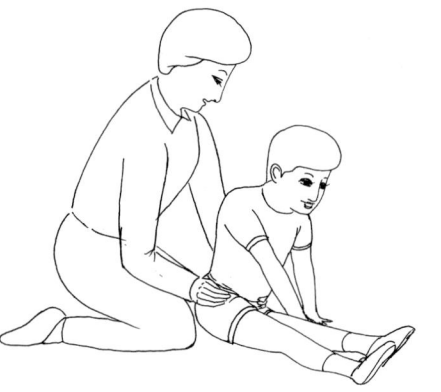	I lean to the left　　1　2　3　4　5	
3. Bend the knees. 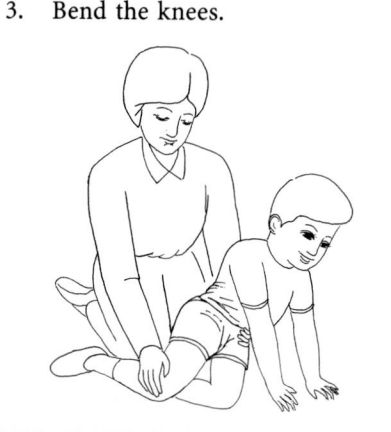	I bend my knees　　1　2　3　4　5	

4. Kneel up and get onto all fours.

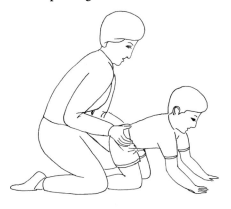

I kneel up   1 2 3 4 5

5. Stretch the elbows.

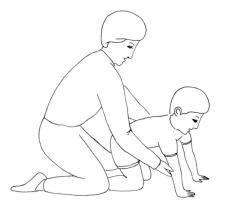

I stretch my elbows   1 2 3 4 5

6. Lift up the head to look at the care-giver.

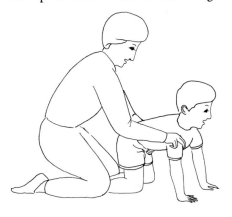

Puppy/Kitten

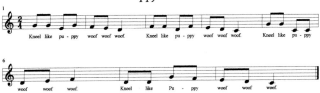

Task 19A Sitting to Standing Task Series: *Transferring from Kneeling on the Floor to Standing Using the Ladderback Chair*

Levels 2–4

Analysis of Motor Task	*Speech/Songs/Rhymes*	*Guidelines*
1. Sit to the side. 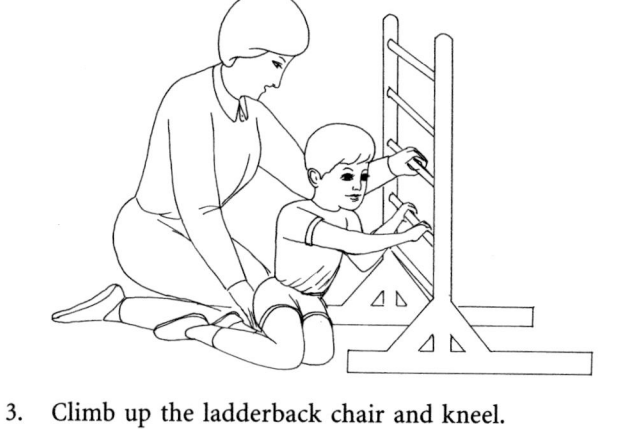	I sit to my left 1 2 3 4 5	1. This task teaches the children to get up from the floor to standing. Children may also use plinth/bed/wall rail/furniture to do this task.
2. Grasp the rung of the chair.	I grasp the chair 1 2 3 4 5	2. Children at level 2 may need help to initiate standing up. They will also need help to sustain their grasp as they stand up. The care-giver may also need to help them fixate their feet on the floor by placing her foot on their feet.
3. Climb up the ladderback chair and kneel.	I kneel up straight 1 2 3 4 5	3. Children at level 3 may also need a little help. However, children at level 4 should learn to do it independently.

Guidelines (continued):

4. When learning to stand up do not allow the children to climb up the ladderback chair and then pull up with their hands. Pushing the chair forward will ensure the children bring their body weight over their feet before they attempt to stand up.

5. Make sure the children learn to keep their weight over their feet and do not allow them to pull backwards in extension.

6. Give the children sufficient time to do the task and encourage them to use speech to guide their movements.

7. In this position the children are ready for walking training (see Chapter 11, Task 20, levels 2–4).

4. Put the left foot flat.

My left foot flat   1   2

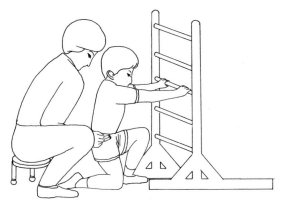

5. Push the ladderback chair forward.

I push the chair   push   push   push

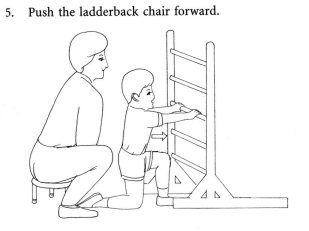

6. Stand up.

I stand up   1   2   3   4   5

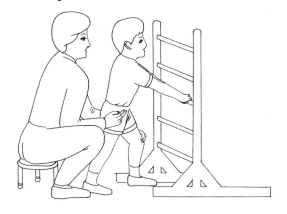

Analysis of Motor Task	*Speech/Songs/Rhymes*	*Guidelines*

1. Grasp the sides of the stool.

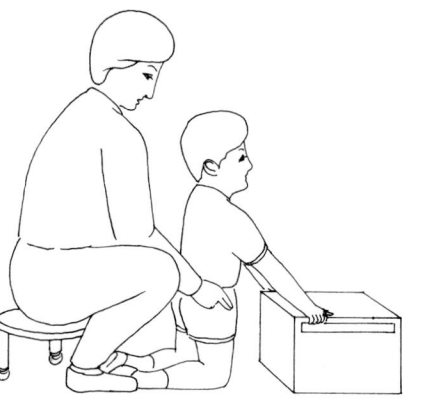

I grasp the stool   1   2

2. Kneel up straight.

I kneel up straight   1   2   3   4   5

3. Put the right foot flat.

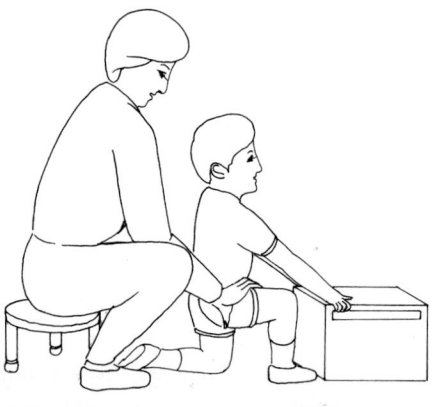

I put my right foot flat   1   2   3   4   5

Guidelines

1. Children at level 3 should begin to learn to stand up using a stool.

2. Children at level 4 may use a stool to stand or may learn to stand up using vertical pole/quadripods/quoit independently.

3. The care-giver should place the vertical pole/quadripod within easy reach for the children to grasp.

4. In the standing position, the children are ready for walking training (see Chapter 11, Task 20, Levels 2–4).

4. Lean forward.

I lean forward   1   2   3   4   5

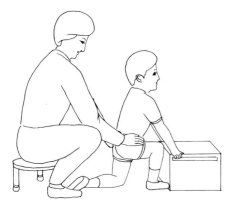

5. Stand up.

I stand up   1   2   3   4   5

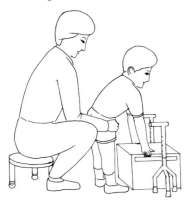

6. Grasp the vertical pole/quadripods/quoit to stand.

I grasp the quadripod   1   2   3   4   5

Look at me

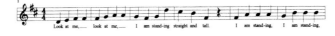

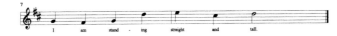

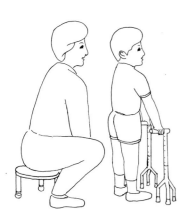

Analysis of Motor Task	*Speech/Songs/Rhymes*	*Guidelines*

1. Sitting task.

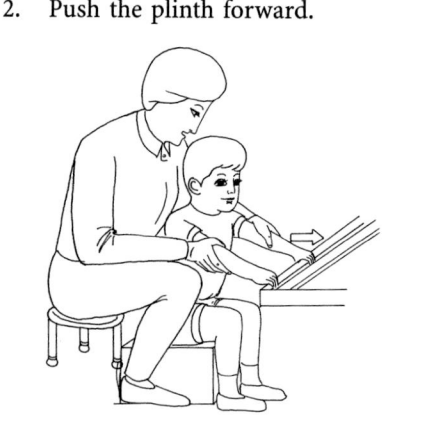

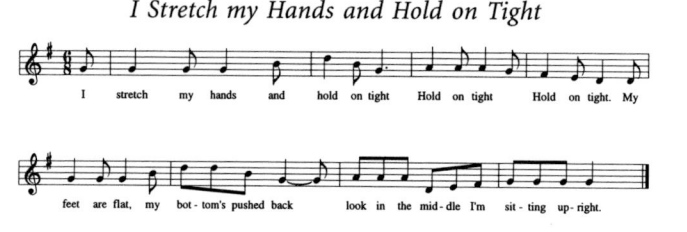

I Stretch my Hands and Hold on Tight

I stretch my hands and hold on tight Hold on tight Hold on tight. My

feet are flat, my bot- tom's pushed back look in the mid-dle I'm sit-ting up-right.

2. Push the plinth forward.

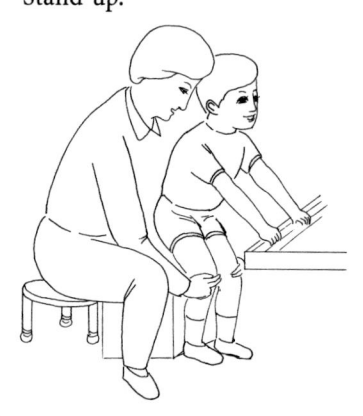

I push the plinth   push push push

3. Stand up.

I stand up   1 2 3 4 5

1. When using speech the care-giver should employ a slow even tempo, this is particularly important for children with spasticity.

2. When doing the steps children with athethosis should learn to hold, fixate and maintain the position. This is crucial in order to help them function in daily life.

3. Roll call helps the children become familiar with one another and encourages interaction in the group.

4. The children may answer to their photograph, their written name or their name when called. The care-giver may vary the manner in which she conducts roll call e.g. she may invite a child who is standing well to give roll call or the class monitor for the day may give it. She may also invite a child in the group to count the number of children.

5. Encourage the children to stand to answer roll call. Children at level 2 will need help to push the plinth forward and sustain grasp as they stand up. They may also need gaiters to stretch the elbows and for stability however, remove the gaiters when the children are sitting. Children at levels 3 may need minimal assistance, children at level 4 should try and learn to stand up independently.

6. Encourage the children at levels 3 and 4 to raise their hands high. Children at level 4 should learn to answer roll call standing independently.

7. It is important the standing well routine (see Chapter 12, Task 21, Levels 2–4) is carried out before the children answer roll call.

8. Give the children sufficient time to answer to their name.

4. Grasp the plinth with one hand and raise the other hand above the head answer to name.

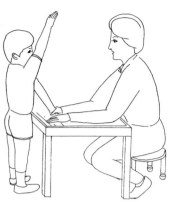

| I grasp the plinth | 1 2 3 4 5 |
| I raise my hand | 1 2 3 4 5 |

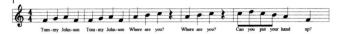

Good Morning

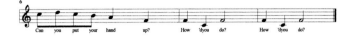

5. Lower the hand and grasp the plinth.

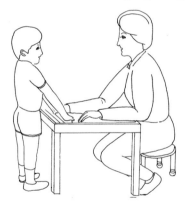

6. Sit down.

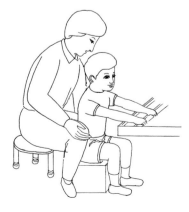

I sit down   1 2 3 4 5

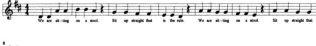

Sit up Straight

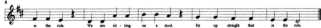

Analysis of Motor Task	*Speech/Songs/Rhymes*	*Guidelines*
1. Look at the stick. 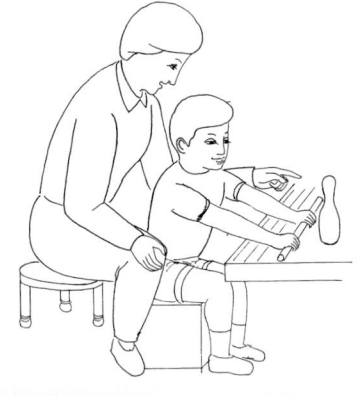	I look at the stick look look look	1. A ball may be used instead of a skittle or any other object that gives the children visual and auditory feedback.
2. Grasp the stick. 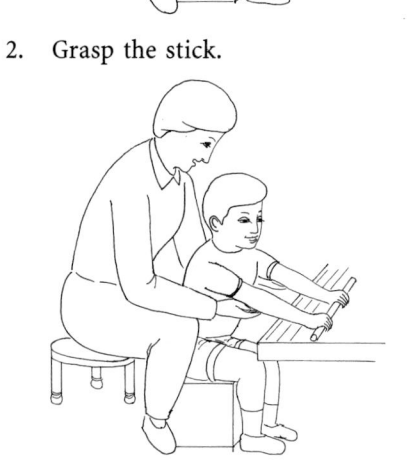	I grasp the stick 1 2 3 4 5	2. Use skittles with different colours to encourage the children to actively participate. Invite the children to choose a colour and to take the skittles and the sticks out of the basket and pass them along to one another. Make sure the children stretch the elbows when doing this.
3. Look at the skittle. 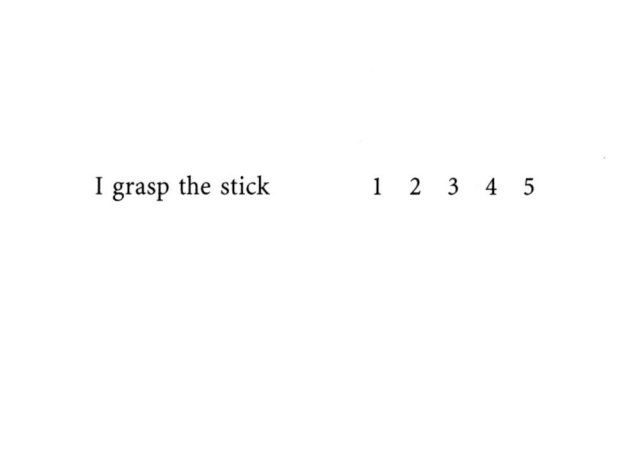	I look at the skittle look look look	3. Children at level 2 will need help. Children at level 3 should learn to do it independently. Encourage the children at level 4 to learn to clasp their hands and push the skittle.

4. Always check children's sitting posture after each game. When children with spasticity try to learn to use the upper part of the body the lower part of the body becomes more spastic and will result in an abnormal sitting posture.

5. If the skittles are different colours the children should learn to name the colours. |

4. Bend the elbows.

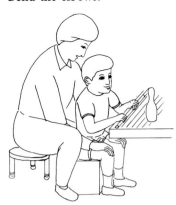

I bend the elbows   1 2 3 4 5

5. Push the skittle and knock it. (Repeat)

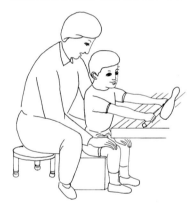

I push the skittle   push push push

Analysis of Motor Task	*Speech/Songs/Rhymes*	*Guidelines*
1. Grasp the stick. 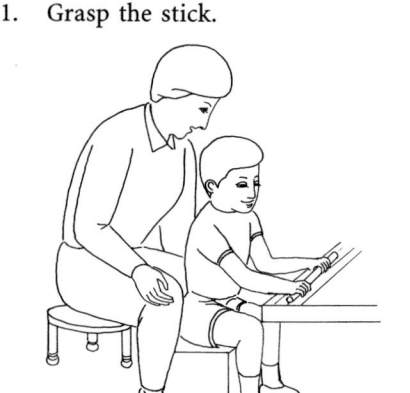	I grasp the stick grasp grasp grasp	1. This task offers the children the opportunity to socialise, make choices learn body image/up/down/behind.
2. Push the stick forward. 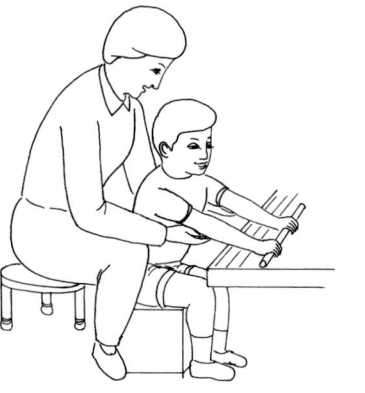	I push the stick push push push	2. Use sticks of different colours to motivate the children to actively participate. The care-giver invites the children choose a colour and learn to take the stick out of the basket. She may also invite a child who is sitting very well to pass along the sticks. This helps the children learn to socialise with one another. If possible the children should begin to learn to name the colour of the stick.
3. Raise the stick. 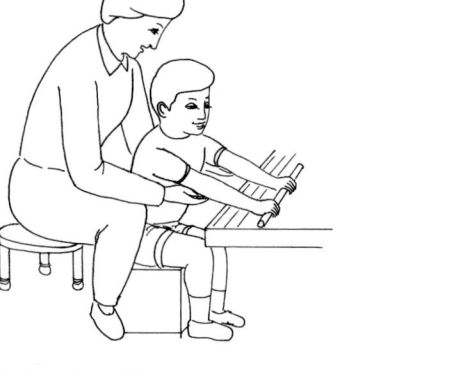	Stick above my head 1 2 3 4 5	3. Children at level 2 will need help to raise up the stick and place it behind their head. At this level they may still need ankle and thigh straps to fixate them in sitting and facilitate them when using their trunk and upper limbs. Encourage the children at levels 3 and 4 to stretch their elbows and shoulders to facilitate them to place the stick behind their head. Make sure they are sitting well with the bottom pushed well back to prevent them slipping forward on the stool when doing this task.
		4. If possible children at levels 3 and 4 may try to learn to grasp the stick with both hands supinated. Some children at level 3 may need help. However, children at level 4 should try and learn to do it independently.

4. Lower the stick behind the head.

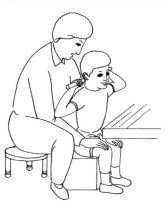

Stick behind my head   1 2 3 4 5

5. Raise the stick above the head.

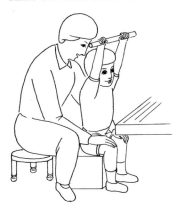

Stick above my head   1 2 3 4 5

6. Bring the stick down to the plinth.

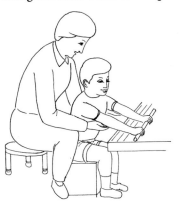

Stick down   1 2 3 4 5

Analysis of Motor Task	*Speech/Songs/Rhymes*	*Guidelines*

1. Sitting task.

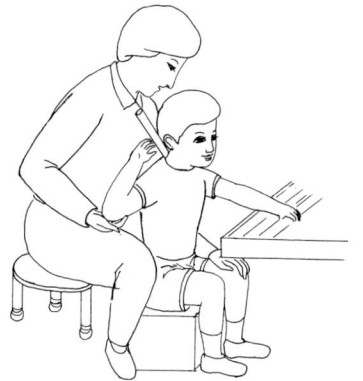

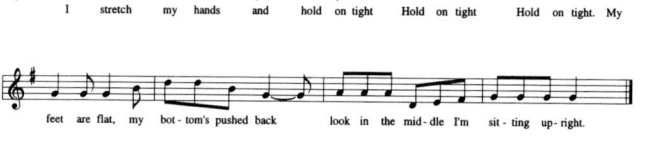

I Stretch my Hands and Hold on Tight

I stretch my hands and hold on tight Hold on tight Hold on tight. My

feet are flat, my bot-tom's pushed back look in the mid-dle I'm sit-ting up-right.

2. Raise one hand and grasp the stick which is placed at the back of the neck.

Hand behind my neck   1 2 3 4 5

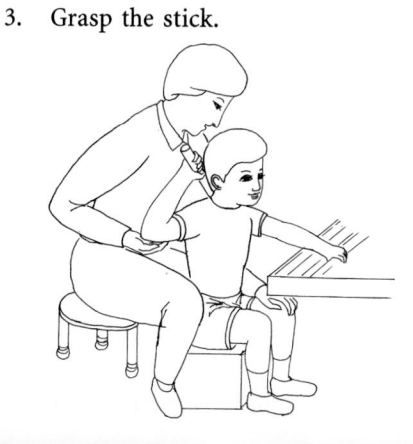

3. Grasp the stick.

I grasp the stick   1 2 3 4 5

1. The children should learn to disassociate the upper limbs e.g. one hand moving, one hand holding as this is a basis for functional activities in daily life.

2. Children at level 2 will need help to raise their hand, grasp the stick and raise it above their heads. Make sure the children maintain their grasp of the plinth with the other hand. Children at level 4 should learn to keep the palm of the hand flat on the plinth. This is a preparation for writing.

3. Children at level 2 may still need ankle and thigh straps for fixation when using their trunk and upper limbs.

4. Encourage the children to push their bottoms well back to prevent them from slipping forward on the stool while doing the task.

5. Give the children sufficient time to do each step and encourage them to use speech to guide their movements.

4. Pull the stick.

I pull the stick   1 2

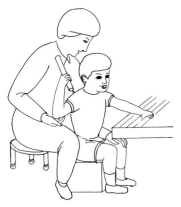

5. Raise the stick above the head.

Stick above my head   1 2 3 4 5

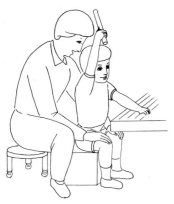

6. Bring the stick down to the plinth.

Stick down   1 2 3 4 5

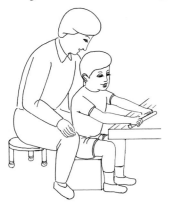

7. Repeat with the other hand.

Analysis of Motor Task	*Speech/Songs/Rhymes*	*Guidelines*

1. Look at the prints.

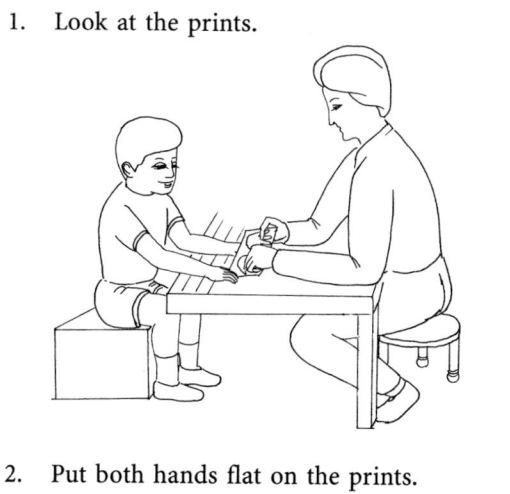

I look at the prints   look look look

1. Use different coloured hand prints to encourage the children to actively take part in the task. Invite the children to choose a colour. Where possible the children should learn to name the colours.

2. It is important the children learn to stretch their fingers and maintain flat hands with the thumb out, especially children with hemiplegia.

3. Children at levels 2 and 3 may find it difficult to separate the movement of their fingers. Give the children sufficient time to do the step and do not hurry them. Use a song with a strong rhythm. This task may be incorporated into a musical session using cymbals.

2. Put both hands flat on the prints.

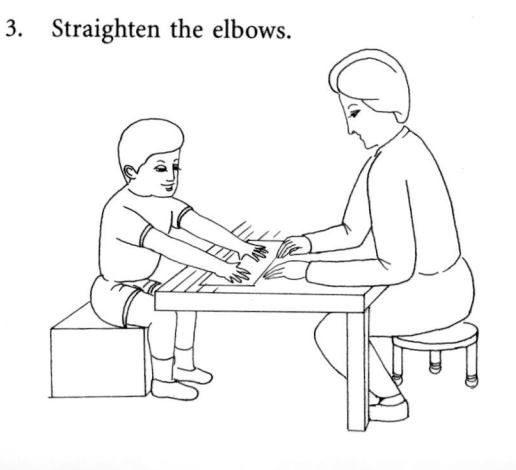

I make two flat hands   1 2 3 4 5

4. Children with athetosis may find it difficult to hold the movement. A strong rhythm is necessary.

5. Always encourage the children to maintain a good sitting position and stretch their elbows at all times to facilitate them while doing the task.

3. Straighten the elbows.

I stretch my elbows   1 2 3 4 5

4. Raise one hand up and down.

My hand up and down   1   2

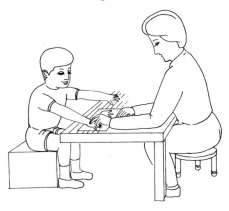

5. Raise the other hand up and down.

My hand up and down   1   2

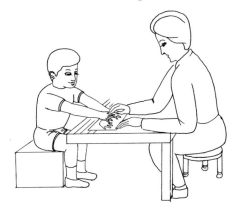

6. Repeat.

Pit-a-pat-a-pit-a-pat

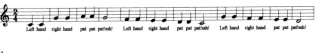

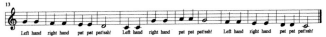

Analysis of Motor Task	*Speech/Songs/Rhymes*	*Guidelines*

1. Grasp the plinth with one hand.

I grasp the plinth   1 2 3 4 5

1. Use washable paints and A4 paper for this task. The shapes for the children to colour should be appropriate to their levels e.g. children at level 2 may need a bigger shape than children at levels 3 and 4. Invite the children to choose a colour.

2. Children at level 2 will need help. Children at level 4 should learn to keep within the lines of the shape/picture. Encourage them to learn to keep the other hand flat on the plinth.

3. Make sure the children with hemiplegia use their affected hand.

2. Make a fist with the other hand.

I make a fist   1 2 3 4 5

4. When the task is complete the children grasp the painting with both hands and hold it up for the care-giver and the other children to look at and admire.

5. The care-giver explains to the children the necessity to show appreciation for one another's work and if appropriate encourage the children to clap.

6. If possible, encourage the children to discuss their effort and when finished attach them to the group's notice board.

3. Point with the index finger.

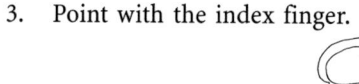

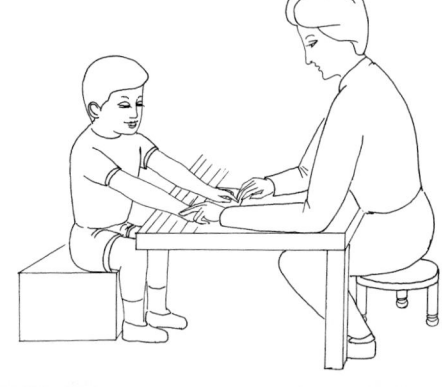

I point with my finger   1 2 3 4 5

4. Dip the index finger in the paint.

I dip my finger   1 2 3 4 5

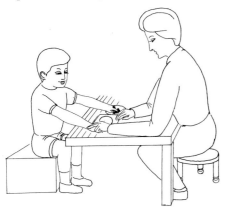

5. Colour the circle.

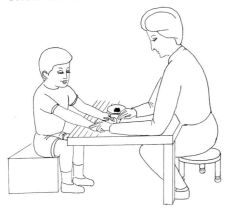

6. Wash the hands.

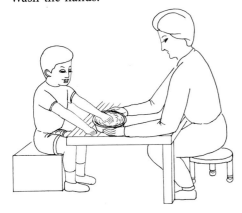

Grooming Song

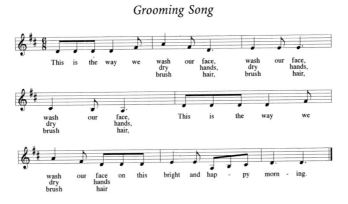

This is the way we wash our face, wash our face,
(dry hands, dry hands,)
(brush hair, brush hair,)

wash our face, This is the way we
dry hands,
brush hair,

wash our face on this bright and hap - py morn - ing.
dry hands
brush hair

461

Analysis of Motor Task	*Speech/Songs/Rhymes*	*Guidelines*

1. Put one hand flat on the print.

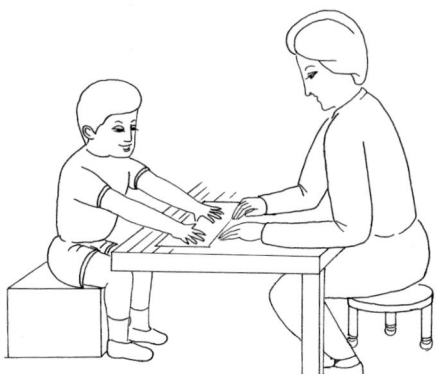

I make one flat hand   1 2 3 4 5

1. This task teaches the children right/left/counting/colours.

2. The painting task (which encourages the children to use the index finger) prepares the children for this task.

3. This task also encourages the children with hemiplegia to use both hands. It teaches children with athetosis to keep one hand flat while moving the other hand.

4. Use different coloured hand prints to encourage the children to actively participate.

5. Children at level 2 will need help, and children at level 3 may need some help. However, children at level 4 should learn to do it independently.

2. Make a fist with the other hand.

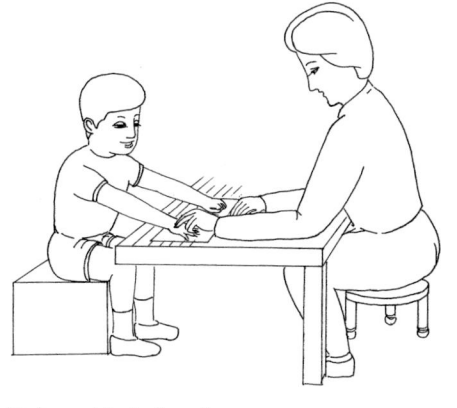

I make one fist   1 2 3 4 5

3. Point with index finger.

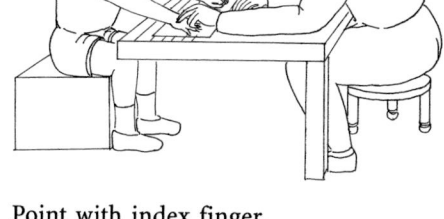

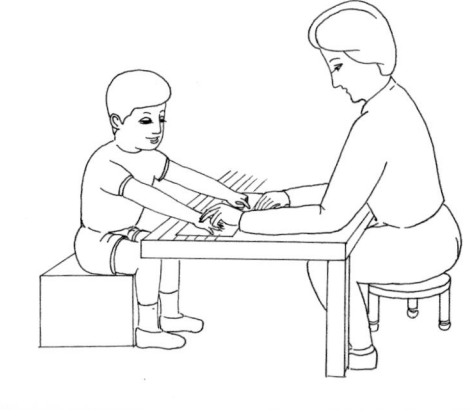

I point my finger   1 2 3 4 5

4. Look at the hands.

I look at my hands   look   look   look

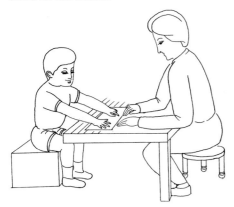

5. Count with the index finger.

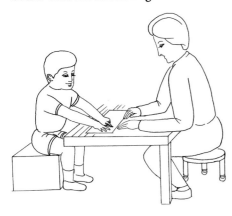

Ten Little Fingers

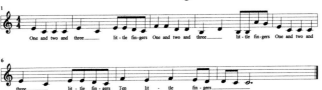

One and two and three_____ lit-tle fin-gers One and two and three_____ lit-tle fin-gers One and two and

three_____ lit-tle fin-gers Ten lit-tle fin-gers_____

Analysis of Motor Task	*Speech/Songs/Rhymes*	*Guidelines*

1. Look at the quoit.

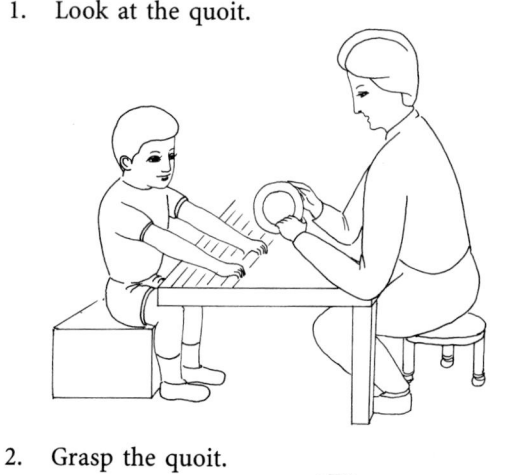

I look at the quoit   look   look   look

1. This task teaches the children to cross the midline.

2. Use quoits or coloured elastic bands for this task.

3. Invite the children to take the quoits from the basket and pass them along to one another.

4. Children at level 2 will need help with the task, children at level 3 may need a little help. However, children at level 4 should learn to do it independently.

5. Make sure the children look at what they are doing.

6. Give the children sufficient time to do each step and encourage them to use speech/song to guide their movements.

2. Grasp the quoit.

I grasp the quoit   1   2   3   4   5

7. Always make sure the children maintain a good sitting posture.

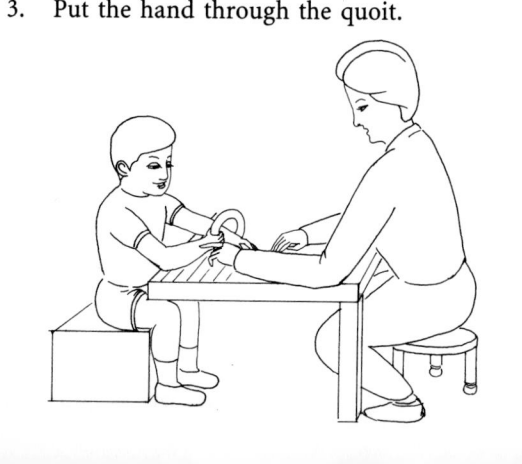

3. Put the hand through the quoit.

I put hand through the quoit   1   2   3   4   5

4. Pull the quoit up to the shoulder.

I pull up the quoit   1 2 3 4 5

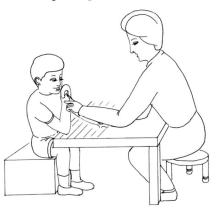

5. Pull the quoit down and remove.

I pull off the quoit   1 2 3 4 5

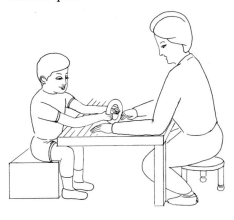

6. Repeat with the other hand.

Analysis of Motor Task	*Speech/Songs/Rhymes*	*Guidelines*

1. Look at the sleeve.

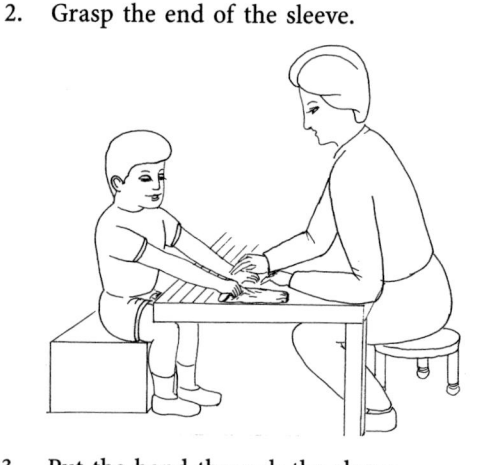

I look at the sleeve   look   look   look

2. Grasp the end of the sleeve.

I grasp the sleeve   1   2   3   4   5

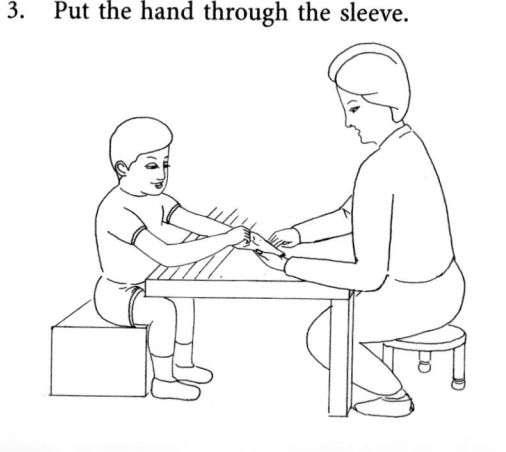

3. Put the hand through the sleeve.

I put on the sleeve   1   2   3   4   5

Guidelines

1. This task prepares the children for dressing/undressing.

2. Use brightly coloured sleeves to motivate the children to actively participate. They should always be worn before the art class to protect the children's clothing.

3. Invite the children to take the sleeves from the basket and to pass them along.

4. Always use every opportunity to teach the children to look/grasp/release and stretch their elbows.

5. Make sure that children with hemiplegia use their affected hand.

6. Children at levels 2 and 3 will need some help. However, children at level 4 should learn to do the task independently.

7. Always make sure the children maintain a good sitting posture.

4. Pull up the sleeve.

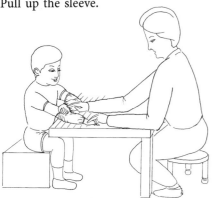

I pull up the sleeve   1 2 3 4 5

5. Raise up both hands and wave.

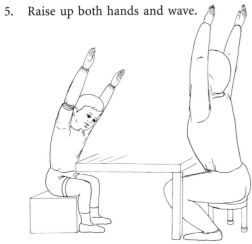

Up to the Sky

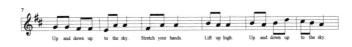

Stretch your hand.   Lift up high.   Up and down up   to the sky.   Stretch your hands and   lift up high.

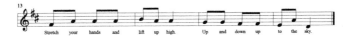

Up and down up   to the sky.   Stretch your hands.   Lift up high.   Up and down up   to the sky.

Stretch   your   hands   and   lift   up   high.   Up   and   down   up   to   the   sky.

6. Grasp the sleeve and pull off.

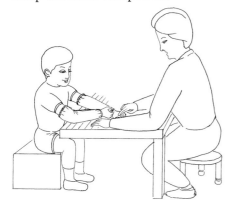

I grasp the sleeve and pull off   1 2 3 4 5

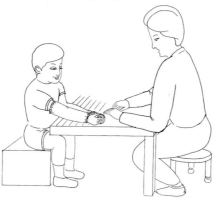

Chapter 17

Advanced Groups

- ADVANCED WALKING TASK SERIES

- ADVANCED HAND TASK SERIES
  (TASKS 1—7)

ADVANCED WALKING TASK SERIES

This advanced walking task series does not focus on a detailed analysis of each task as the children have reached the level where many of their movements have become automatic. The theme is "going to the market to buy fruit and vegetables" and gives the children the opportunity to cope with obstacles and develop their own initiative in solving problems. Although the children are in a group, each child works at his own level. The cognitive input is designed to suit children at different cognitive levels, i.e. some children may be matching fruit while other children are matching the Chinese character with a picture of the fruit.

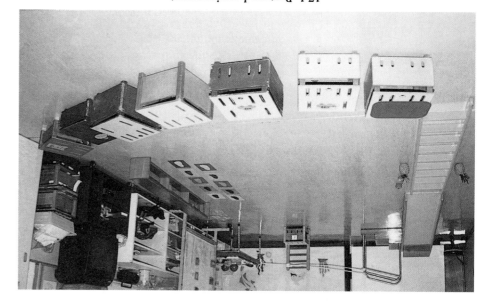

17.1 Prepared environment

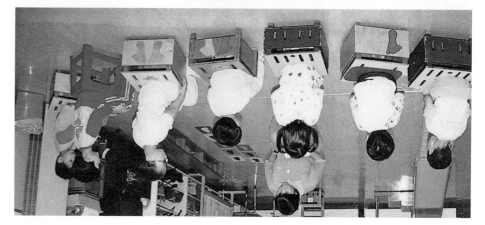

17.2 Sitting well task

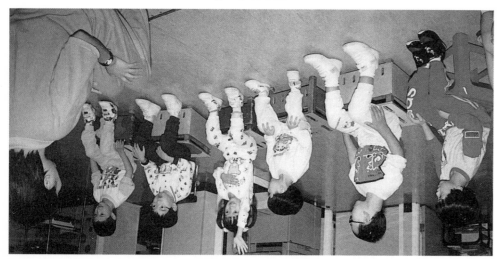

17.3 Roll call

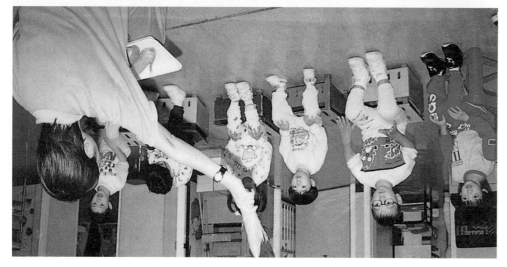

17.4 The care-giver tells the children what they will learn during the task series

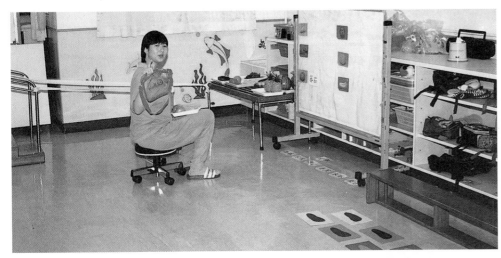

17.5 *The care-giver demonstrates the tasks the children have to do during the series, i.e., when the children buy the fruit they have to put it into the bag. Some children may need help to do this task*

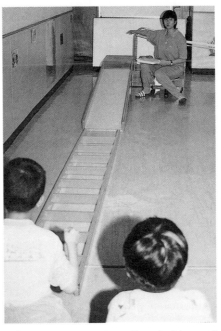

17.7 *Obstacles such as floor ladder and ramp are part of the problems the children will have to solve on their way to the market*

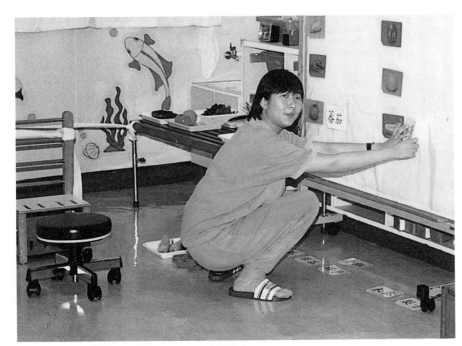

17.6 *The care-giver explains that some children learn to match objects with pictures while others match Chinese characters with pictures*

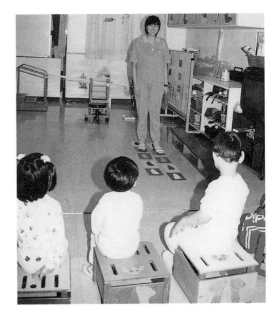

17.8 *She demonstrates the normal walking pattern*

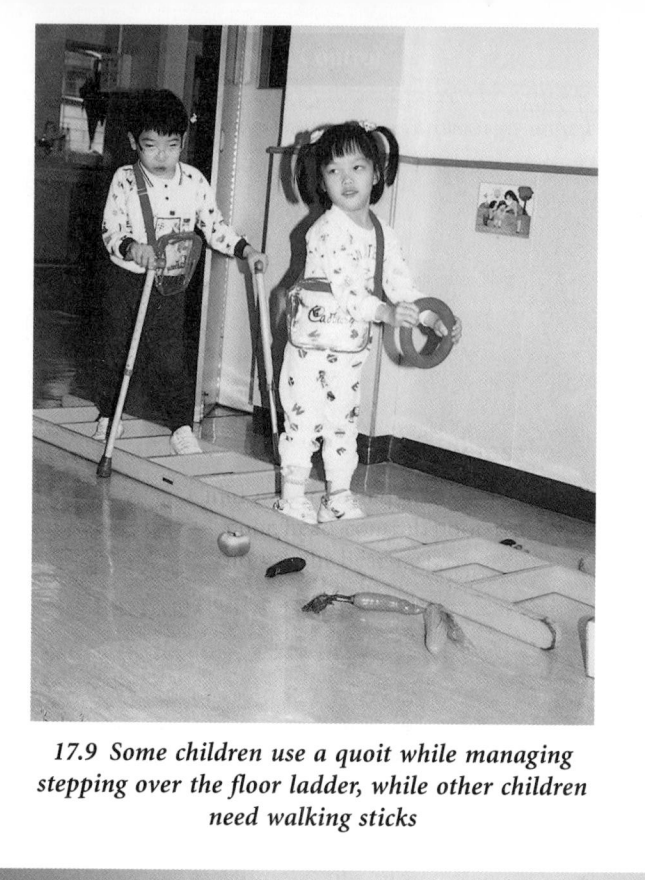

17.9 Some children use a quoit while managing stepping over the floor ladder, while other children need walking sticks

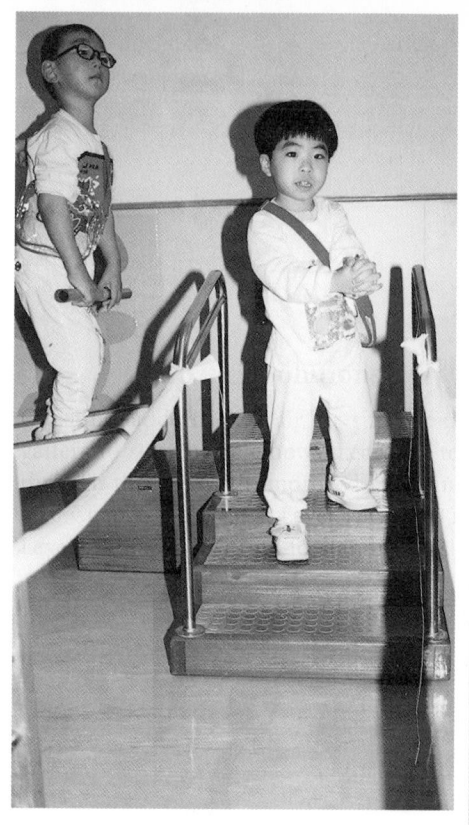

17.11 Learning to walk downstairs

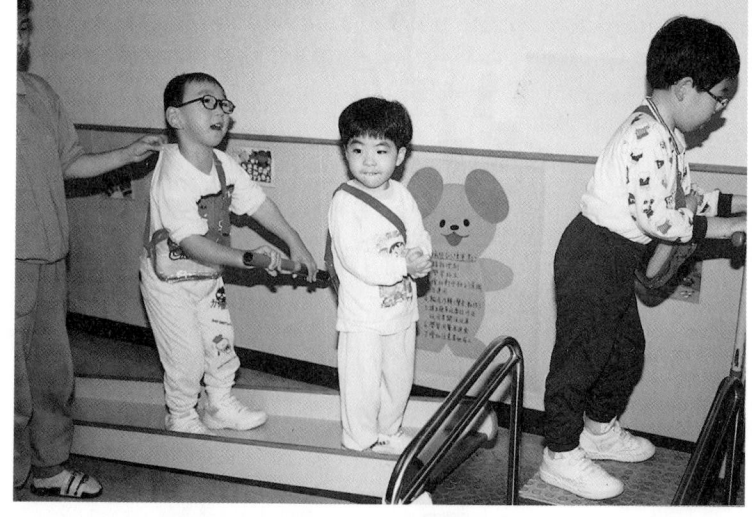

17.10 Some children need minimal assistance while others manage with clasped hands

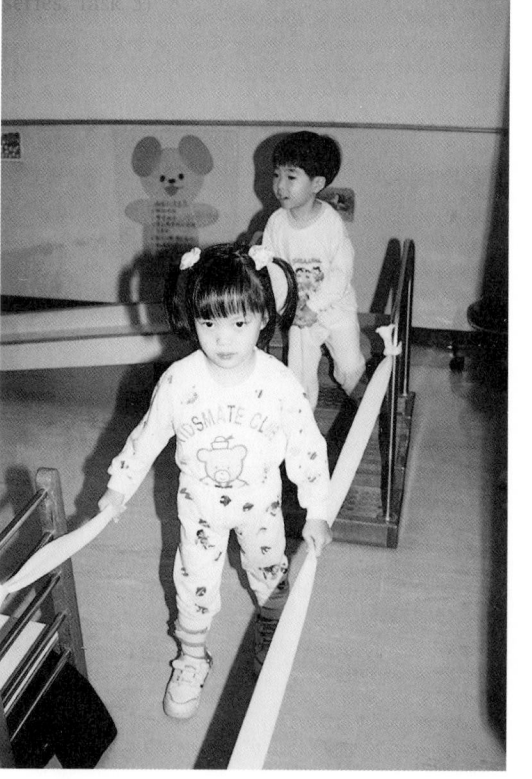

17.12 Learning walking balance between parallel ropes. The planned instability of the ropes challenges the child to improve his balance

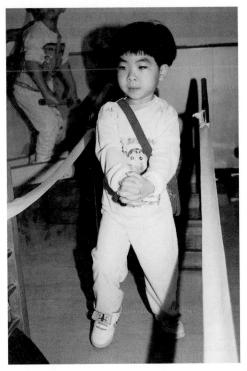

17.13 *Practising walking balance facilitated by the visual security of the parallel ropes*

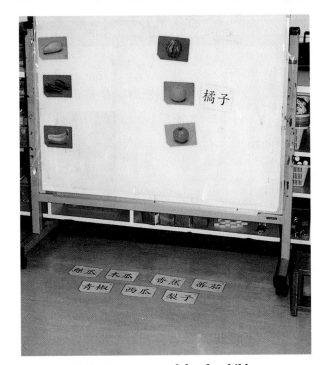

17.15 *Area prepared for the children*

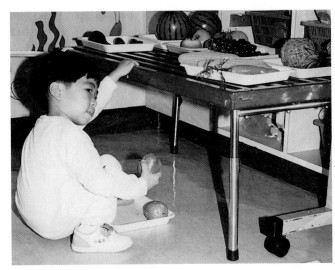

17.14 *Squatting to pick up vegetables from the floor*

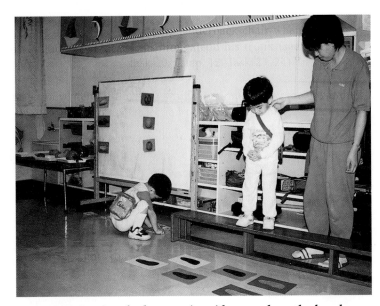

17.16 *Parting the legs moving sideways along the bench*

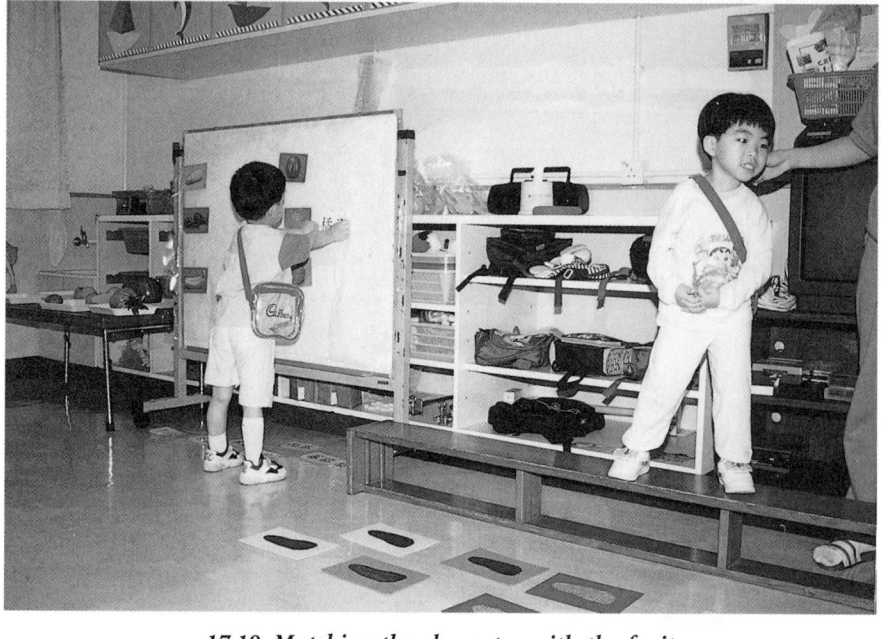

17.19 *Matching the character with the fruit*

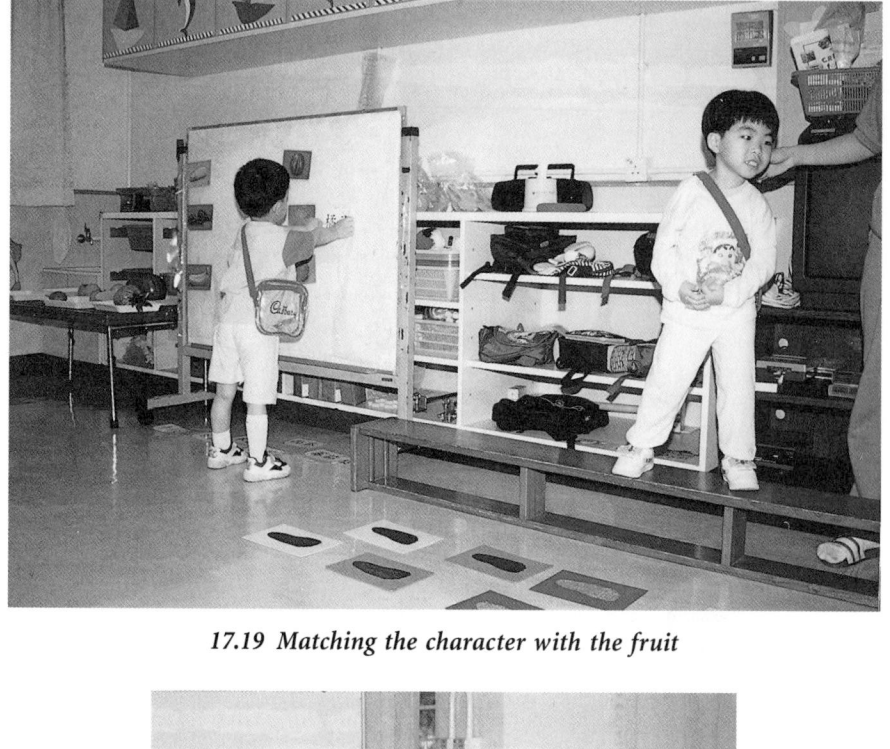

17.17 *Encouragement and minimal assistance from the care-giver*

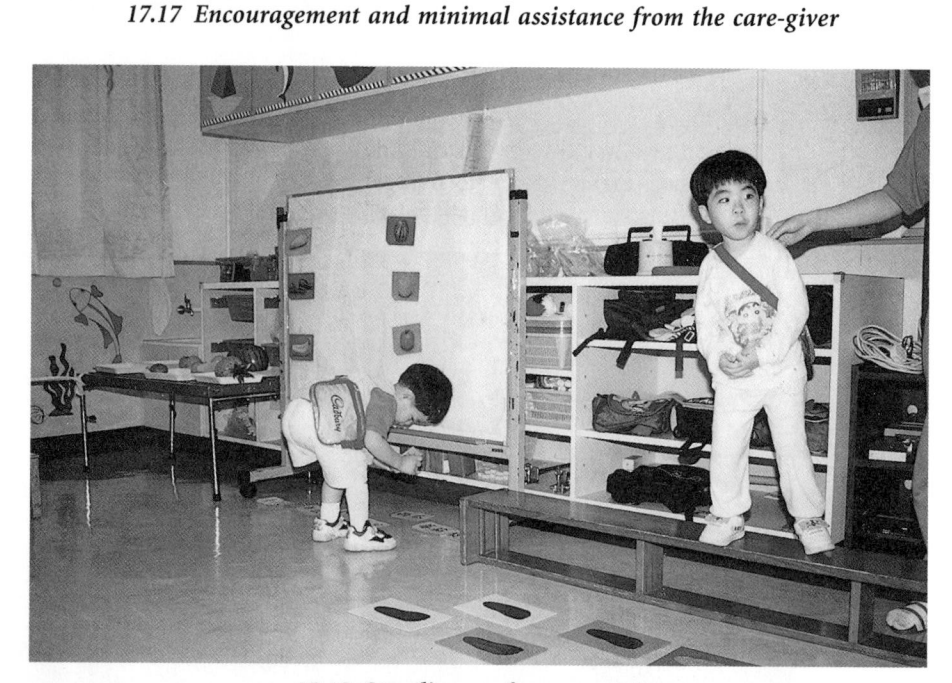

17.18 *Standing up from squatting*

17.20 *Walking up stairs*

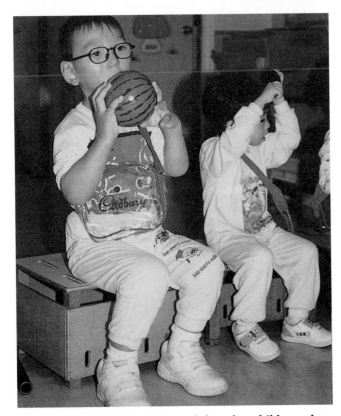

17.21 *Telling the care-giver and the other children what they bought and naming it*

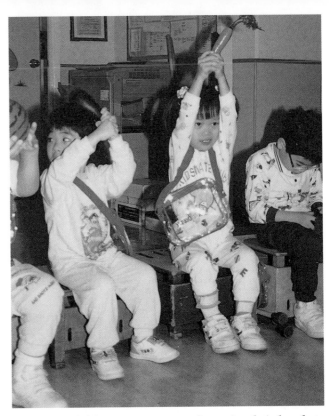

17.22 *The children are encouraged to raise their hands to display their purchases*

Analysis of Motor Task	*Speech/Songs/Rhymes*	*Guidelines*

1. Sit well.

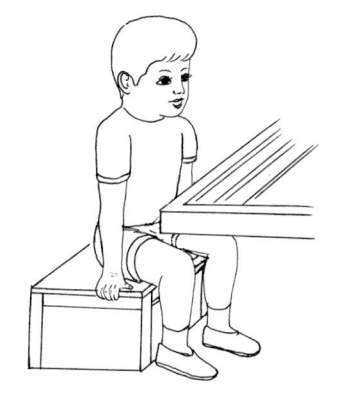

2. Put both hands flat on the table.

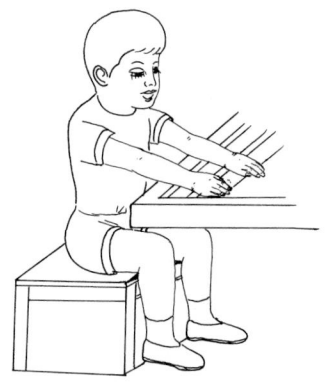

3. With wrists resting on the table, pat the table with alternate hands.

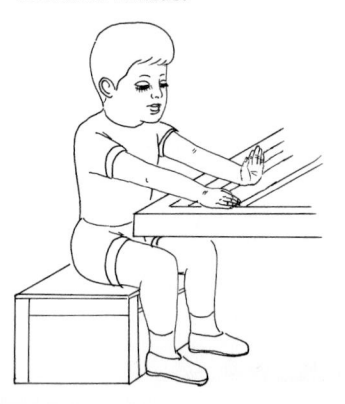

Pit-a-pat-a-pit-a-pat

Left hand right hand pat pat pat!ssh! Left hand right hand pat pat pat!ssh! Left hand right hand pat pat pat!ssh!

Left hand right hand pat pat pat!ssh! Left hand right hand pat pat pat!ssh! Left hand right hand pat pat pat!ssh!

1. While doing this movement make sure the children's wrists are on the table.

2. This is a suitable game for encouraging "standing up" the wrist.

Task 2 **Advanced Hand Task Series:** *Making Fist (Suggested Game: Catching Flies/Mosquitoes)*

Analysis of Motor Task	*Speech/Songs/Rhymes*	*Guidelines*
1. One hand lies flat on the plinth, the other hand reaches out to different positions to catch the imaginary fly. 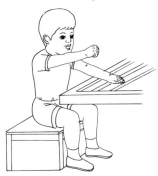	catch…	1. Children at this level are encouraged to engage in imaginary play, e.g., pretending to catch a fly. 2. The game can be repeated with the other hand. 3. Ask the children to catch the fly on either side, above their head and at their feet to give them the opportunity to stretch their arms.
2. Resting one hand on the table, bring the other hand which caught the imaginary fly near the mouth. Supinate the hand and open it slowly. 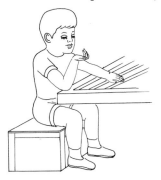		
3. Blow onto the open hand. 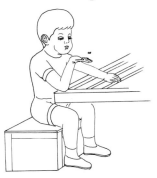	"Bloo…"	

Analysis of Motor Task	*Speech/Songs/Rhymes*	*Guidelines*

1. Rest both elbows on the table and make a ring with the index finger and thumb of each hand.

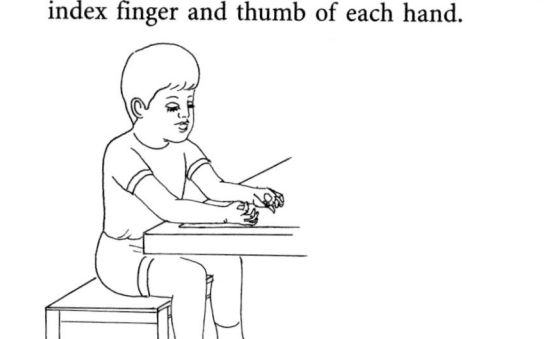

2. Place both rings in front of the eyes and pretend to look around.

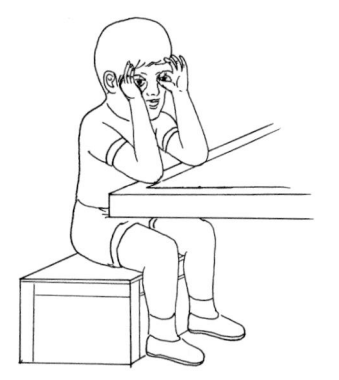

3. Put both hands flat on the table. Repeat.

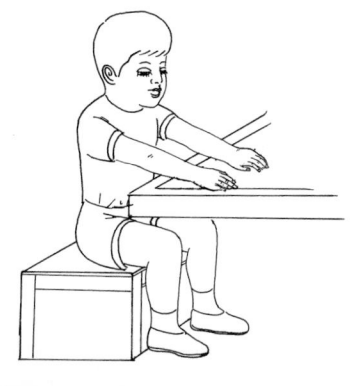

Guidelines

1. At this level children enjoy imaginary play.

2. Ask the children to look at one another when they wear the spectacles.

3. Repeat this game with the middle finger and thumb, the ring finger and thumb and the little finger and thumb respectively.

Task 4   Advanced Hand Task Series: *Climbing a Stick with 2 Fingers (Suggested Game: Pretend to be a Monkey Climbing a Tree)*

Analysis of Motor Task	*Speech/Songs/Rhymes*	*Guidelines*

1. Hold a narrow stick between thumb and index finger of each hand. Stand the stick up.

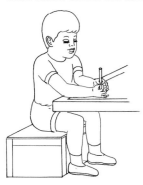

2. With the fingers, climb up the stick using alternate hands.

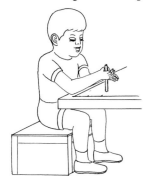

3. Climb down the stick.

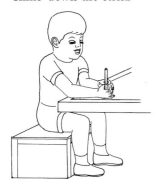

I climb up/down

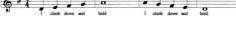

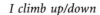

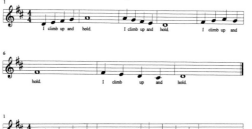

1. Pretend the stick is a tree and each hand represents a monkey. Small leaves may be attached to the top of the stick.

2. Use a small stick somewhat like a pencil.

3. The stick may be painted different colours, each of which occupies approximately 1 inch of the stick. Encourage the children to name the colours as the fingers climb the stick.

Task 5 Advanced Hand Task Series: *Unscrewing Small Bottle Lid (Suggested Game: To Open Bottle)*

Analysis of Motor Task	*Speech/Songs/Rhymes*	*Guidelines*

1. Hold the bottle with one hand.

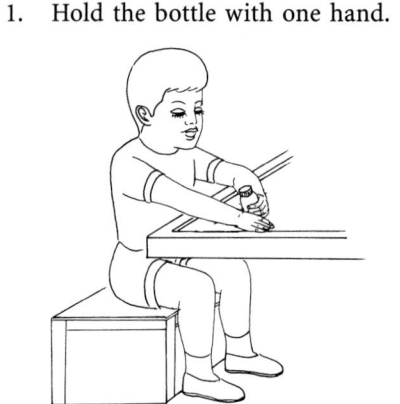

2. Unscrew the bottle lid with the index finger and thumb of the other hand.

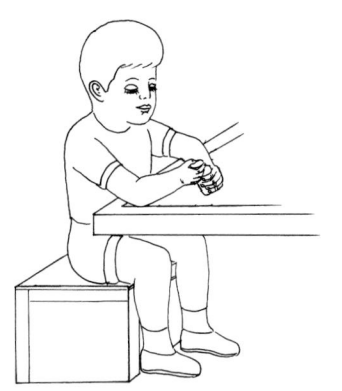

3. Pour out the contents of the bottle.

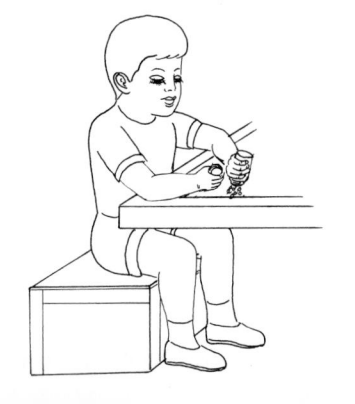

1. The bottle may be coloured, ask the children to name the colour.

Analysis of Motor Task	*Speech/Songs/Rhymes*	*Guidelines*

1. Pick up a bead with one hand and the thread with the other.

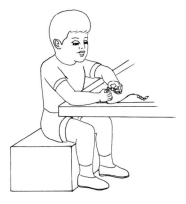

2. Thread the beads.

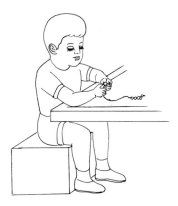

1. Beads may be of different colours and encourage them to follow a pattern of colours as they thread.

2. The children may like to make a necklace. When they have finished, encourage them to put it on and look in the mirror.

Analysis of Motor Task	*Speech/Songs/Rhymes*	*Guidelines*

1. Hold the chopsticks with one hand and pick up the cotton ball.

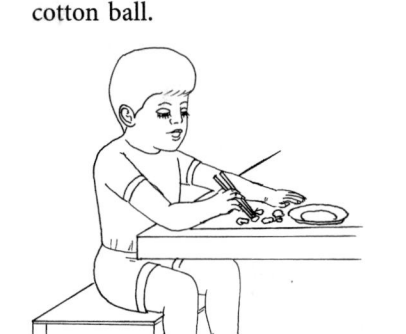

2. Release the cotton ball into a container.

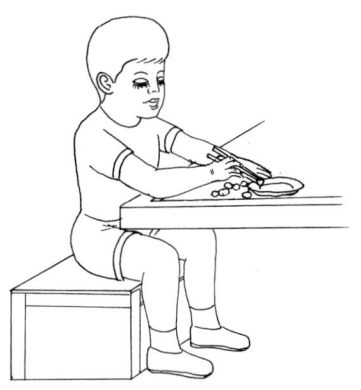

1. Upgrade by picking up:

   a) cotton ball,

   b) crumbs of paper,

   c) marshmallow,

   d) peanuts,

   e) unshelled peanuts.

Problems Which Care-Givers May Encounter

Problems

1. Internal rotation of the upper limb

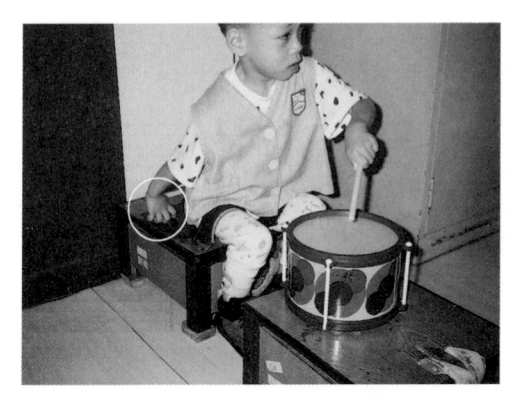

Solutions

Stretching both upper limbs when pulling up the plinth
(see chap. 13, Task 25, 26, chap. 16, lying task series Task 5)

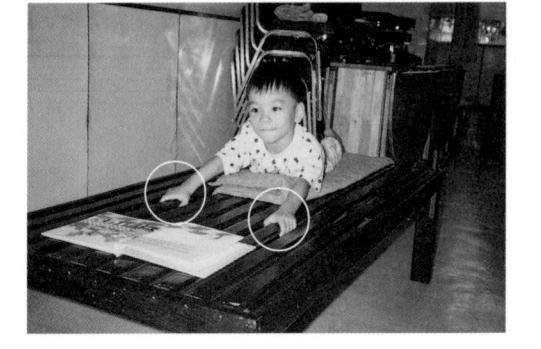

Problems

2. Flexed wrist

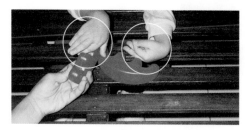

Solutions

Hands — wrist extended when pushing the plinth forward (see Chap. 12, Task 21, Chap. 16, lying task series, Task 2, hand task series, Task 1, sitting to standing task series, Tasks 9, 13, 15, 19A,B)

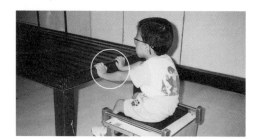

Holding a stick with extended wrist and thumb out (see Chap. 6, Tasks 3, 4, Chap. 9, Task 17, Chap. 11, Tasks 19, 20, Chap. 12, Tasks 23, 24, Chap. 16, lying task series, Tasks 9, 10, sitting to standing task series, Tasks 9–16, 19A)

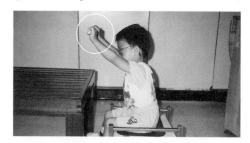

Holding a cup with extended wrist and thumb out (see Chap. 5, Task 2)

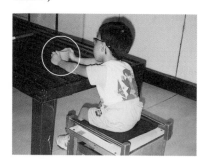

Pulling up the plinth with wrist extended and thumb out (see Chap. 13, Tasks 25, 26, Chap. 16, lying task series, Task 5)

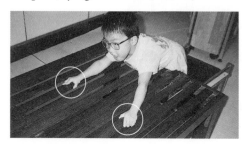

Clasping hands with thumb out and wrist extended (see Chap. 11, Tasks 19, 20, Chap. 12, Tasks 21–24)

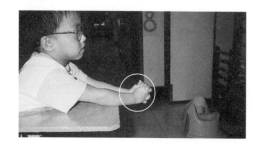

485

Problems

1. No fixation of arms and legs

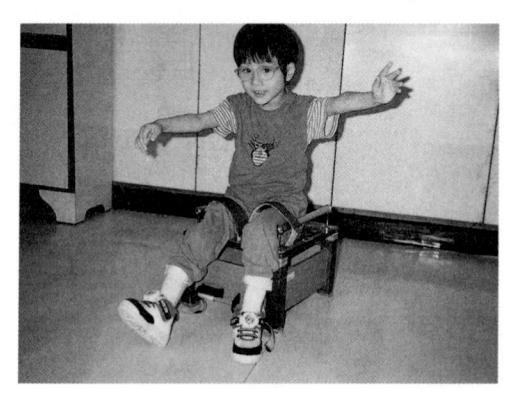

Solutions

Learning to fixate hands and feet and weight bear in standing and walking (see Chap. 6, Task 4, Chap. 7, Task 6, Chap. 11, Tasks 19, 20, Chap. 12, Tasks 21, 23, 24, Chap. 13, Tasks 25, 26, Chap. 16, sitting to standing task series, Tasks 9–13)

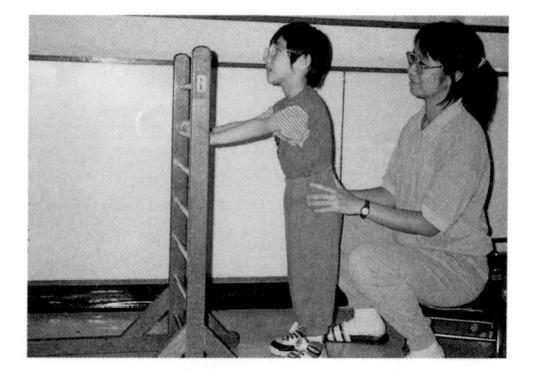

Learning to fixate hands and feet when sitting (see Chap. 6, Task 3, Chap. 7, Tasks 5, 7, 8, Chap. 9, Task 7, Chap. 10, Task 18, Chap. 12, Task 22, Chap. 16, lying task series, Tasks 1, 2, hand task series, Task 1)

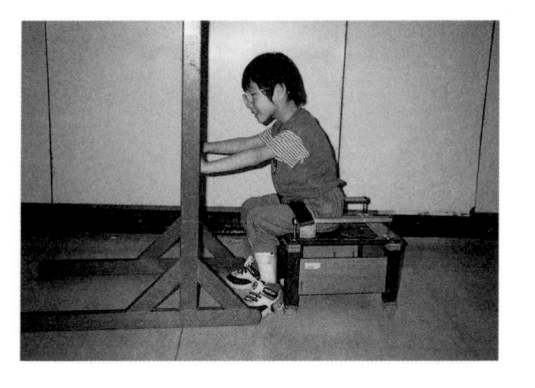

Problems

Child with poor head and trunk control

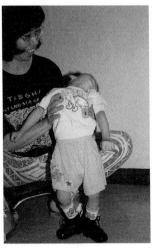

↓

Solutions

Learning to sit at plinth using gaiters to stretch the elbows, thigh and ankle straps for fixation (see Chap. 10, Task 18, Level 1, Chap. 15, hand task series, Tasks 1–5)

Sitting on stool with better head and trunk control using ankle and thigh straps for fixation (see Chap. 15, sitting to standing task series, Tasks 1–4, hand task series, Tasks 1–5)

Sitting on potty learning to maintain grasp of ladderback chair. Able to sustain head in midline position momentarily (see Chap. 6, Tasks 3, 4, Level 1)

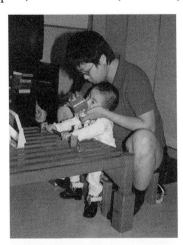

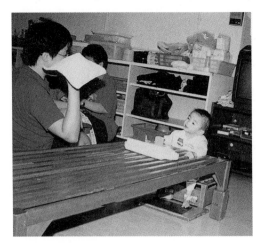

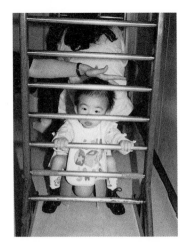

Problems

Child in supported standing
— poor head control, poor trunk extension and no weight bearing

Solutions

Grasping ladderback chair for support using elbow gaiters to stretch the elbows. Learning to bear weight through the legs with improved head and trunk control (see Chap. 6, Tasks 3, 4, Level 1, Chap. 11, Tasks 19, 20, Level 1, Chap. 15, sitting to standing task series, Task 5)

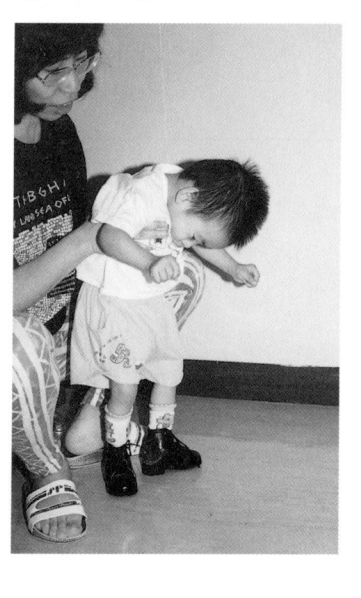

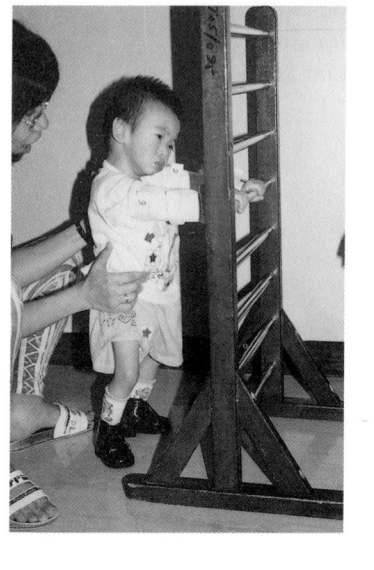

Problems

Child cannot sit with back straight and
consistently leans to one side

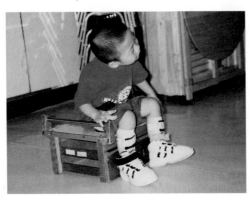

Solutions

Practising active trunk extension when
pulling up/pushing down plinth and when
pushing himself up using extended arms
when lying on tummy (see Chap. 13, Tasks 25,
26, Chap. 16, lying task series, Task 5, 6, 21–23)

Grasping the sides of the stool
for better trunk extension (see
Chap. 16, sitting to standing
task series, Tasks 1, 2)

Grasping ladderback chair when walking
helps him extend his trunk (see Chap. 11,
Task 20, Chap. 12, Task 23, 24)

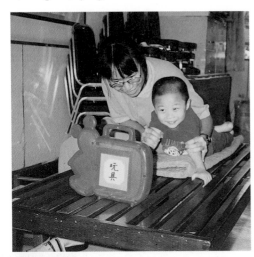

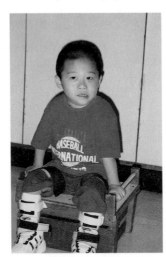

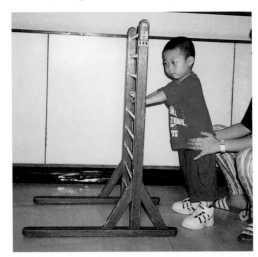

Problems

Child cannot sit with feet flat on the floor
and hips well flexed

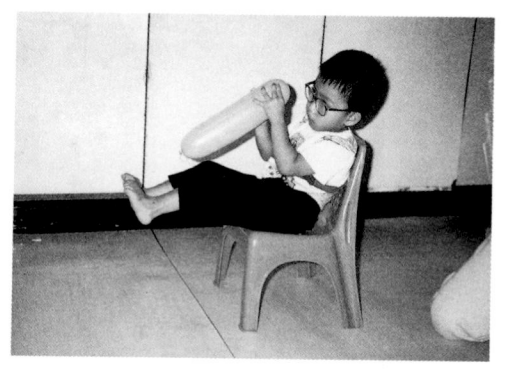

Solutions

Sitting on potty grasping ladderback
chair in front with hips well bent and
feet flat on the floor (see Chap. 6,
Tasks 3, 4, Chap. 12, Tasks 21–24)

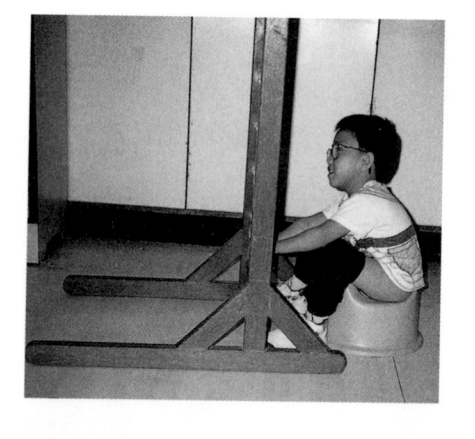

Sitting on stool grasping ladderback chair in
front with feet flat on floor and hips well
bent (see Chap. 7, Tasks 5–8, Chap. 9, Task 7,
Chap. 11, Task 18, Chap. 12, Tasks 21, 22,
Chap. 16, sitting to standing task series, Task 9)

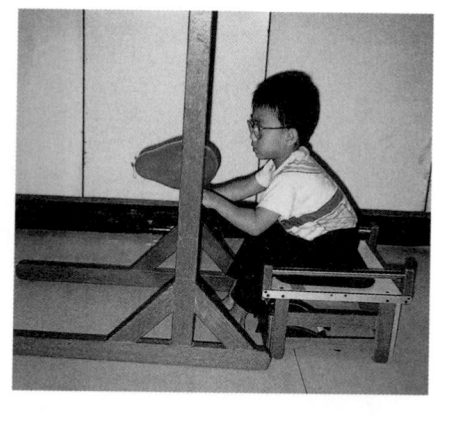

Problems

Child walks in scissoring gait

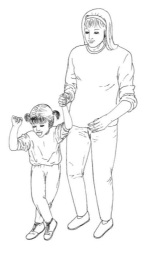

Solutions

Care-giver facilitates parting of knees (see Chap. 11, Tasks 19, 20)

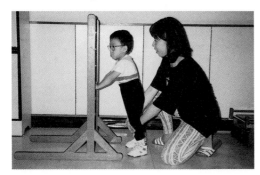

The hands of the care-giver when parting the child's knees

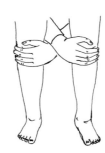

Problems

Child 'w' sits on the floor. This can easily cause hip dislocation

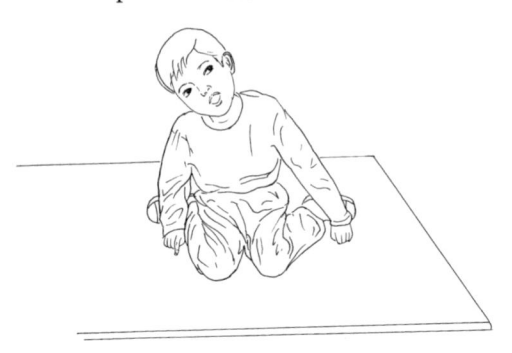

Solutions

Do not encourage the child to sit on floor. Preferably child sits on a stool with knees parted and both hands grasping in the middle of the stool

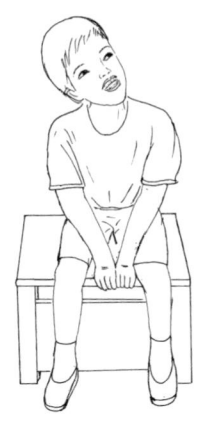

Problems

Child with tight heel cords.

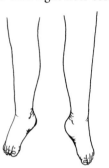

Solutions

Stretching can be done which involves his active participation

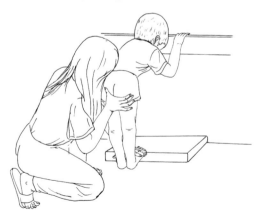

Child learns to sit on potty with elbow gaiters. She learns to grasp the ladderback chair, and sits with hips well bent, feet flat and apart, back straight and head in the midline (see Chap. 6, Tasks 3, 4)

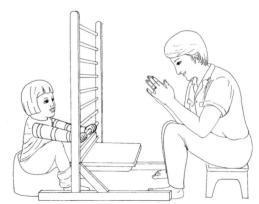

Squatting also helps to stretch tight heel cords (see Chap. 16, sitting to standing task series, Tasks 12, 13)

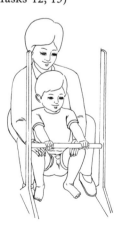

Walking up a ramp (see Chap. 17, Fig. 17.10)

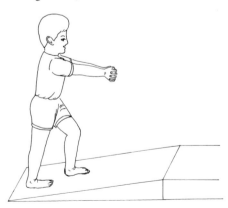

Problems

Child with spastic quadriplegia lying on a mat

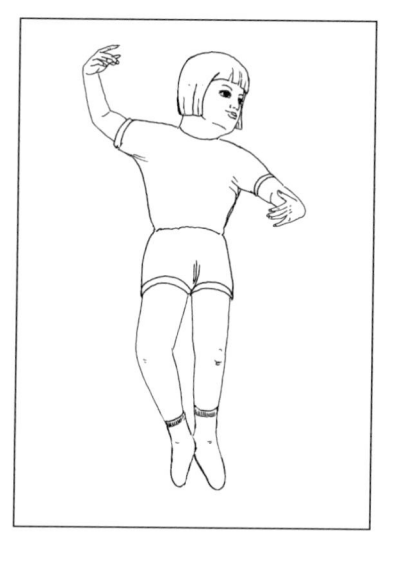

Child sits in a special chair with
— head support
— trunk support
— groin strap
— shoulder strap
— ankle strap and
— a removable table top (not shown in drawing)

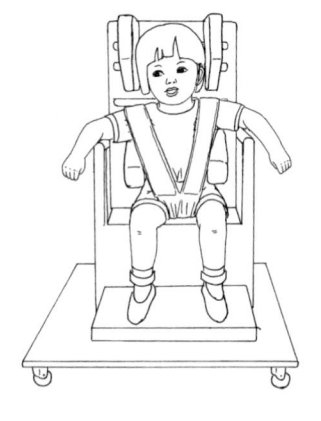

Child sits on a reclining bath chair with trunk leaning to one side, elbows flexed, wrists flexed

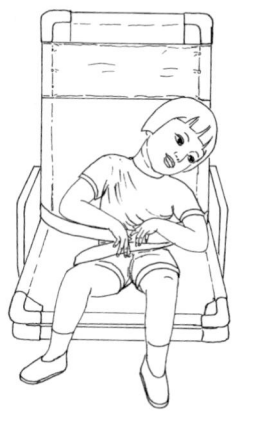

Solutions

Child learns to sit on a stool grasping plinth in front with thumb out. She sits with hips well bent, feet flat and head in midline (see Chap. 10, Task 18, Chap. 15, hand task series, Tasks 1–5)

Child learns to sit on a stool grasping ladderback chair in front. She sits with hips flexed, feet flat and apart, back straight and head in midline (see Chap. 15, sitting to standing task series, Tasks 1–5)

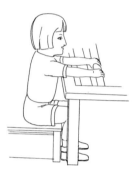

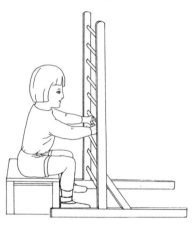

Child learns to take weight over her feet. She practises standing in a standing frame and grasps a horizontal bar in front to give her better trunk extension

Child stands independently grasping a ladderback chair in front (see Chap. 6, Tasks 3, 4, Chap. 11, Tasks 19, 20, Chap. 12, Tasks 23, 24, Chap. 16, sitting to standing task series, Task 9, Chap. 15, sitting to standing task series, Task 5)

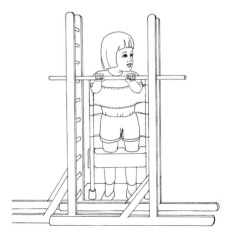

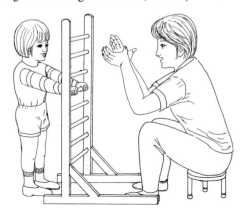

Teachings Aids

The teaching aids illustrated in the following pages are some examples frequently used in the task series.

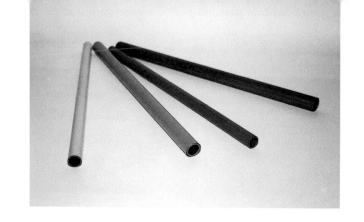

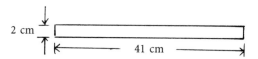

Two different colours

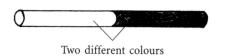

2 cm

41 cm

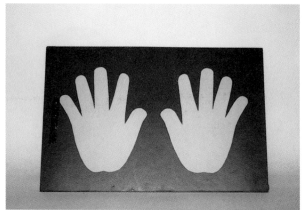

cardboard paper

Handprints made of different tactile materials

Handprints

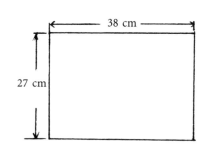

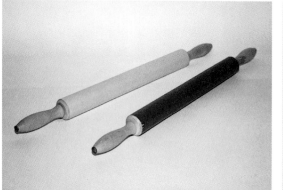

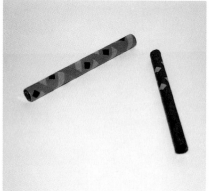

Stick/Rolling Pin

497

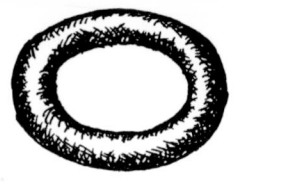

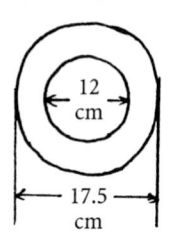

Quoit

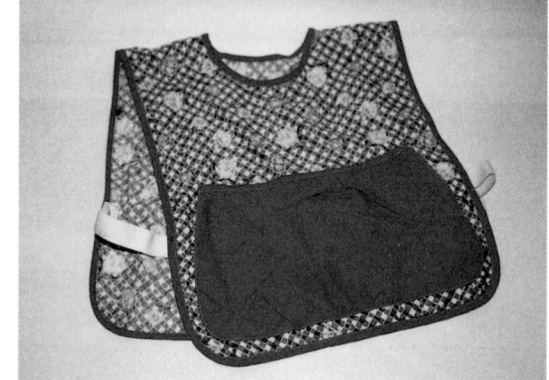

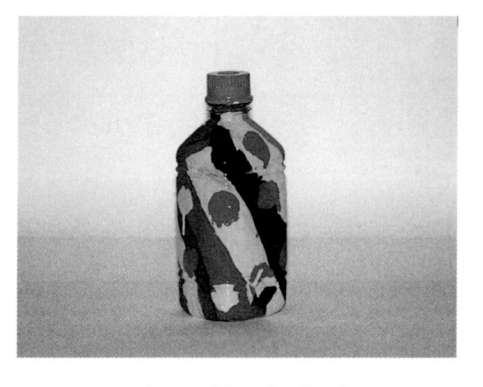

Coloured bottle/skittle

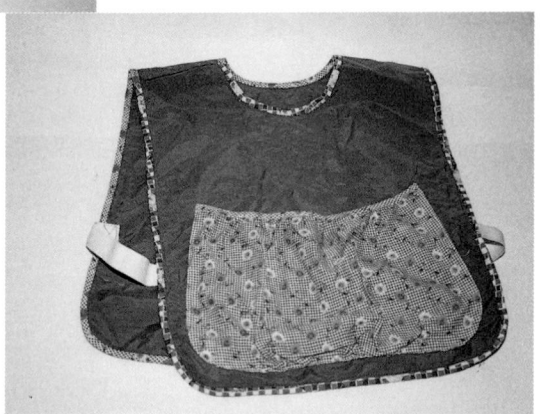

Apron — for pre-dressing activities, messy play during hand task series, with a large pocket in front for holding toys during walking task series

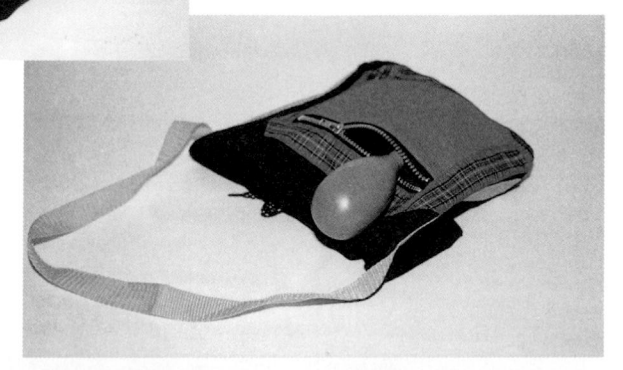

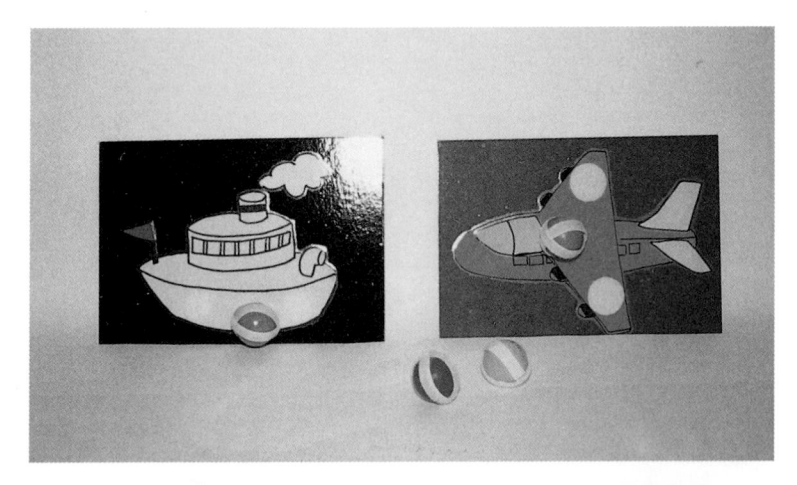

Pictures attached to white/blackboard and coloured ping pong balls with attached

Furniture

The furniture illustrated in the following pages has been found useful when working for children with cerebral palsy. The measurements are for children aged from 3 – 5 years old. Measurements will need to be adapted when working with older children.

Plinth

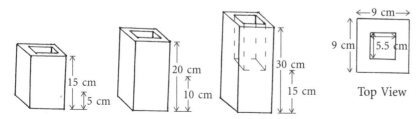

The plinth helps the children learn to grasp and release. It facilitates them to sit upright, stand up, take steps and work for themselves.

Extension blocks

15 cm / 5 cm
20 cm / 10 cm
30 cm / 15 cm

Top View
9 cm / 5.5 cm / 9 cm

Extension blocks added to the legs of the plinth adjusts the height to suit children of different height in sitting, standing and cruising.

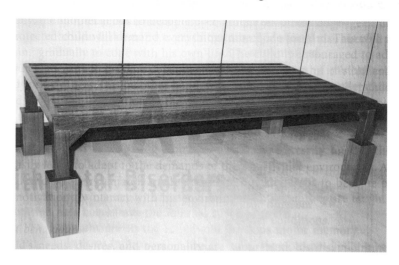

Table top

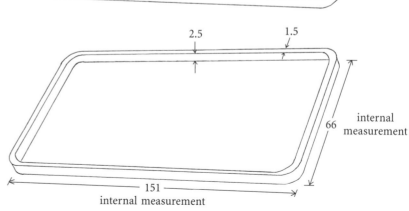

A removable table top fitted over the plinth changes it to an ordinary table.

499

Ladderback chair

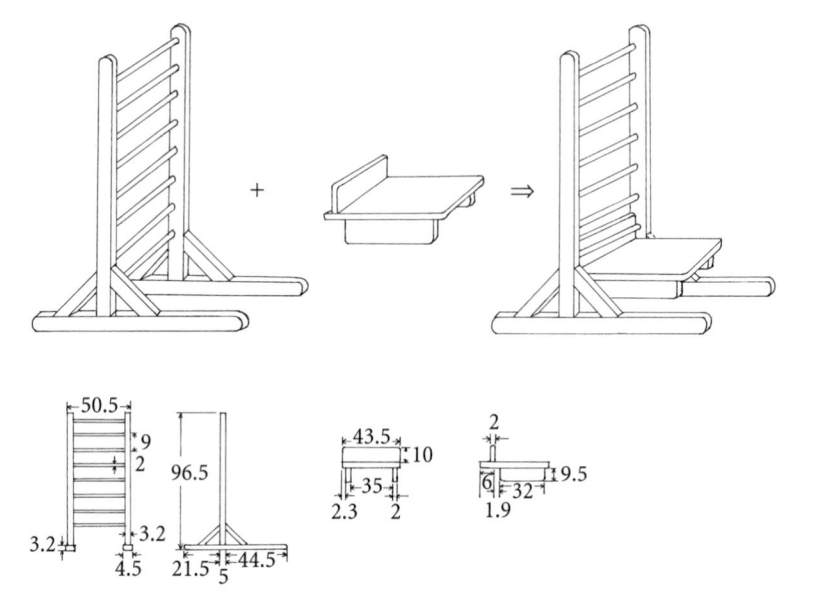

The ladderback chair with height adjustable seat to suit children of different heights. Can be used as a chair, a small table top, for walking and for support when sitting and standing.

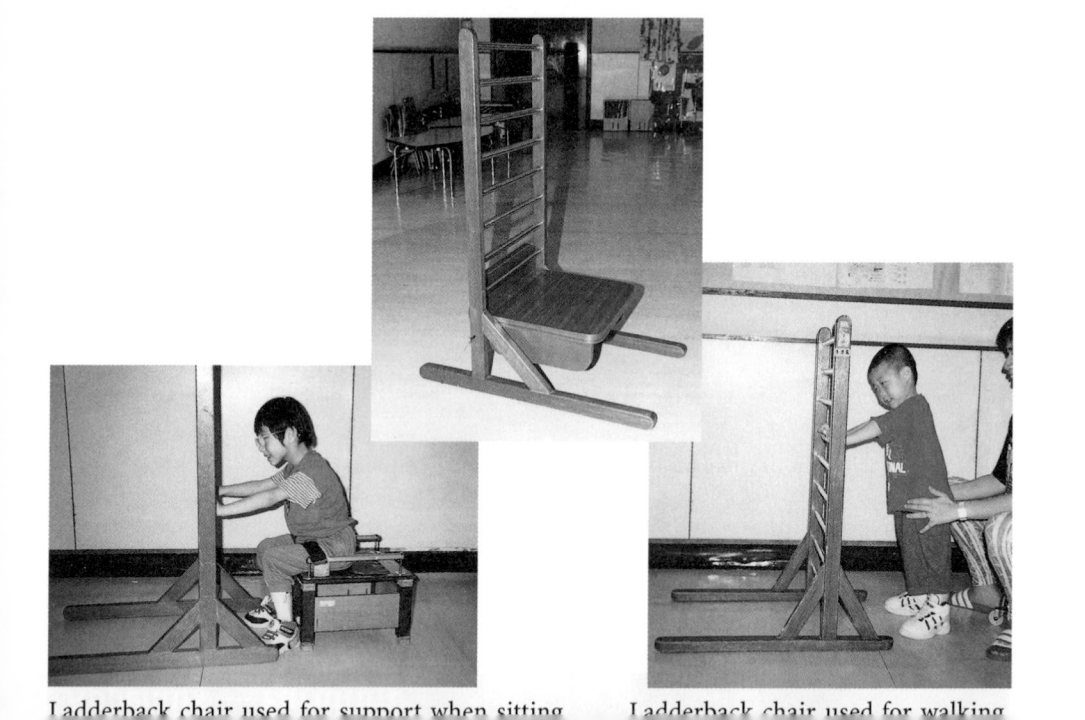

Ladderback chair used for support when sitting   Ladderback chair used for walking

A small ladderback chair with armrests

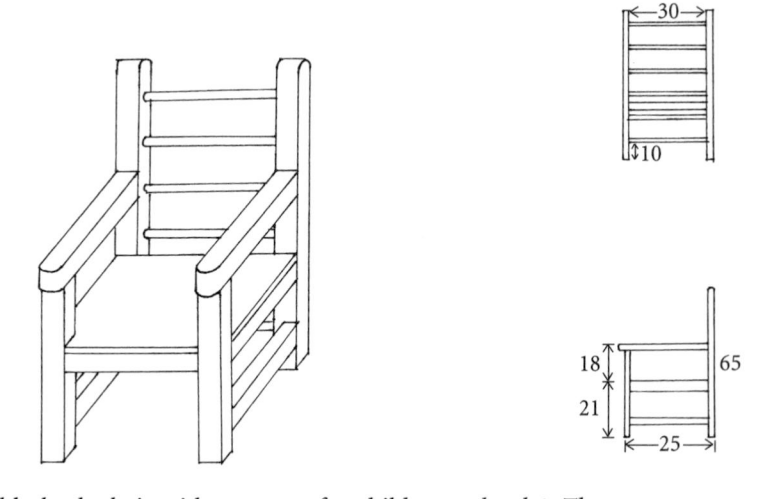

Small ladderback chair with armrests for children at level 1. The measurements shown in the above drawing are for children 2 – 3 years old.

Stool

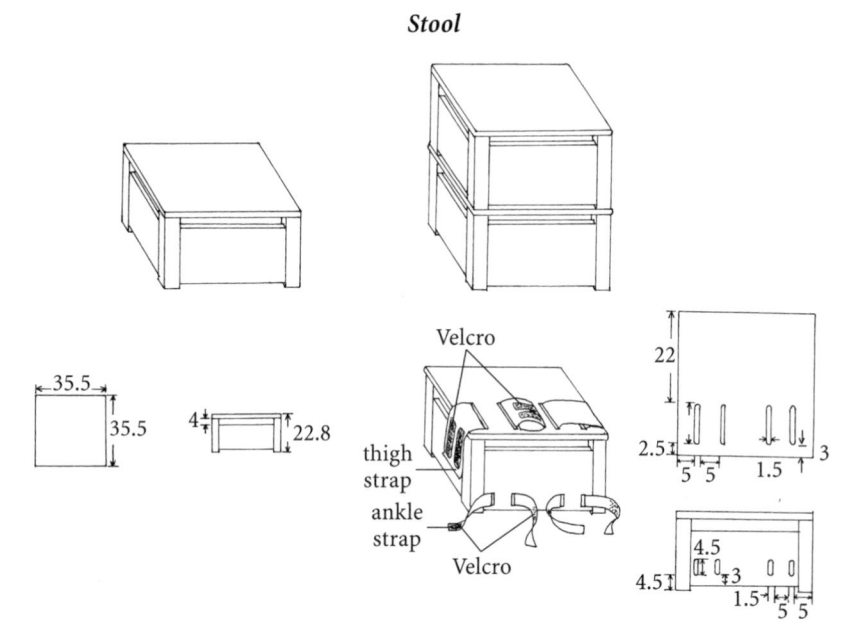

The stool with horizontal slits along the four sides provides a ledge for the children to grasp when sitting. Slits on the seating part and one side should be wide enough to allow the thigh straps and ankle straps to slip through easily. When the stools are not being used, they can be stacked together for storage.

Equipment and Aids

The equipment and aids illustrated in the following pages has been found useful when working for children with cerebral palsy. The measurements are suitable for children ages 3 – 5 years old and will need to be adapted when working with older children.

Arm gaiter

strips of 0.2 cm thick aluminium bar inside

made from denim cloth

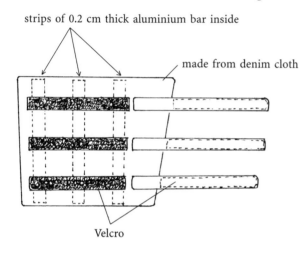

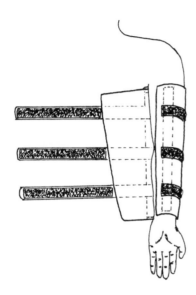

Velcro

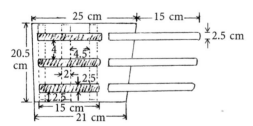

The arm gaiter is used to maintain a limb in the stretched/straight position and for stability. It is made of thick cloth eg. denim, with pockets for strips of aluminium used as stiffeners. It is wrapped firmly around the elbow to keep it straight. Make sure the gaiter is not wrapped too tight, otherwise it may hinder blood circulation to the limb resulting in the fingers becoming blue and cold. If it is wrapped too loosely the elbow will bend and the aluminium bars will hurt the arm.

Flexion mitt

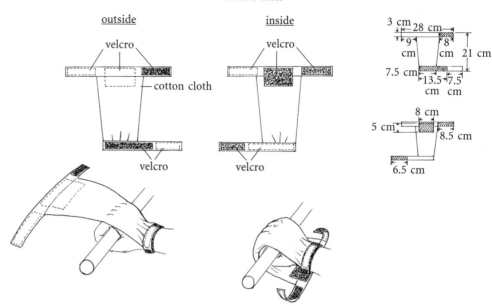

outside inside

velcro velcro

cotton cloth

velcro velcro

The flexion mitt is used to facilitate sustained hand grasp. It is made of thick cotton with velcro attachment. Children who cannot sustain grasp of an object, can have the hand grasping the object enveloped in a flexion mitt. The use of the flexion mitt should be discontinued as soon as the child has learned the concept of sustained grasp.

Horizontal hand bar

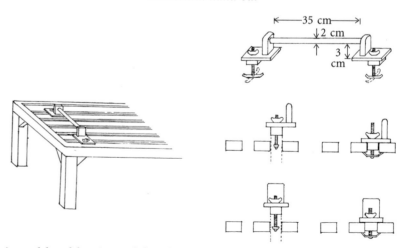

The horizontal hand bar is used for children who have difficulty sustaining grasp of the plinth. Circular in shape, it facilitates grasp. It can be easily attached to the plinth.

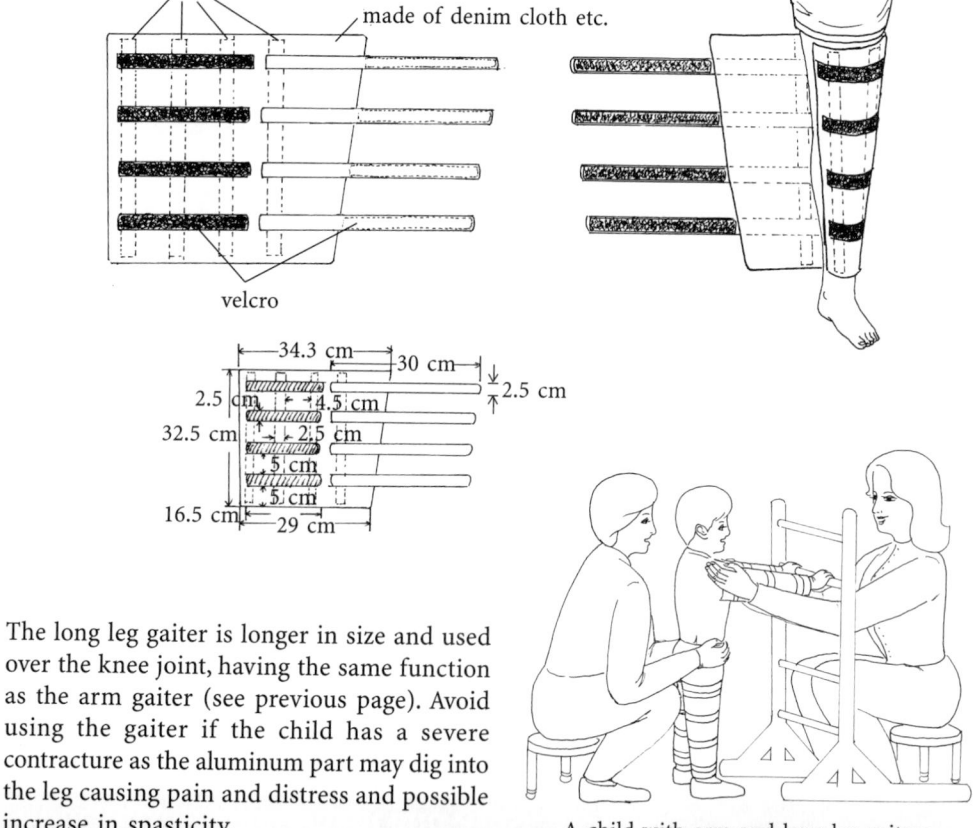

Ankle-foot orthosis (AFO)

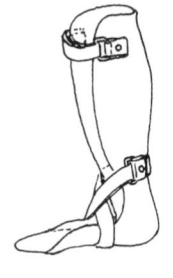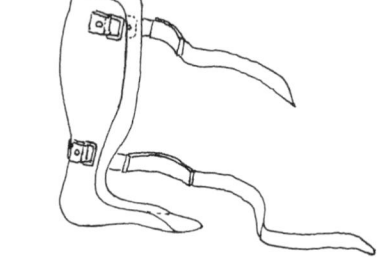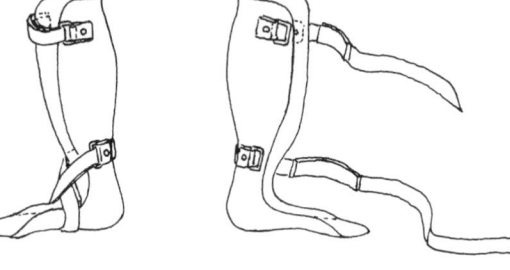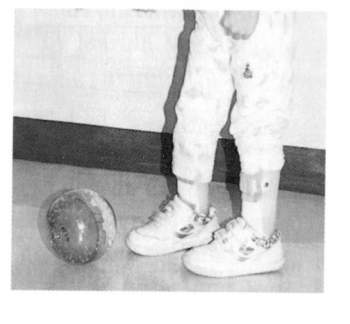

The ankle-foot orthosis (AFO) is useful for some children with cerebral palsy. It helps them stabilise the ankle joint, facilitates better control of the lower limbs and prevents tip-toe gait. Seek advice from the rehabilitation doctor for indications on necessity and use.

Long leg gaiter

strips of 0.2 cm thick aluminium bar inside

made of denim cloth etc.

velcro

34.3 cm — 30 cm — 2.5 cm

2.5 cm — 4.5 cm

32.5 cm — 2.5 cm

5 cm

16.5 cm — 29 cm — 5 cm

The long leg gaiter is longer in size and used over the knee joint, having the same function as the arm gaiter (see previous page). Avoid using the gaiter if the child has a severe contracture as the aluminum part may dig into the leg causing pain and distress and possible increase in spasticity.

A child with arm and long leg gaiters.

Standing frame

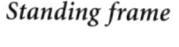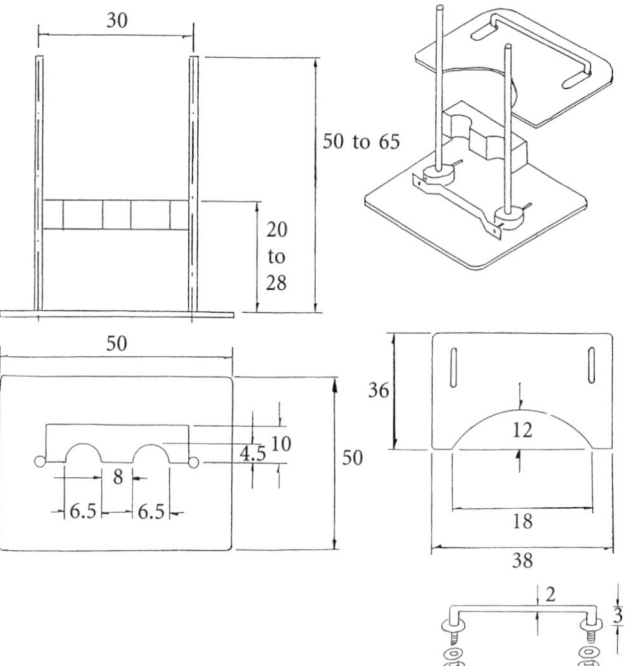

30

50 to 65

20 to 28

50

4.5 10

8

6.5 6.5

36

12

50

18

38

2

3

The standing frame is made of a wooden base with a wooden table. The major frame is made of stainless steel bars and straps made from durable denim cloth or artificial leather. The standing frame provides an opportunity for the child to have the experience of standing in the upright position weight bearing through his legs. The child can play in this position. However, the child should not be left standing in the frame continuously for more than one hour.

Stackable stairs

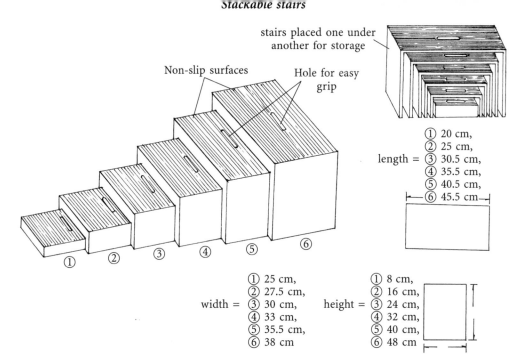

Non-slip surfaces

Hole for easy grip

stairs placed one under another for storage

① ② ③ ④ ⑤ ⑥

length =
① 20 cm,
② 25 cm,
③ 30.5 cm,
④ 35.5 cm,
⑤ 40.5 cm,
⑥ 45.5 cm

width =
① 25 cm,
② 27.5 cm,
③ 30 cm,
④ 33 cm,
⑤ 35.5 cm,
⑥ 38 cm

height =
① 8 cm,
② 16 cm,
③ 24 cm,
④ 32 cm,
⑤ 40 cm,
⑥ 48 cm

The stackable stairs are used for training children in stairs management. They can be stacked together for storage.

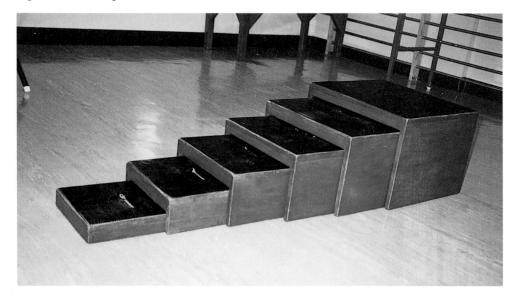

Floor ladder

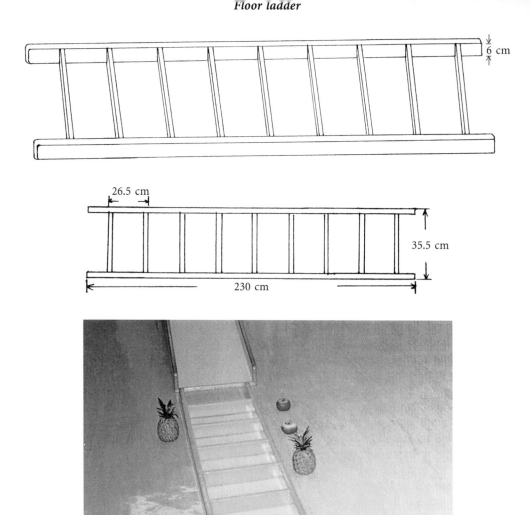

6 cm

26.5 cm

35.5 cm

230 cm

The floor-ladder helps to improve walking balance. It encourages the child to clear his foot off the ground at each step.

Ramp

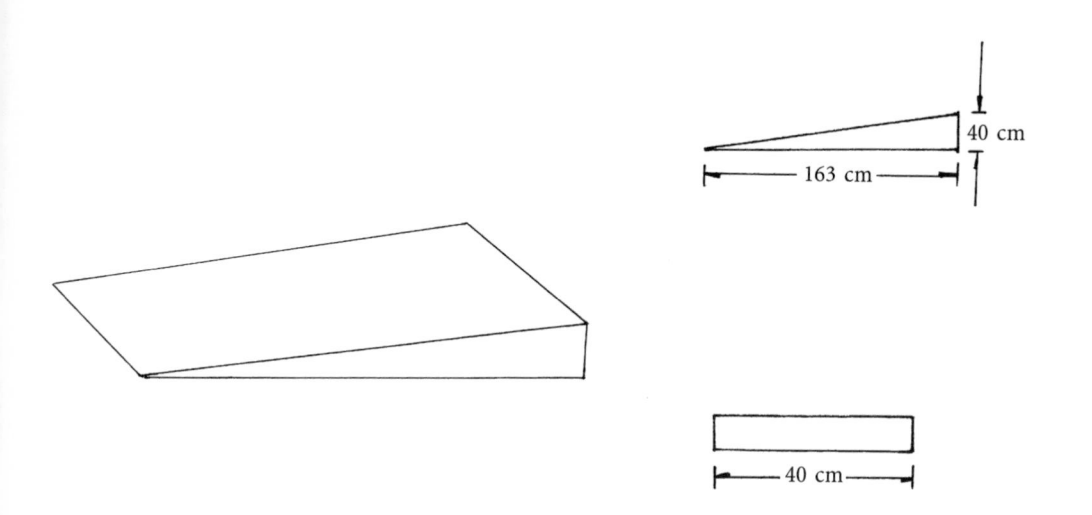

The ramp helps the children improve their balance and teaches them stretch at the ankle joints.

The parallel bar

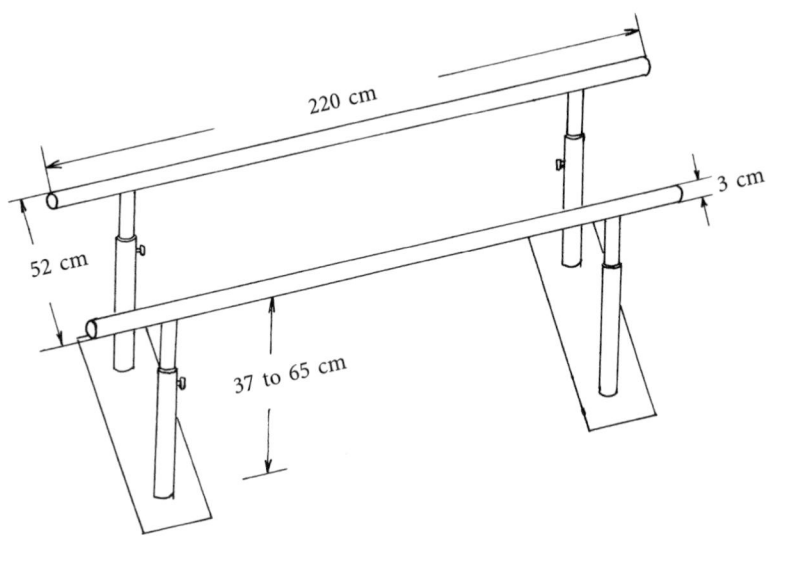

The parallel bar is used for walking training. The bars provide opportunity for the children to learn grasp for support when walking, cruising or learning to squat.

Bench

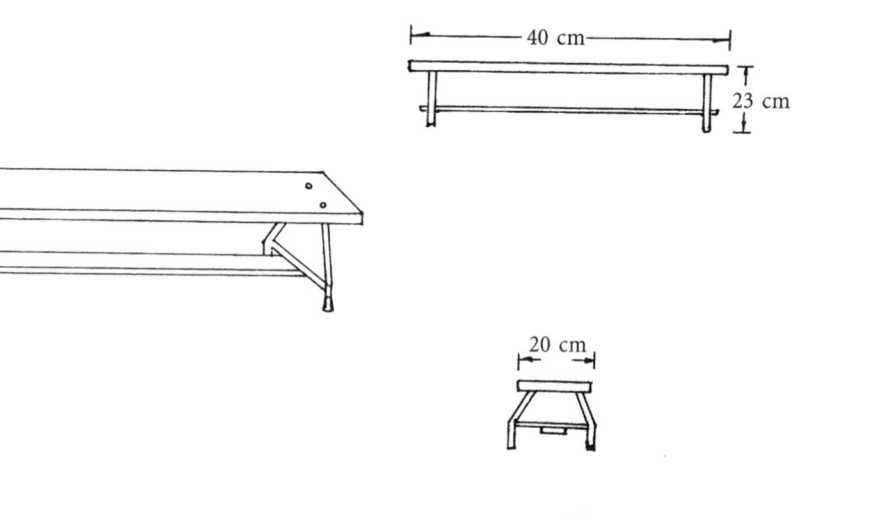

The bench is commonly used for older children. The measurements shown above are for children aged 4 – 7 years. Children learn to part their legs as they slide forwards/backwards.

The wedge

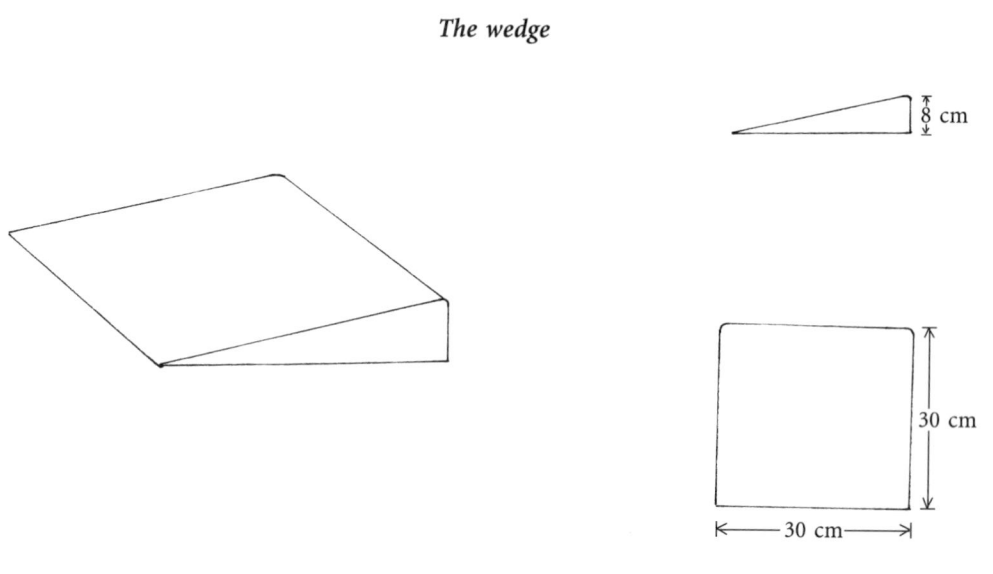

The wedge helps the children to sit with straight back when putting on/taking off shoes and socks in the long sitting position on the floor. The wedge is made of hard foam and covered with artifical leather. Corners and edges should be rounded.

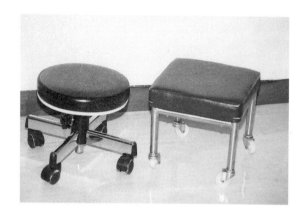

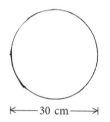
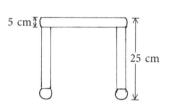

5 cm

25 cm

← 30 cm →

The stool on castors used by the care-giver facilitates her work, and ensures she has eye contact with the child. Using the appropriate height also helps prevent strain on the back.

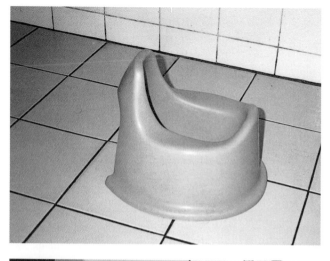

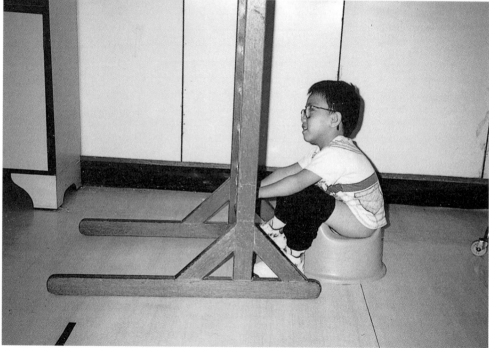

Sandbag

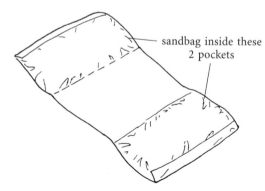

sandbag inside these 2 pockets

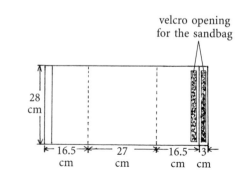

velcro opening for the sandbag

28 cm

← 16.5 cm → ← 27 cm → ← 16.5 cm → ← 3 cm →

As well as its functional use for toiletting, sitting on the potty also helps the child flex the hips, keep the feet apart and flat on the floor and prepares for sitting.

The sandbag hung on the lower rung of the ladderback chair adds weight and prevents the ladderback chair tilting forward.

Songs

1. Apart and Together _____ pivoting on the stool in the sitting position
2. Big Red Ball _____ pushing a ball
3. Finger Exercise _____ individual finger movement
4. Go to Sleep _____ lying still
5. Good Morning _____ raising the hand
6. Grooming Song_____ washing/drying/brushing face/hands/hair
7. Hold on Tight _____ pulling up the plinth
8. I Climb Up/down _____ climbing up/down ladderback chair
9. I Stretch my Hands and Hold on Tight _____ sitting on a chair/stool/plinth
10. Jack in the Box _____ squatting
11. Lie on my Tummy _____ pivoting in the prone position
12. London Bridge is Falling Down _____ bridging
13. Look at Me _____ standing
14. Now we are Going to Say Goodbye _____ goodbye
15. Pass Your Toy _____ passing toys
16. Pit-a-Pat-Pit-a-Pat_____ patting objects
17. Puppy and Kitten _____ four point kneeling
18. Push off Plinth _____ pushing off the plinth
19. Right Hand First_____ cruising
20. Rolling Over _____ continuous rolling
21. Row the Boat _____ raising/lowering a stick using the upper limbs
22. Sit up Straight_____ sitting
23. Stand up Tall_____ standing
24. Stretch your Arms _____ rolling
25. Ten Little Fingers _____ counting fingers
26. Touch my Head _____ learning body parts
27. Up to the Sky _____ raising the upper limbs/sitting balance

1. Apart and Together

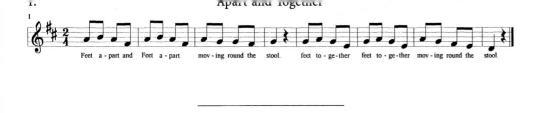

Feet a-part and Feet a-part mov-ing round the stool. feet to-ge-ther feet to-ge-ther mov-ing round the stool.

2. Big Red Ball

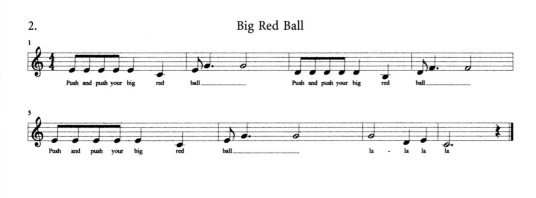

Push and push your big red ball _____ Push and push your big red ball _____

Push and push your big red ball _____ la - la la la

3. Finger Exercise

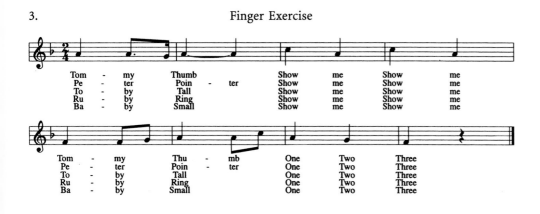

Tom	-	my	Thumb		Show	me	Show	me
Pe	-	ter	Poin	- ter	Show	me	Show	me
To	-	by	Tall		Show	me	Show	me
Ru	-	by	Ring		Show	me	Show	me
Ba	-	by	Small		Show	me	Show	me

Tom	-	my	Thu	- mb	One	Two	Three
Pe	-	ter	Poin	- ter	One	Two	Three
To	-	by	Tall		One	Two	Three
Ru	-	by	Ring		One	Two	Three
Ba	-	by	Small		One	Two	Three

4. Go to Sleep

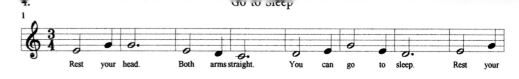

Rest your head. Both arms straight. You can go to sleep. Rest your

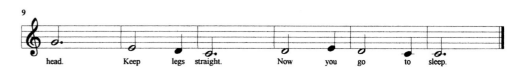

head. Keep legs straight. Now you go to sleep.

5. Good Morning

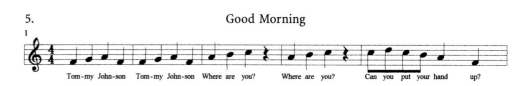

Tom-my John-son Tom-my John-son Where are you? Where are you? Can you put your hand up?

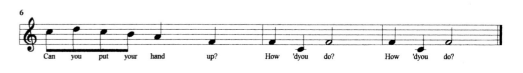

Can you put your hand up? How 'dyou do? How 'dyou do?

6. Grooming Song

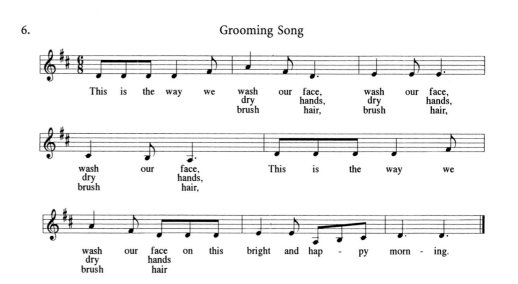

This is the way we wash our face, wash our face,
dry hands, dry hands,
brush hair, brush hair,

wash our face, This is the way we
dry hands,
brush hair,

wash our face on this bright and hap-py morn-ing.
dry hands
brush hair

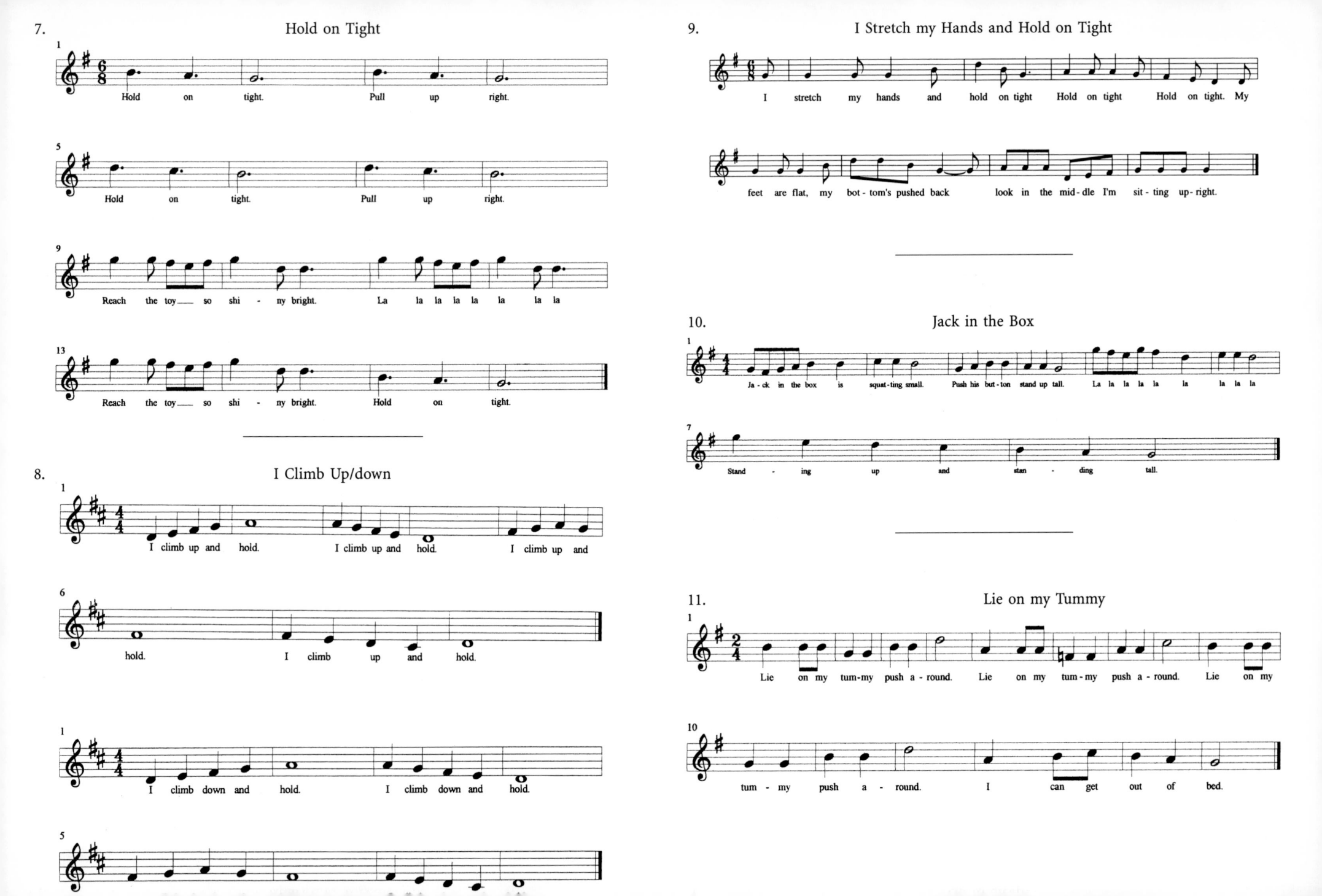

7. Hold on Tight

8. I Climb Up/down

9. I Stretch my Hands and Hold on Tight

10. Jack in the Box

11. Lie on my Tummy

12.

London Bridge is Falling Down

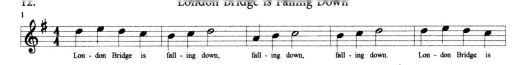

Lon - don Bridge is fall - ing down, fall - ing down, fall - ing down. Lon - don Bridge is

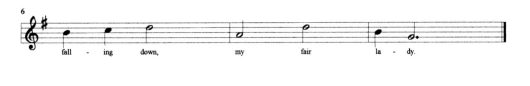

fall - ing down, my fair la - dy.

13.

Look at Me

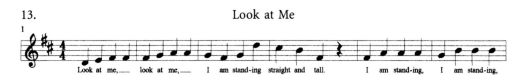

Look at me, look at me, I am stand-ing straight and tall. I am stand-ing, I am stand-ing,

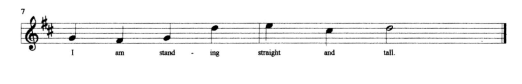

I am stand - ing straight and tall.

14.

Now We are Going to Say Goodbye

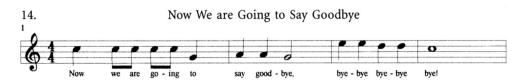

Now we are go - ing to say good - bye, bye - bye bye - bye bye!

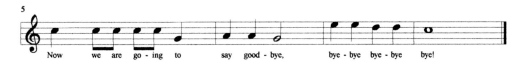

Now we are go - ing to say good - bye, bye - bye bye - bye bye!

15.

Pass Your Toy

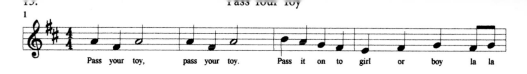

Pass your toy, pass your toy. Pass it on to girl or boy la la

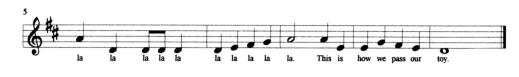

la la la la la la la la la. This is how we pass our toy.

16.

Pit-a-Pat-Pit-a-Pat

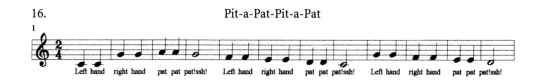

Left hand right hand pat pat pat!ssh! Left hand right hand pat pat pat!ssh! Left hand right hand pat pat pat!ssh!

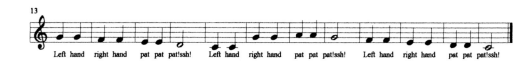

Left hand right hand pat pat pat!ssh! Left hand right hand pat pat pat!ssh! Left hand right hand pat pat pat!ssh!

17.

Puppy/Kitten

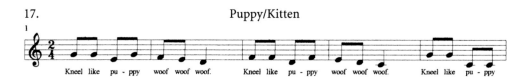

Kneel like pu - ppy woof woof woof. Kneel like pu - ppy woof woof woof. Kneel like pu - ppy

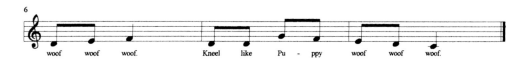

woof woof woof. Kneel like Pu - ppy woof woof woof.

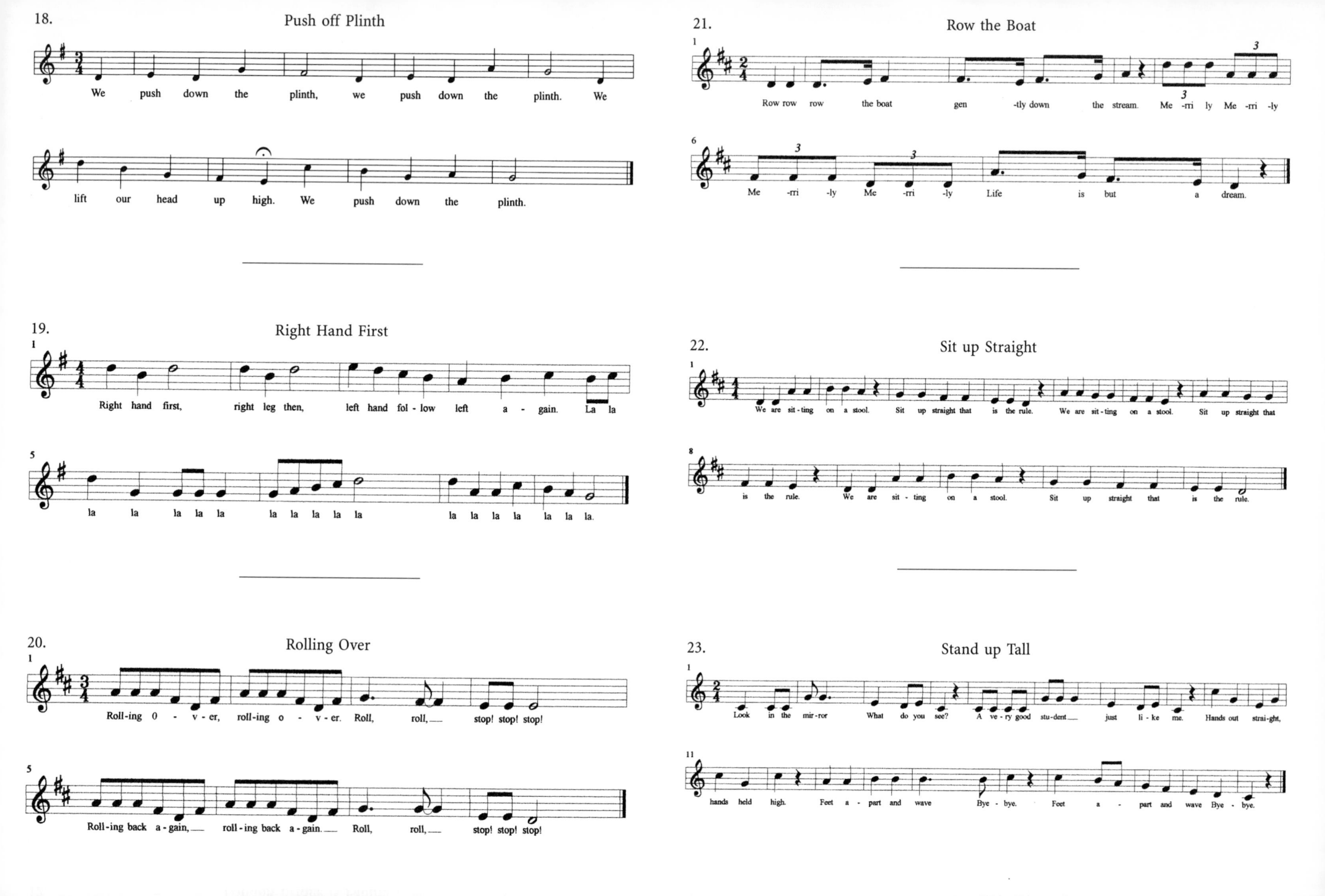

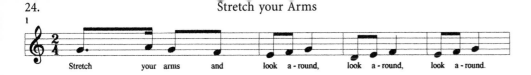

24. Stretch your Arms

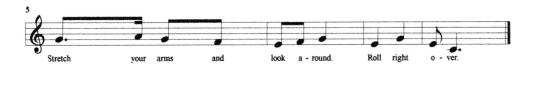

Stretch your arms and look a-round, look a-round, look a-round.

Stretch your arms and look a-round. Roll right o - ver.

25. Ten Little Fingers

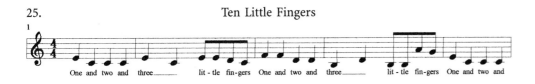

One and two and three____ lit - tle fin-gers One and two and three____ lit - tle fin-gers One and two and

three____ lit - tle fin - gers Ten lit - tle fin - gers____

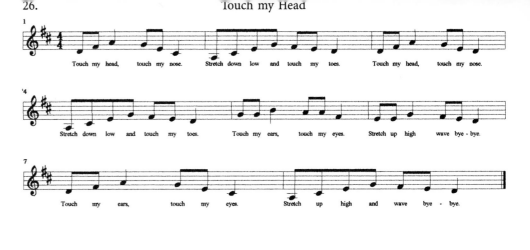

26. Touch my Head

Touch my head, touch my nose. Stretch down low and touch my toes. Touch my head, touch my nose.

Stretch down low and touch my toes. Touch my ears, touch my eyes. Stretch up high wave bye - bye.

Touch my ears, touch my eyes. Stretch up high and wave bye - bye.

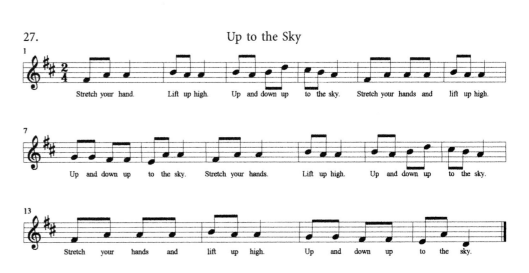

27. Up to the Sky

Stretch your hand. Lift up high. Up and down up to the sky. Stretch your hands and lift up high.

Up and down up to the sky. Stretch your hands. Lift up high. Up and down up to the sky.

Stretch your hands and lift up high. Up and down up to the sky.

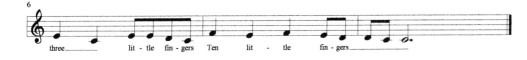

Glossary of Terms

Abduction
— movement of the limbs away from the midline of the body.
— parting of the legs/hands.

Bite reflex
— sudden, uncontrolled bite.

Body awareness
— alertness and knowledge of one's body parts — in terms of the body's different parts and their relation to one another.

Cruising
— walking sideways.

Dorsiflexion
— flexing the ankle joint/wrist to bring the foot/hand towards the body.

Extension
— straightening of any part of the body.

Facilitation
— ways of making movement possible.

Flexion
— bending of any part of the body.

Head control
— the ability to control the position and movement of the head in space.

Midline orientation
— awareness of and the ability to relate to the midline of the body.

Object permanence
— the knowledge that an object still exists even though it is out of sight.

Perception
— the process of organising, integrating and interpreting the sensations received from the environment.

Prone
— lying on the tummy.

Tongue thrust
— sudden, uncontrolled forceful protruding of the tongue.

Trunk rotation
— twisting of the trunk to either left or right.

Spatial concept
— the relationship of one object to another in space.

Supine
— lying on the back.

Symmetry
— the two sides of the body are equal.

Tactile
— the sense of touch.

Trunk
— the body excluding the head and the limbs.

Vestibular
— the sense of movement of the body which is stimulated by the position of the head and is sensitive to the speed and direction of the movement.

Visual
— the sense of seeing.

Weight bearing
— the ability to take the weight through the limbs.

Weight shifting
— transferring the weight from one part of the body to another part.

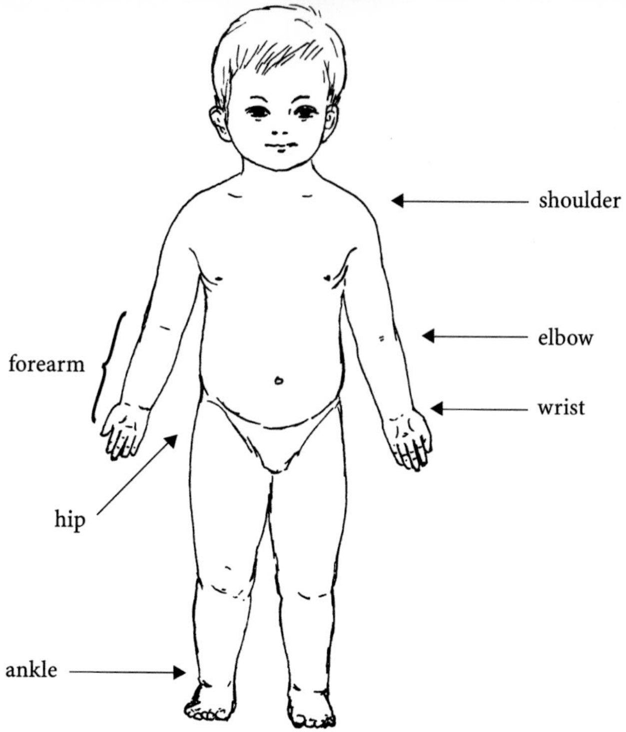

shoulder

elbow

forearm

wrist

hip

ankle

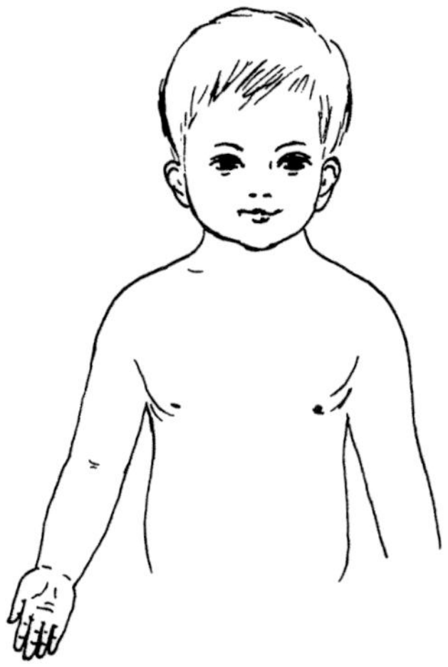

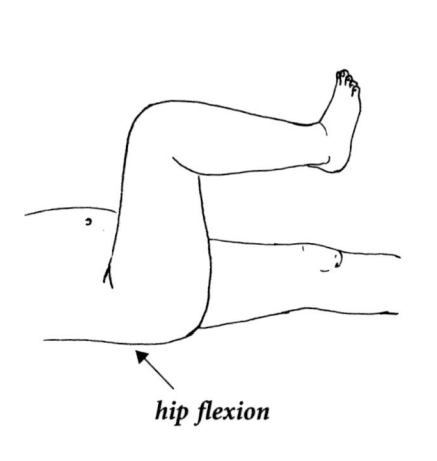

external rotation of
upper limb

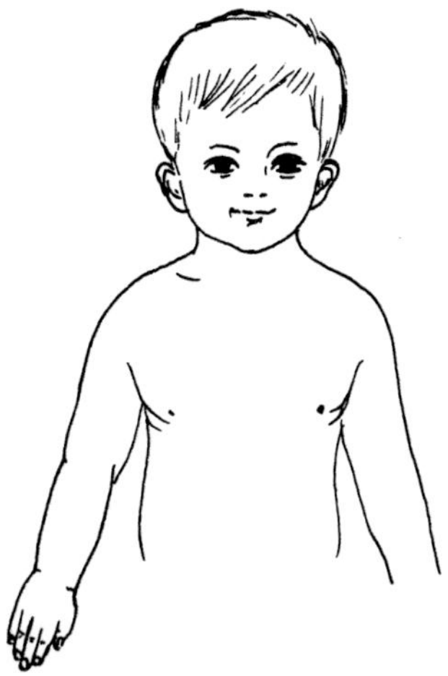

internal rotation of
upper limb

hip flexion

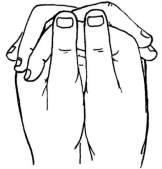

clasped hand

palmar grasp

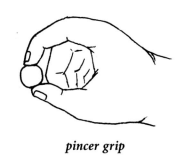

pincer grip

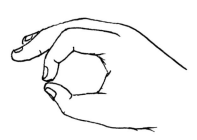

opposition with index finger

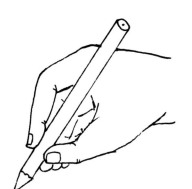

tripod grip

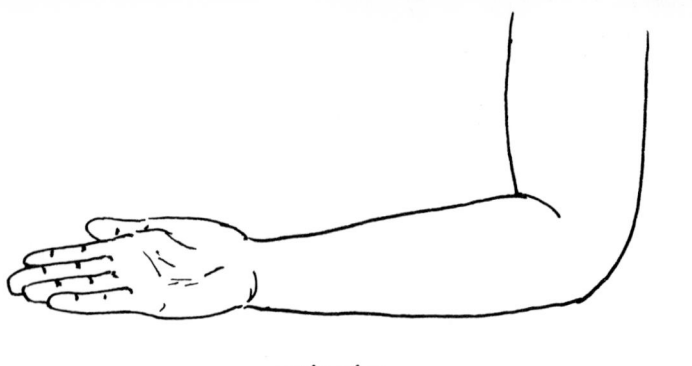

supination

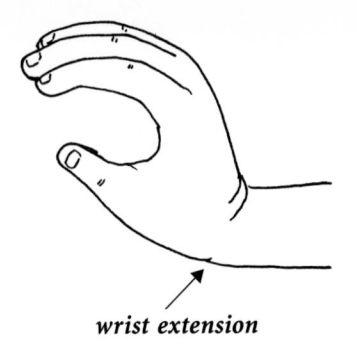

wrist extension

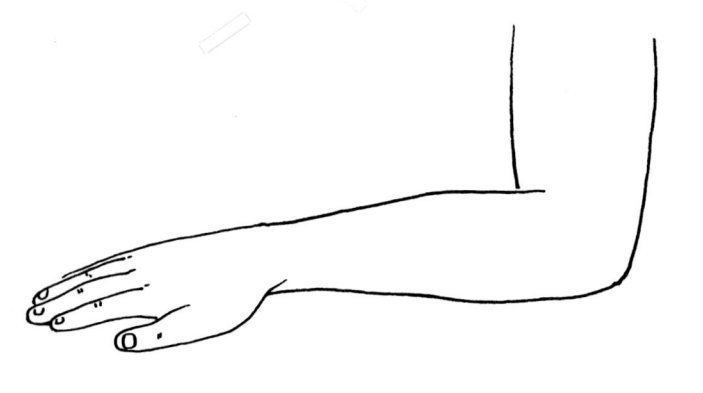

pronation

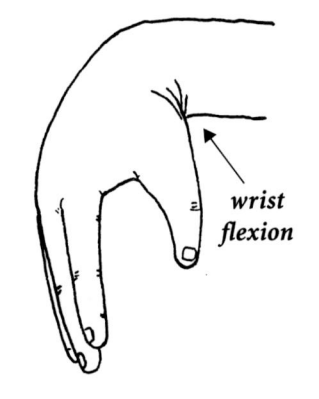

wrist flexion

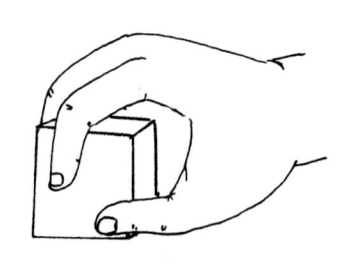

radial grasp

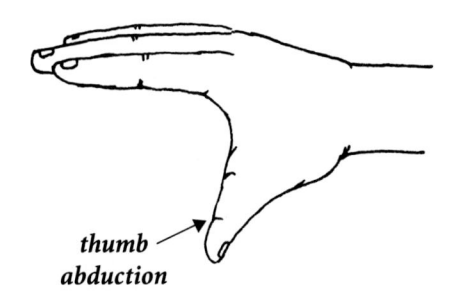

thumb abduction

Berk, L. E. (1994) "Why children talk to themselves" Scientific American, November 1994, 60–65.

Bleck, E. E. (1987) Orthopaedic Management in Cerebral Palsy. London/Cambridge: Mackelth Press with Cambridge University Press.

Bobath, B. (1971) "Motor development: its effect on general development and application to the treatment of cerebral palsy." Physiotherapy, 57: 526–532.

Bobath, B. (1975) Motor Development in the Different Types of Cerebral Palsy. London: Heinemann Medical.

Bobath, K. B. (1964) "The facilitation of normal postural reactions and movements in the treatment of cerebral palsy." Physiotherapy 50: 246–262.

Campion, M. (1979) Conductive Education — the Petö method. Aust L. Physio Paed mono. December 1979.

Carr, J. H. & Shepherd, R. B. (1987) "A motor learning model for rehabilitation" in Carr, J. H. & Shepherd, R.B. (Eds.) Movement Science — Foundations for Physical Therapy in Rehabilitation (31–35). USA, Maryland: Aspen Publication.

Chan, E. (1990) "Conductive Education for a Group of Cerebral Palsied Adolescents in the John F. Kennedy Centre, Hong Kong," The Proceedings of the 3rd International Physiotherapy Congress, Hong Kong, 574–578.

Clarke, J., Evans, E. (1973) "Rhythmical intention as a method of treatment for the cerebral palsied patient." Australian Journal of Physiotherapy 19: 57–64.

"Conductive Education and School Education." (1988) Lecture by Maria Gyorgyi at the Six-Week Course on Conductive Education, Pëto Institute, Budapest.

Cotter, C. (1990) "Behaviour development in the group programmes" in The Conductive Education News, 5(4): 11–13.

Cotton, E. (1975) Conductive Education and Cerebral Palsy. London: The Spastics Society.

Cotton, E. (1970) "Integration of treatment and education in cerebral palsy". *Physiotherapy*, 56: 143–147.

Cotton, E. (1981) The Hand as a Guide to Learning. London: The Spastics Society.

Cotton, E. (1980) The Basic Motor Pattern. London: The Spastics Society.

Cotton E. and Parnwell, M. (1967) "From Hungary the Petö method" British Journal of Special Education, 56(4): 7–11.

Finnie, N. R. (1974) Handling the Cerebral Palsied Child at Home, 2nd ed. London: Heinemann Medical.

Fung, S. (1987) "Physiotherapy — eclectic approach" in Louis C. S. Hsu (Ed.) Cerebral Palsy, Proceedings of a Symposium held on 8th March (1987), 17.

Gentile, A. M. (1987). Skill Acquisition: Action, Movement, and Neuromotor Processes in J. H. Carr & R. B. Sheperd (Eds.), Movement Science: Foundations for Physical Therapy in Rehabilitation (93–154). Rockville, MD: Aspen Publishers.

Gesell, A. et al. (1940) The First 5 years of Life, A Guide to the Study of the Pre-school Child. New York: Harper & Brothers Publishers.

Ginsburg, H. & Opper, S., (1978) Piaget's Theory of Intellectual Development, 2nd ed. New Jersey: Prentice-Hall.

Guide to the Primary Curriculum, the Curriculum Development Council, the Education Department, Hong Kong (1993).

Hari, M. (1975) "The Idea of Learning in Conductive Pedagogy" in Akos, K. (Ed.), Scientific Studies on Conductive Pedagogy. Conductors' College, Budapest.

Hari, M. (1988). "The Human Principle in Conductive Education." Reprinted in Tatlow, A. (Ed.). The 1988 Budapest Report by the Hong Kong Delegates (1990). Hong Kong Conductive Education Project Team, Joint Council for the Physically and Mentally Disabled (Rehabilitation Division, Hong Kong Council of Social Service).

Hari, M. (1991) "Intendation: the principle hypothesis for CE" *Lege Artis Medicinae*, 1(9–10): 544–550.

Hari, M. (1993) "The conductor, training, preparation and practice." Paper presented at Conductive education Conference, Queen Margaret College, Edinburgh, Scotland.

Hari, M. (1988) "The Principle and Essence of Conductive Education". Lecture notes from the Six-Week Course on Conductive Education, December 1998. Pető Institute, Budapest.

Hari, M. and Akos, K. (1971) Conductive Education. London and New York: Routledge; transl. By N. Horton Smith and J. Stevens, (1988).

Hari, M. & Akos, K. (1988). Conductive Education. London: Routledge.

Hari, M. and Tillemans, T. (1984) "Conductive education" in Scrutton D. (Ed.) Management of the Motor Disorders of Children with Cerebral Palsy. Chapter 2. Clinics in Developmental Medicine, No. 90. London: SIMP/Blackwell Scientific; Philadelphia, Penn.: Lippincott, 19–35.

Haskell, S. H. and Barrett, E. K. (1989) The Education of Children with Motor & Neurological Disabilities 2nd ed. New York: Nichols Publishing, 172.

Hong Kong Delegates (1988) The Six-Week International Course on Conductive Education at the Pető Andras State Institute for Conductive Education of the Motor Disabled and Conductors' College, Budapest, Hungary, 1987. Whitehill, T. (Ed.). Working Group on Conductive Education: Hong Kong Council of Social Service, 8–11.

Hong Kong Delegates (1990). The Six-Week International Course on Conductive Education at the Pető Andras State Institute for Conductive Education of the Motor Disabled and Conductors' College, Budapest, Hungary (1988). Tatlow, A. (Ed.). Conductive Education Project Team: Hong Kong Council of Social Service, 3.

Illingworth, R. S. (1960) The Development of the Infant and Young Child, Normal and Abnormal. Edinburgh: E. and S. Livingstone.

"Introduction to the Parents' School" (1988). Lecture by Erzsebet Korispatheky at the Six-Week Course on Conductive Education, Pëto Institute, Budapest.

Jernqvist, L. (1986) "The Use of Speech Regulation of Motor Acts in Conductive Education" in A. Tatlow (Ed.), Hong Kong Physiotherapy Journal, Special Issue: Conductive Education, Vol. 8.

Jernqvist, L. (1986), Rhythmical Intention — the use of speech in a regulative function. Conductive Education Interest Group Newsletter (1984), 5.

Kay, H. (1970) "Analysing Motor Skill Performance" in K. Conolly (Ed.), Mechanisms of Motor Skill Development. London and New York: Academic Press.

Kokuti, M. (1988) "Teaching Handwriting in Conductive Education" Lecture notes from the Six-Week Course on Conductive Education, December 1988. Pető Institute, Budapest.

Kozma, I. (1995) "The basic principles and present practice of conductive education" in European Journal of Special Needs Education, 10(2): 111–123.

Levitt, S. (1977) Treatment of Cerebral Palsy and Motor Delay. Oxford: Blackwell.

Li, H. & Chan, E. (1992) "Integrating the Activity Approach with Conductive Education in Hong Kong" in Tatlow, A. (Ed.), Conductive Education in Hong Kong, Joint Issues 5 & 6. Hong Kong Conductive Education Project Team, Hong Kong Joint Council for the Physically & Mentally Disabled (Rehabilitation Division, Hong Kong Council of Social Service).

Luria, A. R. (1961) The Role of Speech in the Regulation of Normal and Abnormal Behaviour, London: Pergamon Press.

Luria, A. R. (1973), The Working Brain: An Introduction to Neuropsychology. New York: Penguin Books.

Marx, M. and Ferren, J. (1989) "Conductive education as observed in Australia and Hong Kong", World Rehabilitation Fund, Inc., International Exchange of Experts and Information in Rehabilitation (unpublished material).

McCarthy, G. T. (1992) "Cerebral Palsy — Clinical" in Downie P. A. (Ed.), Cash's Textbook of Neurology for Physiotherapists. London: Wolfe Publishing Ltd.

Ng, J., Kwan, W., Thornhill, D., Nam, E., Tatlow, A. & Wong, L., (1987). "Conductive Education Furniture" in Tatlow, A. (Ed.), Conductive Education in Hong Kong, Issue No. I. Working Group on Conductive Education, Hong Kong Joint Council for the Physically & Mentally Disabled (Rehabilitation Division, Hong Kong Council of Social Service).

Parnwell, M. (1970) "Conductive Education of the Cerebral Palsied Child." Proceedings of the 5th International Congress, WFOT, 166–70.

Phelps W. M. (1949) Description and differentiation of types of cerebral palsy. Nerv. Child, 8: 107.

Penfield, W. and Roberts, L. (1959), Speech and Brain Mechanisms. Princeton: Princeton University Press.

Rooke P. and Opel P., (1983) "An approach to teaching profoundly multiple handicapped children — based on certain principles of Conductive Education." Mental Handicap, Vol. II (June), 73–74.

Scherzer A. L. and Tscharnuter I. (1982) Early Diagnosis and Therapy in Cerebral Palsy. New York: Marcel Dekker, Inc.

Shumway C. (1992), "Cerebral Palsy — Management" in Downie, P. A. (Ed.), Cash's Textbook of Neurology for Physiotherapists. London: Wolfe Publishing Ltd.

Sutton, A. (1986) "The 'Practice'" in P. Cottam and A. Sutton (Eds.). Conductive Education: A System for Overcoming Motor Disorder. London: Croom Helm.

Tatlow, A. (1987) "Conductive Education" in Louis C. S. Hsu (Ed.) Cerebral Palsy, Proceedings of a symposium held on 8th March (1987), 17.

Tatlow, A. (1991) "Conductive education: the stick — for cerebral palsied children". Course material, Introductory Course on Conductive Education, Tongji University/Hospital, Wuhan, China.

Tatlow, A. (1993) "The Petö-System (Conductive Education): Facilitation of Movements/ Actions of the Cerebral Palsied Child. In Tatlow, A. (Ed.) The Hong Kong Conductive Education Source Book 144–158. The Hong Kong Council of Social Service.

Thornhill, D. and Nam, E. (1987). 'Furniture for Severely Disabled Adolescents', in "Conductive Education Furniture". Tatlow, A (Ed.) Conductive Education in Hong Kong, Issue No. 1. Working Group on Conductive Education, Hong Kong, Joint Council for the Physically & Mentally Disabled (Rehabilitation Division, Hong Kong Council of Social Service).

Tsang, K. L. V. (1990) "Discussion on applying conductive education to the context of Hong Kong, Part I" in A Tatlow and A. Wong (Eds.). Conductive Education in Hong Kong, Issue No. 4, 15–26. Hong Kong Conductive Education Project Team. Hong Kong: Joint Council for the Physically and Mentally Disabled (Rehabilitation Division, Hong Kong Council of Social Service).

Tsang, K. L. V. (1992) "Discussion on applying conductive education to the context of Hong Kong, Part II: an attempt to construct an integrative educational model" in A. Tatlow (Ed.), Conductive Education in Hong Kong, Focus: Education, Nos. 5 & 6. English/Chinese/Hong Kong Conductive Education Project Team. Working Group on Conductive Education. Hong Kong: Joint Council for the Physically and Mentally Disabled (Rehabilitation Division, Hong Kong Council of Social Service).

Vygotsky, L. S. (1963), "Learning and mental development at school age," in Simon, B. (Ed.), Educational Psychology in the U.S.S.R., Routledge and Kegan Paul.

Wedell, K. (1960b), "The visual perception of cerebral palsied children," Journal of Child Psychology and Psychiatry, 1: 217–27.

Wedell, K. (1964), "Some aspects of perceptual-motor development in young children," in Loring, J. (Ed.), Learning Problems of the Cerebral Palsied, Spastics Society.

Wedell, K. (1968), "Perceptual-motor difficulties," Special Education, 57(4), 25–30.

Wedell, K. (1973), Learning and Perceptual-Motor Disabilities in Children. London: John Wiley.

Yen, N. (1988) "The Lying Task Series and the Multiply Handicapped Child" in Gallagher, S. (Ed.). Conductive Education in Hong Kong, Issue No. 2. Working Groups on Conductive Education. Hong Kong: Joint Council for the Physically & Mentally Disabled (Rehabilitation Division, Hong Kong Council of Social Service).

Your Child has Cerebral Palsy (1991). London: The Spastics Society.

Akos, K. and Akos, M. (1991) Dina: A Mother Practises Conductive Education. The Foundation for Conductive Education.

Allport, G. W. (1961) Pattern and Growth in Personality. New York: Holt, Rinehart and Winston.

Bernstein, N. (1967). The Coordination and Regulation of Movements. London: Pergamon Press.

Cotton E. and Kinsman R. (1983) Conductive Education for Adult Hemiplegia. Churchill Livingstone.

Hilgard, E. R. and Atkinson, R. C. (1967). Introduction to Psychology (4th Ed.). New York: Harcourt Brace and World Inc.

Hurlock, E. B. (1974). Personality Development. New Delhi: Tata McGraw-Hill.

Kielhofner, G. (1980) A Model of Human Occupation: Theory and Application 2–11 Williams & Wilkins.

Lamb, M. E. (1978). Social and Personality Development. New York: Holt, Rinehart and Winston.

Piaget, J. (1977) The Origins of Intelligence in the Child. London: Penguin Educational.

Piaget, J. (1956) The Psychology of Intelligence, Paris: Librarie Arnand Colin.

Russell A., (1994) The Cerebral Palsy Entities. Research and Neurodevelopmental Overveiw Acorn Foundation Publications.

Russell A. & Cotton E. (1994) The Petö System and its Evolution in Britain. Acorn Foundation Publications.

Su, I. (1992), "Conductive Education for cerebral palsied adults at Chai Wan workshop: learning through personality development" in Conductive Education in Hong Kong, Issue Nos. 5 & 6, A. Tatlow (Ed.), Hong Kong Conductive Education Project Team, Joint Council for the Physically and Mentally Disabled, Hong Kong Council of Social Service.